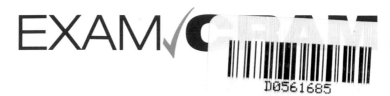

EXAM✓CRAM

D0561685

The NCLEX-RN® Cram Sheet

This cram sheet contains the distilled, key facts about the licensure exam. Review this information just before you enter the testing center, paying special attention to those areas where you feel you need the most review. You can transfer any of these facts from your head onto a blank sheet provided by the testing center. We also recommend reading the glossary as a last-minute cram tool before entering the testing center. Good luck.

GENERAL TEST INFORMATION

1. **Minimum 75/maximum 265**—The maximum time allotted for the test is 6 hours. Don't get frustrated if you need to take the entire number of items or take the entire allotted time. Get up and move around and take breaks if you need a time-out.

2. **Take deep breaths and imagine yourself studying in your favorite location**—Take a small item with you that you have had with you during your study time.

3. **Read the question and all answers carefully**—Don't jump to conclusions or make wild guesses.

4. **Look for keywords**—Avoid answers that include *always, never, all, every, only, must, no, except,* or *none.*

5. **Watch for specific details**—Avoid vague answers. Look for adjectives and adverbs.

6. **Eliminate answers that are clearly wrong or incorrect**—Eliminating any incorrect answer increases the probability of selecting the correct answer by 25%.

7. **Look for information given within the question and the answers**—For example, the phrase "client with *diabetic ketoacidosis" should* bring to mind the range of 7.35–7.45 or normal pH.

8. **Look for the same or similar wording in the question and the answers.**

9. **Watch for grammatical inconsistencies**—Subjects and verbs should agree, meaning singular subject, singular verb or plural subject, plural verb. If the question is an incomplete sentence, the correct answer should complete the question in a grammatically correct manner.

10. **Don't read into questions**—Reading into the question can create errors in judgment. If the question asks for an immediate response or prioritization of action, choose the answer that is critical to the life and safety of the client.

11. **Make an educated guess**—If you are unsure after carefully reading the question and all the answers, choose C or the answer with the most information.

NORMAL LAB VALUES

12. **Serum electrolytes**—It is important for you to remember these normal lab values because they might be included in questions throughout the test.

   ▶ Sodium: 135–145 mEq/L
   ▶ Potassium: 3.5–5.5 mEq/L
   ▶ Calcium: 8.5–10.9 mg/L
   ▶ Chloride: 95–105 mEq/L
   ▶ Magnesium: 1.5–2.5 mEq/L
   ▶ Phosphorus: 2.5–4.5 mg/dL

13. **Hematology values**

   ▶ RBC: 4.5–5.0 million
   ▶ WBC: 5,000–10,000
   ▶ Plt.: 200,000–400,000
   ▶ Hgb: 12–16 gms women; 14–18 gms men

14. **ABG values**

   ▶ HCO_3: 24–26 mEq/L
   ▶ CO_2: 35–45 mEq/L
   ▶ PaO_2: 80%–100%
   ▶ SaO_2: > 95%

15. **Chemistry values**

   ▶ Glucose: 70–110 mg/dL
   ▶ Specific gravity: 1.010–1.030
   ▶ BUN: 7–22 mg/dL
   ▶ Serum creatinine: 0.6–1.35 mg/dL (< 2 in older adults)

   *Information included in laboratory test may vary slightly according to methods used

Review common legal terms: tort, negligence, malpractice, slander, assault, battery.

Legalities—The RN and the physician institute seclusion protection. The MD or the hospice nurse can pronounces the client dead.

39. **Types of drugs**

   *The generic name is listed first with the trade name in parentheses.

   ▶ **Angiotensin-converting agents**: Benazepril (Lotensin), lisinopril (Zestril), captopril (Capoten), enalapril (Vasotec), fosinopril (Monopril), moexipril (Univas), quinapril (Acupril), ramipril (Altace)

   ▶ **Beta adrenergic blockers**: Acebutolol (Monitan, Rhotral, Sectral), atenolol (Tenormin, Apo-Atenol, Nova-Atenol), esmolol (Brevibloc), metaprolol (Alupent, Metaproterenol), propanolol (Inderal)

   ▶ **Anti-infective drugs**: Gentamicin (Garamycin, Alcomicin, Genoptic), kanamycin (Kantrex), neomycin (Mycifradin), strepto-mycin (Streptomycin), tobramycin (Tobrex, Nebcin), amikacin (Amikin)

   ▶ **Benzodiazepine drugs**: Clonazepam (Klonopin), diazepam (Valium), chlordiazepoxide (Librium), lorazepam (Ativan), flurazepam (Dalmane)

   ▶ **Phenothiazine drugs**: Chlopromazine (Thorazine), prochlorperazine (Compazine), trifluoperazine (Stelazine), promethazine (Phenergan), hydroxyzine (Vistaril), fluphenazine (Prolixin)

   ▶ **Glucocorticoid drugs**: Prednisolone (Delta-Cortef, Prednisol, Prednisolone), prednisone (Apo-Prednisone, Deltasone, Meticorten, Orasone, Panasol-S), betamethasone (Celestone, Selestoject, Betnesol), dexamethasone (Decadron, Deronil, Dexon, Mymethasone, Dalalone), cortisone (Cortone), hydrocortisone (Cortef, Hydrocortone Phosphate, Cortifoam), methylprednisolone (Solu-cortef, Depo-Medrol, Depopred, Medrol, Rep-Pred), triamcinolone (Amcort, Aristocort, Atolone, Kenalog, Triamolone)

   ▶ **Antivirals**: Acyclovir (Zovirax), ritonavir (Norvir), saquinavir (Invirase, Fortovase), indinavir (Crixivan), abacavir (Ziagen), cidofovir (Vistide), ganciclovir (Cytovene, Vitrasert)

   ▶ **Cholesterol-lowering drugs**: Atorvastatin (Lipitor), fluvastatin (Lescol), lovastatin (Mevacor), pravastatin (Pravachol), simvastatin (Zocar), rosuvastatin (Crestor)

   ▶ **Angiotensin receptor blocker drugs**: Valsartan (Diovan), candesartan (Altacand), losartan (Cozaar), telmisartan (Micardis)

   ▶ **Cox 2 enzyme blocker drugs**: Celecoxib (Celebrex), valdecoxib (Bextra)

   ▶ **Histamine 2 antagonist drugs**: Cimetidine (Tagamet), famotidine (Pepcid), nizatidine (Axid), rantidine (Zantac)

   ▶ **Proton pump inhibitors**: Esomeprazole (Nexium), lansoprazole (Prevacid), pantoprazole (Protonix), rabeprazole (AciPhex)

   ▶ **Anticoagulant drugs**: Heparin sodium (Hepalean), enoxaparin sodium (Lovenox), dalteparin sodium (Fragmin)

40. **Drug schedules**

   ▶ **Schedule I**—Research use only (example LSD)

   ▶ **Schedule II**—Requires a written prescription (example Ritalin)

   ▶ **Schedule III**—Requires a new prescription after six months or five refills (example codeine)

   ▶ **Schedule IV**—Requires a new prescription after six months (example Darvon)

   ▶ **Schedule V**—Dispensed as any other prescription or without prescription if state law allows (example antitussives)

41. **Medication classifications commonly used in a medical/surgical setting**

   ▶ **Antacids**—Reduce hydrochloric acid in the stomach

   ▶ **Antianemics**—Increase red blood cell production

   ▶ **Anticholenergics**—Decrease oral secretions

   ▶ **Anticoagulants**—Prevent clot formation

   ▶ **Anticonvulsants**—Used for management of seizures/bipolar disorder

   ▶ **Antidiarrheals**—Decrease gastric motility and reduce water in bowel

   ▶ **Antihistamines**—Block the release of histamine

   ▶ **Antihypertensives**—Lower blood pressure and increase blood flow

   ▶ **Anti-infectives**—Used for the treatment of infections

   ▶ **Bronchodilators**—Dilate large air passages in asthma/lung disease

   ▶ **Diuretics**—Decrease water/sodium from the Loop of Henle

   ▶ **Laxatives**—Promote the passage of stool

   ▶ **Miotics**—Constrict the pupils

   ▶ **Mydriatics**—Dilate the pupils

   ▶ **Narcotics/analgesics**—Relieve moderate to severe pain

25. **Arab American cultural attributes**—Females avoid eye contact with males; touch is accepted if done by same-sex healthcare providers; most decisions are made by males; Muslims (Sunni), refuse organ donation; most Arabs do not eat pork; they avoid icy drinks when sick or hot/cold drinks together; colostrum is considered harmful to the newborn.

26. **Asian American cultural attributes**—They avoid direct eye contact; feet are considered dirty (the feet should be touched last during assessment); males make most of the decisions; they usually refuse organ donation; they generally do not prefer cold drinks, believe in the "hot-cold" theory of illness.

27. **Native American cultural attributes**—They sustain eye contact; blood and organ donation is generally refused; they might refuse circumcision; may prefer care from the tribal shaman rather than using western medicine.

28. **Mexican American cultural attributes**—They might avoid direct eye contact with authorities; they might refuse organ donation; most are very emotional during bereavement; believe in the "hot-cold" theory of illness.

29. **Religions beliefs**
    - **Jehovah's Witness**—No blood products should be used
    - **Hindu**—No beef or items containing gelatin
    - **Jewish**—Special dietary restrictions, use of kosher foods

30. **Therapeutic diets**
    - **Renal diet**—High calorie, high carbohydrate, low protein, low potassium, low sodium, and fluid restricted to intake = output + 500 ml
    - **Gout diet**—Low purine; omit poultry ("cold chicken") medication for acute episodes: Colchicine; maintenance medication: Zyloprim
    - **Heart healthy diet**—Low fat (less than 30% of calories should be from fat)

31. **Acid/base balance**
    - ROME (respiratory opposite/metabolic equal) is a quick way of remembering that in respiratory acid/base disorders the pH is opposite to the other components. For example, in respiratory acidosis, the pH is below normal and the CO_2 is elevated, as is the HCO_3 (respiratory opposite). In metabolic disorders, the components of the lab values are the same. An example of this is metabolic acidosis. In metabolic acidosis, the pH is below normal and the CO_2 is decreased, as is the HCO_3. This is true in a compensated situation.
    - pH down, CO_2 up, and HCO_3 up = respiratory acidosis
    - pH down, CO_2 down, and HCO_3 down = metabolic acidosis
    - pH up, CO_2 down, and HCO_3 down = respiratory alkalosis
    - pH up, CO_2 up, and HCO_3 up = metabolic alkalosis

32. **Addison's versus Cushing's**—Addison's and Cushing's are diseases of the endocrine system involving either overproduction or inadequate production of cortisol:
    - Treatment for the client with Addison's: increase sodium intake; medications include cortisone preparations.
    - Treatment for the client with Cushing's: restrict sodium; observe for signs of infection.

33. **Treatment for spider bites/bleeding**—RICE (rest, ice, compression, and elevate extremity)

34. **Treatment for sickle cell crises**—HHOP (heat, hydration, oxygen, pain medications)

35. **Five Ps of fractures and compartment syndrome**—These are symptoms of fractures and compartment syndrome:
    - Pain
    - Pallor
    - Pulselessness
    - Paresthesia
    - Polar (cold)

36. **Hip fractures**—Hip fractures commonly hemorrhage, whereas femur fractures are at risk for fat emboli.

37. **Profile of gallbladder disease**—Fair, fat, forty, five pregnancies, flatulent (actually gallbladder disease can occur in all ages and both sexes).

TIPS FOR ASSIGNING STAFF DUTIES

38. **Management and delegation**
    - Delegate sterile skills such as dressing changes to the RN or LPN. Where nonskilled care is required, you can delegate the stable client to the nursing assistant. Choose the most critical client to assign to the RN, such as the client who has recently returned from chest surgery. Clients who are being discharged should have final assessments done by the RN.
    - The PN, like the RN, can monitor clients with IV therapy, insert urinary catheters and feeding tubes, apply restraints, discontinue IVs, drains, and sutures.
    - For room assignments, do not coassign the post-operative client with clients who have vomiting, diarrhea, open wounds, or chest tube drainage. Remember the A, B, Cs (airway, breathing, circulation) when answering questions choices that ask who would you see first. For hospital triage, care for the client with a life-threatening illness or injury first. For disaster triage, choose to triage first those clients who can be saved with the least use of resources.

- LDH: 100–190 U/L
- CPK: 21–232 U/L
- Uric acid: 3.5–7.5 mg/dL
- Triglyceride: 40–50 mg/dL
- Total cholesterol: 130–200 mg/dL
- Bilirubin: < 1.0 mg/dL
- Protein: 6.2–8.1 g/dL
- Albumin: 3.4–5.0 g/dL

16. **Therapeutic drug levels**
   - Digoxin: 0.5–2.0 ng/ml
   - Lithium: 0.8–1.5 mEq/L
   - Dilantin: 10–20 mcg/dL
   - Theophylline: 10–20 mcg/dL

17. **Vital signs (adult)**
   - Heart rate: 80–100
   - Respiratory rate: 12–20
   - Blood pressure: 110–120 (systolic); 60–90 (diastolic)
   - Temperature: 98.6° ?/–1

18. **Maternity normals**
   - FHR: 120–160 BPM.
   - Variability: 6–10 BPM.
   - Contractions: normal frequency 2–5 minutes apart; normal duration < 90 sec.; intensity < 100 mm/hg.
   - Amniotic fluid: 500–1200 ml (nitrozine urine-litmus paper green/amniotic fluid-litmus paper blue).
   - Apgar scoring: A = appearance, P = pulses, G = grimace, A = activity, R = reflexes (Done at 1 and 5 minutes with a score of 0 for absent, 1 for decreased, and 2 for strongly positive.)
   - AVA: The umbilical cord has two arteries and one vein. (Arteries carry deoxygenated blood. The vein carries oxygenated blood.)

19. **FAB 9**—Folic acid = B9. Hint: *B* stands for brain (decreases the incidence of neural tube defects); the client should begin taking B9 three months prior to becoming pregnant.

20. **Abnormalities in the laboring obstetric client**— Decelerations are abnormal findings on the fetal monitoring strip. Decelerations are classified as
   - **Early decelerations**—Begin prior to the peak of the contraction and end by the end of the contraction. They are caused by head compression. There is no need for intervention if the variability is within normal range (that is, there is a rapid return to the baseline fetal heart rate) and the fetal heart rate is within normal range.

   - **Variable decelerations**—Are noted as V-shaped on the monitoring strip. Variable decelerations can occur anytime during monitoring of the fetus. They are caused by cord compression. The intervention is to change the mother's position; if pitocin is infusing, stop the infusion; apply oxygen; and increase the rate of IV fluids. Contact the doctor if the problem persists.
   - **Late decelerations**—Occur after the peak of the contraction and mirror the contraction in length and intensity. These are caused by uteroplacental insuffiency. The intervention is to change the mother's position; if pitocin is infusing, stop the infusion; apply oxygen;, and increase the rate of IV fluids. Contact the doctor if the problem persists.

21. **TORCHS syndrome in the neonate**—This is a combination of diseases. These include toxoplasmosis, rubella (German measles), cytomegalovirus, herpes, and syphyllis. Pregnant nurses should not be assigned to care for the client with toxoplasmosis or cytomegalovirus.

22. **STOP**—This is the treatment for maternal hypotension after an epidural anesthesia:
   1. Stop pitocin if infusing.
   2. Turn the client on the left side.
   3. Administer oxygen.
   4. If hypovolemia is present, push IV fluids.

23. **Anticoagulant therapy and monitoring**
   - Coumadin (sodium warfarin) PT: 10–12 sec. (control).
   - Antidote: The antidote for Coumadin is vitamin K.
   - Heparin/Lovenox/Dalteparin PTT: 30–45 sec. (control).
   - Antidote: The antidote for Heparin is protamine sulfate.
   - Therapeutic level: It is important to maintain a bleeding time that is slightly prolonged so that clotting will not occur; therefore, the bleeding time with mediication should be 1 1/2–2 times the control.

   *The control is the premedication bleeding time.

24. **Rule of nines for calculating TBSA for burns**
   - Head = 9%
   - Arms = 18% (9% each)
   - Back = 18%
   - Legs = 36% (18% each)
   - Genitalia = 1%

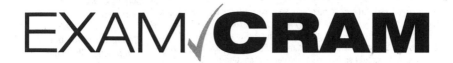

NCLEX-RN®
Practice
Questions

Second Edition

Wilda Rinehart
Diann Sloan
Clara Hurd

NCLEX-RN® Practice Questions
Second Edition

ISBN-13: 978-07897-3704-5

ISBN-10: 0-7897-3704-3

Library of Congress Cataloging-in-Publication Data

Rinehart, Wilda.

NCLEX-RN practice questions / Wilda Rinehart, Diann Sloan, Clara Hurd. -- 2nd ed.

p. ; cm.

ISBN-13: 978-0-7897-3704-5 (pbk. w/CD)

ISBN-10: 0-7897-3704-3 (pbk. w/CD)

1. Nursing--Examinations, questions, etc. 2. National Council Licensure Examination for Registered Nurses--Study guides. I. Sloan, Diann. II. Hurd, Clara. III. Title.

[DNLM: 1. Nursing--Examination Questions. WY 18.2 R579n 2008]

RT55.R565 2008

610.73076--dc22

2007042132

Printed in the United States of America

Second Printing: May 2008

Trademarks

Warning and Disclaimer

Bulk Sales

Que Publishing offers excellent discounts on this book when ordered in quantity for bulk purchases or special sales. For more information, please contact

U.S. Corporate and Government Sales
1-800-382-3419
corpsales@pearsontechgroup.com

For sales outside the U.S., please contact

International Sales
international@pearsoned.com

Associate Publisher
David Dusthimer

Acquisitions Editor
Betsy Brown

Senior Development Editor
Christopher Cleveland

Managing Editor
Patrick Kanouse

Senior Project Editor
San Dee Phillips

Technical Editor
Dr. Catherine Dearman

Publishing Coordinator
Vanessa Evans

Multimedia Developer
Dan Scherf

Book Designer
Gary Adair

Page Layout
TnT Design, Inc.

Rinehart and Associates

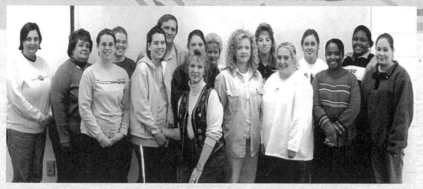

Prepare With the Best
Rinehart and Associates

For Nursing Students and Nursing Graduates- "Rinehart and Associates "NCLEX® Review Seminars", a three or four day seminar that provides a **complete, comprehensive review of nursing theory and practice with emphasis of the "NEW" NCLEX® test plan.**

We will come to your school and conduct a mini-review for you:

"Pharmacology Made Easy", a mini workshop for students reviewing commonly prescribed drugs as well as **hints** for remembering drug categories and nursing implications.

"Testing for Nursing School and NCLEX® Success", a mini workshop for nursing students to enhance success in nursing school and beyond.

"Fluid and Electrolytes- A Practical Approach", a mini workshop to increase the student's knowledge of Fluid and Electrolytes and Acid Base Disorders.

Pass the Licensure Exam the First Time

For more information on these and other workshops call:
662-728-4622
662-416-3340

Visit our web site at www.nclexreview.net
e-mail wrinehar@tsixroads.com or visit www.nclexreview.net
N CLEX is a registered trademark of the N ational Council of State Boards of Nursing

Contents at a Glance

Table of Contents

About the Authors

Wilda Rinehart received her associate degree in nursing from Northeast Mississippi Community College in Booneville, Mississippi. After working as a staff nurse and charge nurse, she became a public health nurse and served in that capacity for a number of years. In 1975, she received her Nurse Practitioner Certification in obstetric-gynecology from the University of Mississippi Medical Center in Jackson, Mississippi. In 1979, she completed her bachelor of science degree in nursing from Mississippi University for Women and the following year completed her master's degree in nursing from the same university. In 1980, Ms. Rinehart accepted a faculty position at Northeast Mississippi Community College where she taught medical-surgical nursing and obstetrical nursing. In 1982, she founded Rinehart and Associates Educational Consults. For the past 22 years, she and her associates have worked with nursing graduates and schools of nursing to assist graduates to pass the National Council Licensure Exam for Nursing. She has also worked with faculty who want to improve their item writing skills and as a curriculum consultant. Ms. Rinehart has served as a convention speaker throughout the southeastern United States and as a reviewer of medical-surgical and obstetric texts. She has coauthored NCLEX review materials and is presently working on DVD and CD review programs. As president of Rinehart and Associates, she serves as coordinator of a company dedicated to improving the quality of health through nursing education.

Dr. Diann Sloan holds an associate degree in nursing from Northeast Mississippi Community College, a bachelor's degree in nursing from the University of Mississippi, and a master's degree in nursing from Mississippi University for Women. In addition to her nursing degrees, she holds a master of science in education degree in counseling psychology from Georgia State University and a doctor of philosophy degree in counselor education. She has minors in both psychology and educational psychology, from Mississippi State University. She has completed additional graduate studies in healthcare administration at Western New England College and the University of Mississippi.

As a nurse educator, Dr. Sloan has taught pediatric nursing, psychiatric mental health nursing, and medical surgical nursing in both associate degree and baccalaureate nursing programs. As a member of Rinehart and Associates Nursing Review, Dr. Sloan has conducted test construction workshops for faculty and nursing review seminars for both registered and practical nurse graduates. She has coauthored materials used in the item writing workshops for nursing faculty and Rinehart and Associates Nursing Review. She is a member of Sigma Theta Tau nursing honor society.

Clara Hurd is an associate degree nurse graduate of Northeast Mississippi Community College in Booneville, Mississippi (1975). Her experiences in nursing are clinically based, having served as a staff nurse in medical-surgical nursing. She has worked as an oncology, intensive care, orthopedics, neurological, and pediatric nurse. She received her bachelor of science degree in nursing from the University of North Alabama in Florence, Alabama, and her master's degree in nursing from the Mississippi University for Women in Columbus, Mississippi. She is currently serving as a nurse educator at Northeast Mississippi Community College teaching medical-surgical content. Ms. Hurd has taught in both associate degree and baccalaureate nursing programs. She was a faculty member of Mississippi University for Women; Austin Peay State University in Clarksville, Tennessee; and Tennessee State University in Nashville, Tennessee. Ms. Hurd joined Rinehart and Associates in 1993. She has worked with students in preparing for the National Council Licensure Exam and with faculty as a consultant in writing test items. Ms. Hurd has also been a presenter at nursing conventions on various topics, including item writing for nursing faculty. Her primary professional goal is to prepare the student and graduate for excellence in the delivery of healthcare.

Contributing Authors

Tammy R. Owens, MSN, RN. Master of Science in Nursing, University of Phoenix Online. Associate degree in Nursing, Paducah Kentucky. Tammy is an assistant professor of nursing at Western Kentucky Community and Technical College in Paducah, Kentucky.

Michael W. Rager, MSN, RN. Master of Science in Nursing, University of Southern Indiana. Michael is an assistant professor at Madisonville Community College, a school within West Kentucky Community and Technical College in Paducah, Kentucky.

Susan Taylor, MSN, RN. Master of Science in Nursing, University of Evansville; Bachelor of Science in Nursing, Murray State University. Susan is an assistant professor of nursing at Western Kentucky and Technical College in Paducah, Kentucky.

Rhonda Payne, MSN, RN. Master of Science in Nursing, University of Alabama Mobile; Bachelor of Science in Nursing, Medical College of Georgia. Rhonda is an assistant professor of nursing at Bainbridge College of Nursing in Bainbridge, Georgia.

Linda A. Brown, MSN, RN. Master of Science in Nursing, Seattle Pacific University; Bachelor of Science in Nursing, University of Washington. Linda is a professor of nursing at Southwest Georgia Technical College in Thomasville, Georgia.

Rhonda Lansdell, MSN, RN, EdD., University of Mississippi; Higher Education Administration and Student Personnel, Master of Science in Nursing, University of Alabama, Birmingham; Bachelor of Science in Nursing, University of North Alabama. Rhonda is a professor of nursing at Northeast Mississippi Community College in Booneville, Mississippi.

Rosemary Marecle, MSN, RN. Master of Science in Nursing, University of Mississippi Medical Center College of Nursing; Bachelor of Science in Nursing, University of Alabama, Huntsville. Rosemary is a professor of nursing at Northeast Mississippi Community College in Booneville, Mississippi.

Dedication

We would like to thank our families for tolerating our late nights and long hours. Also, thanks to Gene Sloan for his help without pay. Special thanks to all the graduates who have attended Rinehart and Associates Review Seminars. Thanks for allowing us to be a part of your success.

We Want to Hear from You!

As the reader of this book, *you* are our most important critic and commentator. We value your opinion and want to know what we're doing right, what we could do better, what areas you'd like to see us publish in, and any other words of wisdom you're willing to pass our way.

As an associate publisher for Que Publishing, I welcome your comments. You can email or write me directly to let me know what you did or didn't like about this book—as well as what we can do to make our books better.

Please note that I cannot help you with technical problems related to the topic of this book. We do have a User Services group, however, where I will forward specific technical questions related to the book.

When you write, please be sure to include this book's title and author as well as your name, email address, and phone number. I will carefully review your comments and share them with the author and editors who worked on the book.

Email: feedback@quepublishing.com

Mail: Dave Dusthimer
           Associate Publisher
           Pearson Education
           800 East 96th Street
           Indianapolis, IN 46240 USA

Reader Services

Visit our website and register this book at www.quepublishing.com/register for convenient access to any updates, downloads, or errata that might be available for this book.

Introduction

Welcome to the *NCLEX-RN®* *Practice Questions Exam Cram*

This book helps you get ready to take and pass the Licensure Exam for Registered Nurses. This portion of the book discusses the NCLEX-RN® exam in general and how this Exam Cram can help you prepare for the test. It doesn't matter whether this is the first time you're going to take the exam or whether you have taken it previously; this book gives you the necessary information and techniques to obtain licensure.

The *NCLEX-RN® Practice Questions Exam Cram* helps you practice taking questions that are written in the NCLEX® format. Used with the *NCLEX-RN® Exam Cram*, it will help you understand and appreciate the subjects and materials you need to pass. Both books are aimed at test preparation and review. They do not teach you everything you need to know about the subject of nursing. Instead, they present you with materials that you are likely to encounter on the exam. Using a simple approach, we help you understand the "need to know" information.

To be able to pass the NCLEX®, you must understand how the exam is developed. The NCLEX-RN® consists of questions from the cognitive levels of knowledge, comprehension, application, and analysis. The majority of questions are written at the application and analysis level. Questions incorporate the five stages of the Nursing Process (assessment, diagnosis, planning, implementation, and evaluation) and the four categories of Client Needs. Client Needs are divided into subcategories that define the content within each of the four major categories. These categories and subcategories are:

A. Safe effective care: 8%–14%
   Management of care: 13%–19%
   Safety and infection control: 8%–14%

B. Health promotion and maintenance: 6%–12%

C. Psychosocial integrity: 6%–12%

D. Physiological integrity
Basic care and comfort: 6%–12%
Pharmacological and parenteral therapy: 13%–19%
Reduction of risk: 13%–19%
Physiological adaptation: 11%–17%

Taking the Computerized Adaptive Test

Computer-adaptive testing, commonly known as CAT, offers the candidate several advantages. The graduate can schedule the exam at a time that is convenient for him or her. It's also possible that you will not be tested on the entire 265-question range; if you answer the beginning questions correctly, the CAT might stop early in the session, with far fewer than the 265 questions you were expecting. The first questions will be difficult and should get easier. When the engine has determined your ability level and is satisfied that you are qualified to be a registered nurse, it will stop. The disadvantage of a CAT is that you cannot go back and change answers. When you make a decision and move on, that's it—no second guessing like on a paper exam.

The Pearson Vue testing group is responsible for administering the exam. You can locate a center nearest you by visiting www.pearsonvue.com. Because you might not be familiar with the Pearson Vue testing centers, we recommend that you arrive at least 30 minutes early. If you are late, you will not be allowed to take the test. Bring two forms of identification with you, one of which must be a picture ID. Be sure that your form of identification matches your application. You will be photographed and fingerprinted upon entering the testing site, so don't let this increase your stress. The allotted time is 6 hours, and the candidate can receive results within approximately 7 days (in some states, even sooner). Remember, the exam is written at approximately the tenth-grade reading level, so keep a good dictionary handy during your studies.

The Cost of the Exam

A candidate wanting to write the licensure exam must fill out two applications, one to the National Council and one to the state where he or she wants to be licensed. A separate fee must accompany each application. The fee required by the National Council is $200. State licensing fees vary. Licensure applications can be obtained at www.ncsbn.org. Several states are members of the multistate licensure compact. This means that if you are issued a multistate license, you pay only one fee. This information also can be obtained by visiting the National Council's website.

How to Prepare for the Exam

Judicious use of this book and its sister book, the *NCLEX-RN® Exam Cram*, either alone or with a review seminar such as that provided by Rinehart and Associates, will help you achieve your goal of becoming a registered nurse. As you review for the NCLEX® exam, we suggest that you find a location where you can concentrate on the material each day. A minimum of 2 hours per day for at least 2 weeks is suggested. In the *NCLEX-RN® Exam Cram*, we provide you with exam alerts, tips, notes, and sample questions, both multiple choice and alternate items. Using both books allows you to practice taking hundreds of questions much like those on the actual licensure exam. We have also formulated a "mock" exam with those difficult management and delegation questions that you can score to determine your readiness to test. Pay particular attention to the helpful hints and the Cram Sheet. Using these will help you gain and retain knowledge, and will help reduce your stress as you prepare to test.

What You Will Find in This Book

As seems obvious from the title, this book is all about practice questions! There are five full exams in this book, totaling 1,250 questions. Each chapter is set up with the questions and their possible answers first; the correct answers and rationales appear at the end of each chapter. In the margins next to each question, you will see a quick key to finding the location of its answer and rationales. Here's exactly what you will find in the chapters:

▶ *Practice Questions*—These are the numerous questions that will help you learn, drill, and review.

▶ *Quick Check Answers*—When you have finished answering the questions, you can quickly grade your exam from this section. Only correct answers are given here—no rationales are offered yet.

▶ *Answers and Rationales*—This section offers you the correct answers, as well as further explanation about the content posed in that question. Use this information to learn why an answer is correct and to reinforce the content in your mind for exam day.

You will also find a Cram Sheet at the beginning of this book specifically written for this exam. This is a very popular element that is also found in *NCLEX_RN® Exam Cram* (Que Publishing, ISBN 0-7897-3269-6). This item condenses all the necessary facts found in this exam into one easy-to-handle tearcard. The Cram Sheet is something you can carry with you to the exam location and use as a last-second study aid. Be aware that you can't take it into the exam room, though.

Hints for Using This Book

We suggest that you score your exam by subtracting the missed items from the total and then dividing the total answered correctly by the total number of questions. This gives you the percentage answered correctly. We also suggest that you achieve a score of at least 77% before you schedule your exam.

If you do not, take the exam again until you do. The higher the score, the better your chance to do well on the NCLEX® exam!

You should also take advantage of the CD exam engine; it provides you with a computer-adaptive test, or CAT, very similar to the one you will experience during the NCLEX® exam. Every question in this book is on the CD, including the answer rationales.

Aside from being a test-preparation book, this book is useful if you are brushing up on your nursing knowledge. It is an excellent quick reference for the licensed nurse.

Need Further Study?

If you are having a hard time correctly answering questions, be sure to see the sister book to this one, the *NCLEX-RN® Exam Cram* (Que Publishing, ISBN 0-7897-3269-6). If you still need further study, you might want to take an NCLEX® review seminar or look at one of the many other books available at your local bookstore.

Contact the Author

The authors of this text are interested in you and want you to pass on the first attempt. If after reviewing with this text you would like to contact the authors, you may do so at Rinehart and Associates, PO Box 124, Booneville, MS, 38829, or by visiting www.nclexreview.net. You may also contact them by phone at 662-728-4622.

CHAPTER ONE

Practice Exam 1 and Rationales

1. A client with a diagnosis of passive-aggressive personality disorder is seen at the local mental health clinic. A common characteristic of persons with passive-aggressive personality disorder is:

   ○ **A.** Superior intelligence
   ○ **B.** Underlying hostility
   ○ **C.** Dependence on others
   ○ **D.** Ability to share feelings

2. The client is admitted for evaluation of aggressive behavior and diagnosed with antisocial personality disorder. A key part of the care of such clients is:

   ○ **A.** Setting realistic limits
   ○ **B.** Encouraging the client to express remorse for behavior
   ○ **C.** Minimizing interactions with other clients
   ○ **D.** Encouraging the client to act out feelings of rage

3. An important intervention in monitoring the dietary compliance of a client with bulimia is:

   ○ **A.** Allowing the client privacy during mealtimes
   ○ **B.** Praising her for eating all her meal
   ○ **C.** Observing her for 1–2 hours after meals
   ○ **D.** Encouraging her to choose foods she likes and to eat in moderation

4. Assuming that all have achieved normal cognitive and emotional development, which of the following children is at greatest risk for accidental poisoning?

   ○ **A.** A 6-month-old
   ○ **B.** A 4-year-old
   ○ **C.** A 12-year-old
   ○ **D.** A 13-year-old

5. Which of the following examples represents parallel play?

Quick Answer: **52**
Detailed Answer: **55**

- ○ **A.** Jenny and Tommy share their toys.
- ○ **B.** Jimmy plays with his car beside Mary, who is playing with her doll.
- ○ **C.** Kevin plays a game of Scrabble with Kathy and Sue.
- ○ **D.** Mary plays with a handheld game while sitting in her mother's lap.

6. The nurse is ready to begin an exam on a 9-month-old infant. The child is sitting in his mother's lap. Which should the nurse do first?

Quick Answer: **52**
Detailed Answer: **55**

- ○ **A.** Check the Babinski reflex
- ○ **B.** Listen to the heart and lung sounds
- ○ **C.** Palpate the abdomen
- ○ **D.** Check tympanic membranes

7. In terms of cognitive development, a 2-year-old would be expected to:

Quick Answer: **52**
Detailed Answer: **55**

- ○ **A.** Think abstractly
- ○ **B.** Use magical thinking
- ○ **C.** Understand conservation of matter
- ○ **D.** See things from the perspective of others

8. Which of the following best describes the language of a 24-month-old?

Quick Answer: **52**
Detailed Answer: **55**

- ○ **A.** Doesn't understand yes and no
- ○ **B.** Understands the meaning of words
- ○ **C.** Able to verbalize needs
- ○ **D.** Asks "why?" to most statements

9. A client who has been receiving urokinase has a large bloody bowel movement. Which action would be best for the nurse to take immediately?

Quick Answer: **52**
Detailed Answer: **56**

- ○ **A.** Administer vitamin K IM
- ○ **B.** Stop the urokinase
- ○ **C.** Reduce the urokinase and administer heparin
- ○ **D.** Stop the urokinase and call the doctor

10. The client has a prescription for a calcium carbonate compound to neutralize stomach acid. The nurse should assess the client for:

Quick Answer: 52
Detailed Answer: 56

○ A. Constipation

○ B. Hyperphosphatemia

○ C. Hypomagnesemia

○ D. Diarrhea

11. Heparin has been ordered for a client with pulmonary embolis. Which statement, if made by the graduate nurse, indicates a lack of understanding of the medication?

Quick Answer: 52
Detailed Answer: 56

○ A. "I will administer the medication 1-2 inches away from the umbilicus."

○ B. "I will administer the medication in the abdomen."

○ C. "I will check the PTT before administering the medication."

○ D. "I will need to aspirate when I give Heparin."

12. The nurse is caring for a client with peripheral vascular disease. To correctly assess the oxygen saturation level, the monitor may be placed on the.

Quick Answer: 52
Detailed Answer: 56

○ A. Hip

○ B. Ankle

○ C. Earlobe

○ D. Chin

13. While caring for a client with hypertension, the nurse notes the following vital signs: BP of 140/20, pulse 120, respirations 36, temperature 100.8°F. The nurse's initial action should be to:

Quick Answer: 52
Detailed Answer: 56

○ A. Call the doctor

○ B. Recheck the vital signs

○ C. Obtain arterial blood gases

○ D. Obtain an ECG

14. The nurse is preparing a client with an axillo-popliteal bypass graft for discharge. The client should be taught to avoid:

Quick Answer: 52
Detailed Answer: 56

○ A. Using a recliner to rest

○ B. Resting in supine position

○ C. Sitting in a straight chair

○ D. Sleeping in right Sim's position

15. The doctor has ordered antithrombolic stockings to be applied to the legs of the client with peripheral vascular disease. The nurse knows antithrombolic stockings should be applied:

   ○ **A.** Before rising in the morning
   ○ **B.** With the client in a standing position
   ○ **C.** After bathing and applying powder
   ○ **D.** Before retiring in the evening

Quick Answer: **52**
Detailed Answer: **56**

16. The nurse has just received the shift report and is preparing to make rounds. Which client should be seen first?

   ○ **A.** The client with a history of a cerebral aneurysm with an oxygen saturation rate of 99%
   ○ **B.** The client three days post–coronary artery bypass graft with a temperature of 100.2°F
   ○ **C.** The client admitted 1 hour ago with shortness of breath
   ○ **D.** The client being prepared for discharge following a femoral popliteal bypass graft

Quick Answer: **52**
Detailed Answer: **56**

17. A client with a femoral popliteal bypass graft is assigned to a semiprivate room. The most suitable roommate for this client is the client with:

   ○ **A.** Hypothyroidism
   ○ **B.** Diabetic ulcers
   ○ **C.** Ulcerative colitis
   ○ **D.** Pneumonia

Quick Answer: **52**
Detailed Answer: **57**

18. The nurse is teaching the client regarding use of sodium warfarin. Which statement made by the client would require further teaching?

   ○ **A.** "I will have blood drawn every month."
   ○ **B.** "I will assess my skin for a rash."
   ○ **C.** "I take aspirin for a headache."
   ○ **D.** "I will use an electric razor to shave."

Quick Answer: **52**
Detailed Answer: **57**

19. The client returns to the recovery room following repair of an abdominal aneurysm. Which finding would require further investigation?

   ○ **A.** Pedal pulses regular
   ○ **B.** Urinary output 20mL in the past hour
   ○ **C.** Blood pressure 108/50
   ○ **D.** Oxygen saturation 97%

Quick Answer: **52**
Detailed Answer: **57**

20. The nurse is doing bowel and bladder retraining for the client with paraplegia. Which of the following is not a factor for the nurse to consider?

Quick Answer: **52**
Detailed Answer: **57**

- ○ **A.** Diet pattern
- ○ **B.** Mobility
- ○ **C.** Fluid intake
- ○ **D.** Sexual function

21. A 20-year-old is admitted to the rehabilitation unit following a motorcycle
accident. Which would be the appropriate method for measuring the
client for crutches?

Quick Answer: **52**
Detailed Answer: **57**

- ○ **A.** Measure five finger breadths under the axilla
- ○ **B.** Measure 3 inches under the axilla
- ○ **C.** Measure the client with the elbows flexed 10°
- ○ **D.** Measure the client with the crutches 20 inches from the side
of the foot

22. The nurse is caring for the client following a cerebral vascular accident.
Which portion of the brain is responsible for taste, smell, and hearing?

Quick Answer: **52**
Detailed Answer: **57**

- ○ **A.** Occipital
- ○ **B.** Frontal
- ○ **C.** Temporal
- ○ **D.** Parietal

23. The client is admitted to the unit after a motor vehicle accident with a
temperature of 102°F rectally. The most likely explanations for the elevated temperature is that:

Quick Answer: **52**
Detailed Answer: **57**

- ○ **A.** There was damage to the hypothalamus.
- ○ **B.** He has an infection from the abrasions to the head and face.
- ○ **C.** He will require a cooling blanket to decrease the temperature.
- ○ **D.** There was damage to the frontal lobe of the brain.

24. The client is admitted to the hospital in chronic renal failure. A diet low in
protein is ordered. The rationale for a low-protein diet is:

Quick Answer: **52**
Detailed Answer: **57**

- ○ **A.** Protein breaks down into blood urea nitrogen and other
waste.
- ○ **B.** High protein increases the sodium and potassium levels.
- ○ **C.** A high-protein diet decreases albumin production.
- ○ **D.** A high-protein diet depletes calcium and phosphorous.

25. The client who is admitted with thrombophlebitis has an order for heparin. The medication should be administered using a/an:

- ○ **A.** Buretrol
- ○ **B.** Infusion controller
- ○ **C.** Intravenous filter
- ○ **D.** Three-way stop-cock

26. The nurse is taking the blood pressure of the obese client. If the blood pressure cuff is too small, the results will be:

- ○ **A.** A false elevation
- ○ **B.** A false low reading
- ○ **C.** A blood pressure reading that is correct
- ○ **D.** A subnormal finding

27. A 4-year-old male is admitted to the unit with nephotic syndrome. He is extremely edematous. To decrease the discomfort associated with scrotal edema, the nurse should:

- ○ **A.** Apply ice to the scrotum
- ○ **B.** Elevate the scrotum on a small pillow
- ○ **C.** Apply heat to the abdominal area
- ○ **D.** Administer an analgesic

28. The client with an abdominal aortic aneurysm is admitted in preparation for surgery. Which of the following should be reported to the doctor?

- ○ **A.** An elevated white blood cell count
- ○ **B.** An abdominal bruit
- ○ **C.** A negative Babinski reflex
- ○ **D.** Pupils that are equal and reactive to light

29. If the nurse is unable to elicit the deep tendon reflexes of the patella, the nurse should ask the client to:

- ○ **A.** Pull against the palms
- ○ **B.** Grimace the facial muscles
- ○ **C.** Cross the legs at the ankles
- ○ **D.** Perform Valsalva maneuver

30. The physician has ordered atropine sulfate 0.4mg IM before surgery. The medication is supplied in 0.8mg per milliliter. The nurse should administer how many milliliters of the medication?

- ○ **A.** 0.25mL
- ○ **B.** 0.5mL
- ○ **C.** 1.0mL
- ○ **D.** 1.25mL

Quick Answer: **52**
Detailed Answer: **58**

31. The nurse is evaluating the client's pulmonary artery pressure. The nurse is aware that this test evaluates:

- ○ **A.** Pressure in the left ventricle
- ○ **B.** The systolic, diastolic, and mean pressure of the pulmonary artery
- ○ **C.** The pressure in the pulmonary veins
- ○ **D.** The pressure in the right ventricle

Quick Answer: **52**
Detailed Answer: **58**

32. A client is being monitored using a central venous pressure monitor. If the pressure is 2cm of water, the nurse should:

- ○ **A.** Call the doctor immediately
- ○ **B.** Slow the intravenous infusion
- ○ **C.** Listen to the lungs for rales
- ○ **D.** Administer a diuretic

Quick Answer: **52**
Detailed Answer: **58**

33. The nurse identifies ventricular tachycardia on the heart monitor. The nurse should immediately:

- ○ **A.** Administer atropine sulfate
- ○ **B.** Check the potassium level
- ○ **C.** Prepare to administer an antiarrhythmic such as lidocaine
- ○ **D.** Defibrillate at 360 joules

Quick Answer: **52**
Detailed Answer: **58**

34. The doctor is preparing to remove chest tubes from the client's left chest. In preparation for the removal, the nurse should instruct the client to:

- ○ **A.** Breathe normally
- ○ **B.** Hold his breath and bear down
- ○ **C.** Take a deep breath
- ○ **D.** Sneeze on command

Quick Answer: **52**
Detailed Answer: **58**

35. The doctor has ordered 80mg of furosemide (Lasix) two times per day. The nurse notes the patient's potassium level to be 2.5meq/L. The nurse should:

Quick Answer: **52**
Detailed Answer: **58**

- ○ **A.** Administer the Lasix as ordered
- ○ **B.** Administer half the dose
- ○ **C.** Offer the patient a potassium-rich food
- ○ **D.** Withhold the drug and call the doctor

36. Which of the following lab studies should be done periodically if the client is taking warfarin sodium (Coumadin)?

Quick Answer: **52**
Detailed Answer: **58**

- ○ **A.** Stool specimen for occult blood
- ○ **B.** White blood cell count
- ○ **C.** Blood glucose
- ○ **D.** Erthyrocyte count

37. The client has an order for heparin to prevent post-surgical thrombi. Immediately following a heparin injection, the nurse should:

Quick Answer: **52**
Detailed Answer: **58**

- ○ **A.** Aspirate for blood
- ○ **B.** Check the pulse rate
- ○ **C.** Massage the site
- ○ **D.** Check the site for bleeding

38. The client with AIDS tells the nurse that he has been using acupuncture to help with his pain. The nurse should question the client regarding this treatment because acupuncture uses:

Quick Answer: **52**
Detailed Answer: **59**

- ○ **A.** Pressure from the fingers and hands to stimulate the energy points in the body
- ○ **B.** Oils extracted from plants and herbs
- ○ **C.** Needles to stimulate certain points on the body to treat pain
- ○ **D.** Manipulation of the skeletal muscles to relieve stress and pain

39. The nurse is taking the vital signs of the client admitted with cancer of the pancreas. The nurse is aware that the fifth vital sign is:

Quick Answer: **52**
Detailed Answer: **59**

- ○ **A.** Anorexia
- ○ **B.** Pain
- ○ **C.** Insomnia
- ○ **D.** Fatigue

40. The 84-year-old male has returned from the recovery room following a total hip repair. He complains of pain and is medicated with morphine sulfate and promethazine. Which medication should be kept available for the client being treated with opioid analgesics?

   ○ **A.** Naloxone (Narcan)
   ○ **B.** Ketorolac (Toradol)
   ○ **C.** Acetylsalicylic acid (aspirin)
   ○ **D.** Atropine sulfate (Atropine)

41. The doctor has ordered a patient-controlled analgesia (PCA) pump for the client with chronic pain. The client asks the nurse if he can become overdosed with pain medication using this machine. The nurse demonstrates understanding of the PCA if she states:

   ○ **A.** "The machine will administer only the amount that you need to control your pain without any action from you."
   ○ **B.** "The machine has a locking device that prevents overdosing."
   ○ **C.** The machine will administer one large dose every 4 hours to relieve your pain."
   ○ **D.** "The machine is set to deliver medication only if you need it."

42. The doctor has ordered a Transcutaneous Electrical Nerve Stimulation (TENS) unit for the client with chronic back pain. The nurse teaching the client with a TENS unit should tell the client:

   ○ **A.** "You may be electrocuted if you use water with this unit."
   ○ **B.** "Please report skin irritation to the doctor."
   ○ **C.** "The unit may be used anywhere on the body without fear of adverse reactions."
   ○ **D.** "A cream should be applied to the skin before applying the unit."

43. The nurse asked the client if he has an advance directive. The reason for asking the client this question is:

   ○ **A.** She is curious about his plans regarding funeral arrangements.
   ○ **B.** Much confusion can occur with the client's family if he does not have an advanced directive.
   ○ **C.** An advanced directive allows the medical personnel to make decisions for the client.
   ○ **D.** An advanced directive allows active euthanasia to be carried out if the client is unable to care for himself.

44. A client who has chosen to breastfeed tells the nurse that her nipples became very sore while she was breastfeeding her older child. Which measure will help her to avoid soreness of the nipples?

- ○ **A.** Feeding the baby during the first 48 hours after delivery
- ○ **B.** Breaking suction by placing a finger between the baby's mouth and the breast when she terminates the feeding
- ○ **C.** Applying hot, moist soaks to the breast several times per day
- ○ **D.** Wearing a support bra

45. The nurse is performing an assessment of an elderly client with a total hip repair. Based on this assessment, the nurse decides to medicate the client with an analgesic. Which finding most likely prompted the nurse to decide to administer the analgesic?

- ○ **A.** The client's blood pressure is 130/86.
- ○ **B.** The client is unable to concentrate.
- ○ **C.** The client's pupils are dilated.
- ○ **D.** The client grimaces during care.

46. An obstetrical client decides to have an epidural anesthetic to relieve pain during labor. Following administration of the anesthesia, the nurse should monitor the client for:

- ○ **A.** Seizures
- ○ **B.** Postural hypertension
- ○ **C.** Respiratory depression
- ○ **D.** Hematuria

47. The nurse is assessing the client admitted for possible oral cancer. The nurse identifies which of the following to be a late-occurring symptom of oral cancer?

- ○ **A.** Warmth
- ○ **B.** Odor
- ○ **C.** Pain
- ○ **D.** Ulcer with flat edges

48. The nurse understands that the diagnosis of oral cancer is confirmed with:

- ○ **A.** Biopsy
- ○ **B.** Gram Stain
- ○ **C.** Oral culture
- ○ **D.** Oral washings for cytology

49. The nurse is caring for the patient following removal of a large posterior oral lesion. The priority nursing measure would be to:

    ○ **A.** Maintain a patent airway

    ○ **B.** Perform meticulous oral care every 2 hours

    ○ **C.** Ensure that the incisional area is kept as dry as possible

    ○ **D.** Assess the client frequently for pain

Quick Answer: **52**
Detailed Answer: **60**

50. The registered nurse is conducting an in-service for colleagues on the subject of peptic ulcers. The nurse would be correct in identifying which of the following as a causative factor?

    ○ **A.** *N. gonorrhea*

    ○ **B.** *H. influenza*

    ○ **C.** *H. pylori*

    ○ **D.** *E. coli*

Quick Answer: **52**
Detailed Answer: **60**

51. The patient states, "My stomach hurts about 2 hours after I eat." Based upon this information, the nurse suspects the patient likely has a:

    ○ **A.** Gastric ulcer

    ○ **B.** Duodenal ulcer

    ○ **C.** Peptic ulcer

    ○ **D.** Curling's ulcer

Quick Answer: **52**
Detailed Answer: **60**

52. The nurse is caring for a patient with suspected diverticulitis. The nurse would be most prudent in questioning which of the following diagnostic tests?

    ○ **A.** Abdominal ultrasound

    ○ **B.** Barium enema

    ○ **C.** Complete blood count

    ○ **D.** Computed tomography (CT) scan

Quick Answer: **52**
Detailed Answer: **60**

53. The nurse is planning care for the patient with celiac disease. In teaching about the diet, the nurse should instruct the patient to avoid which of the following for breakfast?

    ○ **A.** Puffed wheat

    ○ **B.** Banana

    ○ **C.** Puffed rice

    ○ **D.** Cornflakes

Quick Answer: **52**
Detailed Answer: **60**

54. The nurse is teaching about irritable bowel syndrome (IBS). Which of the following would be most important?

Quick Answer: **52**
Detailed Answer: **60**

- ○ **A.** Reinforcing the need for a balanced diet
- ○ **B.** Encouraging the client to drink 16 ounces of fluid with each meal
- ○ **C.** Telling the client to eat a diet low in fiber
- ○ **D.** Instructing the client to limit his intake of fruits and vegetables

55. In planning care for the patient with ulcerative colitis, the nurse identifies which nursing diagnosis as a priority?

Quick Answer: **52**
Detailed Answer: **60**

- ○ **A.** Anxiety
- ○ **B.** Impaired skin integrity
- ○ **C.** Fluid volume deficit
- ○ **D.** Nutrition altered, less than body requirements

56. The patient is prescribed metronidazole (Flagyl) for adjunct treatment for a duodenal ulcer. When teaching about this medication, the nurse would include:

Quick Answer: **52**
Detailed Answer: **60**

- ○ **A.** "This medication should be taken only until you begin to feel better."
- ○ **B.** "This medication should be taken on an empty stomach to increase absorption."
- ○ **C.** "While taking this medication, you do not have to be concerned about being in the sun."
- ○ **D.** "While taking this medication, alcoholic beverages and products containing alcohol should be avoided."

57. The nurse is preparing to administer a feeding via a nasogastric tube. The nurse would perform which of the following before initiating the feeding?

Quick Answer: **52**
Detailed Answer: **60**

- ○ **A.** Assess for tube placement by aspirating stomach content
- ○ **B.** Place the patient in a left-lying position
- ○ **C.** Administer feeding with 50% Dextrose
- ○ **D.** Ensure that the feeding solution has been warmed in a microwave for 2 minutes

58. Which is true regarding the administration of antacids?

Quick Answer: **52**
Detailed Answer: **61**

- ○ **A.** Antacids should be administered without regard to mealtimes.
- ○ **B.** Antacids should be administered with each meal and snack of the day.
- ○ **C.** Antacids should not be administered with other medications.
- ○ **D.** Antacids should be administered with all other medications, for maximal absorption.

59. The nurse is caring for a patient with a colostomy. The patient asks, "Will I ever be able to swim again?" The nurse's best response would be:

Quick Answer: **52**
Detailed Answer: **61**

- ○ **A.** "Yes, you should be able to swim again, even with the colostomy."
- ○ **B.** "You should avoid immersing the colostomy in water."
- ○ **C.** "No, you should avoid getting the colostomy wet."
- ○ **D.** "Don't worry about that. You will be able to live just like you did before."

60. The nurse is assisting in the care of a patient who is 2 days post-operative from a hemorroidectomy. The nurse would be correct in instructing the patient to:

Quick Answer: **52**
Detailed Answer: **61**

- ○ **A.** Avoid a high-fiber diet
- ○ **B.** Continue to use ice packs
- ○ **C.** Take a laxative daily to prevent constipation
- ○ **D.** Use a sitz bath after each bowel movement

61. The nurse is assisting in the care of a client with diverticulosis. Which of the following assessment findings must necessitate an immediate report to the doctor?

Quick Answer: **52**
Detailed Answer: **61**

- ○ **A.** Bowel sounds are present
- ○ **B.** Intermittent left lower-quadrant pain
- ○ **C.** Constipation alternating with diarrhea
- ○ **D.** Hemoglobin 26% and hematocrit 32

62. The client is newly diagnosed with juvenile onset diabetes. Which of the following nursing diagnoses is a priority?

Quick Answer: **52**
Detailed Answer: **61**

- ○ **A.** Anxiety
- ○ **B.** Pain
- ○ **C.** Knowledge deficit
- ○ **D.** Altered thought process

63. The nurse is asked by the nurse aide, "Are peptic ulcers really caused by stress?" The nurse would be correct in replying with the following:

Quick Answer: **52**
Detailed Answer: **61**

- ○ **A.** "Peptic ulcers result from overeating fatty foods."
- ○ **B.** "Peptic ulcers are always caused from exposure to continual stress."
- ○ **C.** "Peptic ulcers are like all other ulcers, which all result from stress."
- ○ **D.** "Peptic ulcers are associated with *H. pylori,* although there are other ulcers that are associated with stress."

64. The nurse is assisting in the assessment of the patient admitted with "extreme abdominal pain." The nurse asks the client about the medication that he has been taking because:

Quick Answer: **52**
Detailed Answer: **61**

- ○ **A.** Interactions between medications will cause abdominal pain.
- ○ **B.** Various medications taken by mouth can affect the alimentary tract.
- ○ **C.** This will provide an opportunity to educate the patient regarding the medications used.
- ○ **D.** The types of medications might be attributable to an abdominal pathology not already identified.

65. The nurse is assessing the abdomen. The nurse knows the best sequence to perform the assessment is:

Quick Answer: **52**
Detailed Answer: **61**

- ○ **A.** Inspection, auscultation, palpation
- ○ **B.** Auscultation, palpation, inspection
- ○ **C.** Palpation, inspection, auscultation
- ○ **D.** Inspection, palpation, auscultation

66. The nurse is caring for the client who has been in a coma for 2 months. He has signed a donor card, but the wife is opposed to the idea of organ donation. How should the nurse handle the topic of organ donation with the wife?

Quick Answer: **52**
Detailed Answer: **61**

- ○ **A.** Tell the wife that the hospital will honor her wishes regarding organ donation, but contact the organ-retrieval staff
- ○ **B.** Tell her that because her husband signed a donor card, the hospital has the right to take the organs upon the death of her husband
- ○ **C.** Explain that it is necessary for her to donate her husband's organs because he signed the permit
- ○ **D.** Refrain from talking about the subject until after the death of her husband

67. The client with cancer refuses to care for herself. Which action by the nurse would be best?

Quick Answer: **52**
Detailed Answer: **61**

- ○ **A.** Alternate nurses caring for the client so that the staff will not get tired of caring for this client
- ○ **B.** Talk to the client and explain the need for self-care
- ○ **C.** Explore the reason for the lack of motivation seen in the client
- ○ **D.** Talk to the doctor about the client's lack of motivation

68. The charge nurse is making assignments for the day. After accepting the assignment to a client with leukemia, the nurse tells the charge nurse that her child has chickenpox. Which initial action should the charge nurse take?

Quick Answer: **52**
Detailed Answer: **61**

- ○ **A.** Change the nurse's assignment to another client
- ○ **B.** Explain to the nurse that there is no risk to the client
- ○ **C.** Ask the nurse if the chickenpox have scabbed
- ○ **D.** Ask the nurse if she has ever had the chickenpox

69. The nurse is caring for the client with a mastectomy. Which action would be contraindicated?

Quick Answer: **52**
Detailed Answer: **62**

- ○ **A.** Taking the blood pressure in the side of the mastectomy
- ○ **B.** Elevating the arm on the side of the mastectomy
- ○ **C.** Positioning the client on the unaffected side
- ○ **D.** Performing a dextrostix on the unaffected side

70. The client has an order for gentamycin to be administered. Which lab results should be reported to the doctor before beginning the medication?

Quick Answer: **52**
Detailed Answer: **62**

- ○ **A.** Hematocrit
- ○ **B.** Creatinine
- ○ **C.** White blood cell count
- ○ **D.** Erythrocyte count

71. Which of the following is the best indicator of the diagnosis of HIV?

Quick Answer: **52**
Detailed Answer: **62**

- ○ **A.** White blood cell count
- ○ **B.** ELISA
- ○ **C.** Western Blot
- ○ **D.** Complete blood count

72. The client presents to the emergency room with a "bull's eye" rash. Which question would be most appropriate for the nurse to ask the client?

- ○ **A.** "Have you found any ticks on your body?"
- ○ **B.** "Have you had any nausea in the last 24 hours?"
- ○ **C.** "Have you been outside the country in the last 6 months?"
- ○ **D.** "Have you had any fever for the past few days?"

73. Which client should be assigned to the nursing assistant?

- ○ **A.** The 18-year-old with a fracture to two cervical vertebrae
- ○ **B.** The infant with meningitis
- ○ **C.** The elderly client with a thyroidectomy 4 days ago
- ○ **D.** The client with a thoracotomy 2 days ago

74. The client presents to the emergency room with a hyphema. Which action by the nurse would be best?

- ○ **A.** Elevate the head of the bed and apply ice to the eye
- ○ **B.** Place the client in a supine position and apply heat to the knee
- ○ **C.** Insert a Foley catheter and measure the intake and output
- ○ **D.** Perform a vaginal exam and check for a discharge

75. The client has an order for $FeSo_4$ liquid. Which method of administration would be best?

- ○ **A.** Administer the medication with milk
- ○ **B.** Administer the medication with a meal
- ○ **C.** Administer the medication with orange juice
- ○ **D.** Administer the medication undiluted

76. The client with an ileostomy is being discharged. Which teaching should be included in the plan of care?

- ○ **A.** Using Karaya powder to seal the bag.
- ○ **B.** Irrigating the ileostomy daily.
- ○ **C.** Using stomahesive as the best skin protector.
- ○ **D.** Using Neosporin ointment to protect the skin.

77. Vitamin K is administered to the newborn shortly after birth for which of the following reasons?

- ○ **A.** To stop hemorrhage
- ○ **B.** To treat infection
- ○ **C.** To replace electrolytes
- ○ **D.** To facilitate clotting

78. Before administering Methyltrexate orally to the client with cancer, the nurse should check the:

    - ○ **A.** IV site
    - ○ **B.** Electrolytes
    - ○ **C.** Blood gases
    - ○ **D.** Vital signs

79. The nurse is teaching a group of new graduates about the safety needs of the client receiving chemotherapy. Before administering chemotherapy, the nurse should:

    - ○ **A.** Administer a bolus of IV fluid
    - ○ **B.** Administer pain medication
    - ○ **C.** Administer an antiemetic
    - ○ **D.** Allow the patient a chance to eat

80. The client is admitted to the postpartum unit with an order to continue the infusion of Pitocin. The nurse is aware that Pitocin is working if the fundus is:

    - ○ **A.** Deviated to the left.
    - ○ **B.** Firm and in the midline.
    - ○ **C.** Boggy.
    - ○ **D.** Two finger breadths below the umbilicus.

81. A 5-year-old is a family contact to the client with tuberculosis. Isoniazid (INH) has been prescribed for the client. The nurse is aware that the length of time that the medication will be taken is:

    - ○ **A.** 6 months
    - ○ **B.** 3 months
    - ○ **C.** 1 year
    - ○ **D.** 2 years

82. A 4-year-old with cystic fibrosis has a prescription for Viokase pancreatic enzymes to prevent malabsorption. The correct time to give pancreatic enzyme is:

    - ○ **A.** 1 hour before meals
    - ○ **B.** 2 hours after meals
    - ○ **C.** With each meal and snack
    - ○ **D.** On an empty stomach

83. A client with osteomylitis has an order for a trough level to be done because he is taking Gentamycin. When should the nurse call the lab to obtain the trough level?

   ○ **A.** Before the first dose

   ○ **B.** 30 minutes before the fourth dose

   ○ **C.** 30 minutes after the first dose

   ○ **D.** 30 minutes before the first dose

Quick Answer: **52**
Detailed Answer: **63**

84. A new diabetic is learning to administer his insulin. He receives 10U of NPH and 12U of regular insulin each morning. Which of the following statements reflects understanding of the nurse's teaching?

   ○ **A.** "When drawing up my insulin, I should draw up the regular insulin first."

   ○ **B.** "When drawing up my insulin, I should draw up the NPH insulin first."

   ○ **C.** "It doesn't matter which insulin I draw up first."

   ○ **D.** "I cannot mix the insulin, so I will need two shots."

Quick Answer: **52**
Detailed Answer: **63**

85. The client is scheduled to have an intravenous cholangiogram. Before the procedure, the nurse should assess the patient for:

   ○ **A.** Shellfish allergies

   ○ **B.** Reactions to blood transfusions

   ○ **C.** Gallbladder disease

   ○ **D.** Egg allergies

Quick Answer: **52**
Detailed Answer: **63**

86. Shortly after the client was admitted to the postpartum unit, the nurse notes heavy lochia rubra with large clots. The nurse should anticipate an order for:

   ○ **A.** Methergine

   ○ **B.** Stadol

   ○ **C.** Magnesium sulfate

   ○ **D.** Phenergan

Quick Answer: **52**
Detailed Answer: **63**

87. The client with a recent liver transplant asks the nurse how long he will have to take an immunosuppressant. Which response would be correct?

   ○ **A.** 1 year

   ○ **B.** 5 years

   ○ **C.** 10 years

   ○ **D.** The rest of his life

Quick Answer: **52**
Detailed Answer: **63**

88. The client is admitted from the emergency room with multiple injuries sustained from an auto accident. His doctor prescribes a histamine blocker. The nurse is aware that the reason for this order is to:

- ○ **A.** Treat general discomfort
- ○ **B.** Correct electrolyte imbalances
- ○ **C.** Prevent stress ulcers
- ○ **D.** Treat nausea

89. The physician prescribes regular insulin, 5 units subcutaneous. Regular insulin begins to exert an effect:

- ○ **A.** In 5–10 minutes
- ○ **B.** In 10–20 minutes
- ○ **C.** In 30–60 minutes
- ○ **D.** In 60–120 minutes

90. A 60-year-old diabetic is taking glyburide (Diabeta) 1.25mg daily to treat Type II diabetes mellitus. Which statement indicates the need for further teaching?

- ○ **A.** "I will keep candy with me just in case my blood sugar drops."
- ○ **B.** "I need to stay out of the sun as much as possible."
- ○ **C.** "I often skip dinner because I don't feel hungry."
- ○ **D.** "I always wear my medical identification."

91. A 20-year-old female has a prescription for tetracycline. While teaching the client how to take her medicine, the nurse learns that the client is also taking Ortho-Novum oral contraceptive pills. Which instructions should be included in the teaching plan?

- ○ **A.** The oral contraceptives will decrease the effectiveness of the tetracycline.
- ○ **B.** Nausea often results from taking oral contraceptives and antibiotics.
- ○ **C.** Toxicity can result when taking these two medications together.
- ○ **D.** Antibiotics can decrease the effectiveness of oral contraceptives, so the client should use an alternate method of birth control.

92. The client is taking prednisone 7.5mg po each morning to treat his systemic lupus erythematosis. Which statement best explains the reason for taking the prednisone in the morning?

- ○ **A.** There is less chance of forgetting the medication if taken in the morning.
- ○ **B.** There will be less fluid retention if taken in the morning.
- ○ **C.** Prednisone is absorbed best with the breakfast meal.
- ○ **D.** Morning administration mimics the body's natural secretion of corticosteroid.

93. The client is taking rifampin 600mg po daily to treat his tuberculosis. Which action by the nurse indicates understanding of the medication?

- ○ **A.** Telling the client that the medication will need to be taken with juice
- ○ **B.** Telling the client that the medication will change the color of the urine
- ○ **C.** Telling the client to take the medication before going to bed at night
- ○ **D.** Telling the client to take the medication if the night sweats occur

94. The client is diagnosed with multiple myloma. The doctor has ordered cyclophosphamide (Cytoxan). Which instruction should be given to the client?

- ○ **A.** "Walk about a mile a day to prevent calcium loss."
- ○ **B.** "Increase the fiber in your diet."
- ○ **C.** "Report nausea to the doctor immediately."
- ○ **D.** "Drink at least eight large glasses of water a day."

95. An elderly client is diagnosed with ovarian cancer. She has surgery followed by chemotherapy with a fluorouracil (Adrucil) IV. What should the nurse do if she notices crystals in the IV medication?

- ○ **A.** Discard the solution and order a new bag
- ○ **B.** Warm the solution
- ○ **C.** Continue the infusion and document the finding
- ○ **D.** Discontinue the medication

96. The 10-year-old is being treated for asthma. Before administering
     Theodur, the nurse should check the:

- ○ **A.** Urinary output
- ○ **B.** Blood pressure
- ○ **C.** Pulse
- ○ **D.** Temperature

97. Which information obtained from the mother of a child with cerebral
     palsy correlates to the diagnosis?

- ○ **A.** She was born at 40 weeks gestation.
- ○ **B.** She had meningitis when she was 6 months old.
- ○ **C.** She had physiologic jaundice after delivery.
- ○ **D.** She has frequent sore throats.

98. A 6-year-old with cerebral palsy functions at the level of an 18-month-
     old. Which finding would support that assessment?

- ○ **A.** She dresses herself.
- ○ **B.** She pulls a toy behind her.
- ○ **C.** She can build a tower of eight blocks.
- ○ **D.** She can copy a horizontal or vertical line.

99. A 5-year-old is admitted to the unit following a tonsillectomy. Which of
     the following would indicate a complication of the surgery?

- ○ **A.** Decreased appetite
- ○ **B.** A low-grade fever
- ○ **C.** Chest congestion
- ○ **D.** Constant swallowing

100. The child with seizure disorder is being treated with phenytoin (Dilantin).
     Which of the following statements by the patient's mother indicates to the
     nurse that the patient is experiencing a side effect of Dilantin therapy?

- ○ **A.** "She is very irritable lately."
- ○ **B.** "She sleeps quite a bit of the time."
- ○ **C.** "Her gums look too big for her teeth."
- ○ **D.** "She has gained about 10 pounds in the last six months."

101. The physician has prescribed tranylcypromine sulfate (Parnate) 10mg bid. The nurse should teach the client to refrain from eating foods containing tyramine because it may cause:

Quick Answer: **53**
Detailed Answer: **65**

- ○ **A.** Hypertension
- ○ **B.** Hyperthermia
- ○ **C.** Hypotension
- ○ **D.** Urinary retention

102. The client is admitted to the emergency room with shortness of breath, anxiety, and tachycardia. His ECG reveals atrial fibrillation with a ventricular response rate of 130 beats per minute. The doctor orders quinidine sulfate. While he is receiving quinidine, the nurse should monitor his ECG for:

Quick Answer: **53**
Detailed Answer: **65**

- ○ **A.** Peaked P wave
- ○ **B.** Elevated ST segment
- ○ **C.** Inverted T wave
- ○ **D.** Prolonged QT interval

103. Lidocaine is a medication frequently ordered for the client experiencing:

Quick Answer: **53**
Detailed Answer: **65**

- ○ **A.** Atrial tachycardia
- ○ **B.** Ventricular tachycardia
- ○ **C.** Heart block
- ○ **D.** Ventricular brachycardia

104. The doctor orders 2% nitroglycerin ointment in a 1-inch dose every 12 hours. Proper application of nitroglycerin ointment includes:

Quick Answer: **53**
Detailed Answer: **65**

- ○ **A.** Rotating application sites
- ○ **B.** Limiting applications to the chest
- ○ **C.** Rubbing it into the skin
- ○ **D.** Covering it with a gauze dressing

105. The physician prescribes captopril (Capoten) 25mg po tid for the client with hypertension. Which of the following adverse reactions can occur with administration of Capoten?

Quick Answer: **53**
Detailed Answer: **65**

- ○ **A.** Tinnitus
- ○ **B.** Persistent cough
- ○ **C.** Muscle weakness
- ○ **D.** Diarrhea

106. The client is admitted with a BP of 210/100. Her doctor orders furosemide (Lasix) 40mg IV stat. How should the nurse administer the prescribed furosemide to this client?

Quick Answer: **53**
Detailed Answer: **65**

- ○ **A.** By giving it over 1–2 minutes
- ○ **B.** By hanging it IV piggyback
- ○ **C.** With normal saline only
- ○ **D.** With a filter

107. The client is receiving heparin for thrombophlebitis of the left lower extremity. Which of the following drugs reverses the effects of heparin?

Quick Answer: **53**
Detailed Answer: **65**

- ○ **A.** Cyanocobalamine
- ○ **B.** Protamine sulfate
- ○ **C.** Streptokinase
- ○ **D.** Sodium warfarin

108. The nurse is making assignments for the day. Which client should be assigned to the pregnant nurse?

Quick Answer: **53**
Detailed Answer: **65**

- ○ **A.** The client receiving linear accelerator radiation therapy for lung cancer
- ○ **B.** The client with a radium implant for cervical cancer
- ○ **C.** The client who has just been administered soluble brachytherapy for thyroid cancer
- ○ **D.** The client who returned from placement of iridium seeds for prostate cancer

109. The nurse is planning room assignments for the day. Which client should be assigned to a private room if only one is available?

Quick Answer: **53**
Detailed Answer: **66**

- ○ **A.** The client with Cushing's disease
- ○ **B.** The client with diabetes
- ○ **C.** The client with acromegaly
- ○ **D.** The client with myxedema

110. The charge nurse witnesses the nursing assistant hitting the client in the long-term care facility. The nursing assistant can be charged with:

Quick Answer: **53**
Detailed Answer: **66**

- ○ **A.** Negligence
- ○ **B.** Tort
- ○ **C.** Assault
- ○ **D.** Malpractice

111. Which assignment should not be performed by the licensed practical nurse?

    ○ **A.** Inserting a Foley catheter

    ○ **B.** Discontinuing a nasogastric tube

    ○ **C.** Obtaining a sputum specimen

    ○ **D.** Starting a blood transfusion

Quick Answer: **53**
Detailed Answer: **66**

112. The client returns to the unit from surgery with a blood pressure of 90/50, pulse 132, respirations 30. Which action by the nurse should receive priority?

    ○ **A.** Continue to monitor the vital signs

    ○ **B.** Contact the physician

    ○ **C.** Ask the client how he feels

    ○ **D.** Ask the LPN to continue the post-op care

Quick Answer: **53**
Detailed Answer: **66**

113. The nurse is caring for a client with B-Thalassemia major. Which therapy is used to treat Thalassemia?

    ○ **A.** IV fluids

    ○ **B.** Frequent blood transfusions

    ○ **C.** Oxygen therapy

    ○ **D.** Iron therapy

Quick Answer: **53**
Detailed Answer: **66**

114. The child with a history of respiratory infections has an order for a sweat test to be done. Which finding would be positive for cystic fibrosis?

    ○ **A.** A serum sodium of 135meq/L

    ○ **B.** A sweat analysis of 69 meq/L

    ○ **C.** A potassium of 4.5meq/L

    ○ **D.** A calcium of 8mg/dL

Quick Answer: **53**
Detailed Answer: **66**

115. The nurse caring for the child with a large meningomylocele is aware that the priority care for this client is to:

    ○ **A.** Cover the defect with a moist, sterile saline gauze

    ○ **B.** Place the infant in a supine position

    ○ **C.** Feed the infant slowly

    ○ **D.** Measure the intake and output

Quick Answer: **53**
Detailed Answer: **66**

116. The nurse is caring for an infant admitted from the delivery room. Which finding should be reported?

    ○ **A.** Acyanosis

    ○ **B.** Acrocyanosis

    ○ **C.** Halequin sign

    ○ **D.** Absent femoral pulses

Quick Answer: **53**
Detailed Answer: **66**

117. The nurse is aware that a common mode of transmission of clostridium difficile is:

- ○ **A.** Use of unsterile surgical equipment
- ○ **B.** Contamination with sputum
- ○ **C.** Through the urinary catheter
- ○ **D.** Contamination with stool

118. The nurse has just received the change of shift report. Which client should the nurse assess first?

- ○ **A.** A client 2 hours post-lobectomy with 150ml drainage
- ○ **B.** A client 2 days post-gastrectomy with scant drainage
- ○ **C.** A client with pneumonia with an oral temperature of 102°F
- ○ **D.** A client with a fractured hip in Buck's traction

119. A client has been receiving cyanocobalamine (B12) injections for the past six weeks. Which laboratory finding indicates that the medication is having the desired effect?

- ○ **A.** Neutrophil count of 60%
- ○ **B.** Basophil count of 0.5%
- ○ **C.** Monocyte count of 2%
- ○ **D.** Reticulocyte count of 1%

120. The nurse is providing discharge teaching for a client taking dissulfiram (Antabuse). The nurse should instruct the client to avoid eating:

- ○ **A.** Peanuts, dates, raisins
- ○ **B.** Figs, chocolate, eggplant
- ○ **C.** Pickles, salad with vinaigrette dressing, beef
- ○ **D.** Milk, cottage cheese, ice cream

121. A 70-year-old male who is recovering from a stroke exhibits signs of unilateral neglect. Which behavior is suggestive of unilateral neglect?

- ○ **A.** The client is observed shaving only one side of his face.
- ○ **B.** The client is unable to distinguish between two tactile stimuli presented simultaneously.
- ○ **C.** The client is unable to complete a range of vision without turning his head side to side.
- ○ **D.** The client is unable to carry out cognitive and motor activity at the same time.

122. A client with acute leukemia develops a low white blood cell count. In addition to the institution of isolation, the nurse should:

- ○ **A.** Request that foods be served with disposable utensils
- ○ **B.** Ask the client to wear a mask when visitors are present
- ○ **C.** Prep IV sites with mild soap and water and alcohol
- ○ **D.** Provide foods in sealed, single-serving packages

123. A new nursing graduate indicates in charting entries that he is a licensed registered nurse, although he has not yet received the results of the licensing exam. The graduate's action can result in a charge of:

- ○ **A.** Fraud
- ○ **B.** Tort
- ○ **C.** Malpractice
- ○ **D.** Negligence

124. The nurse is assigning staff for the day. Which client should be assigned to the nursing assistant?

- ○ **A.** A 5-month-old with bronchiolitis
- ○ **B.** A 10-year-old 2-day post-appendectomy
- ○ **C.** A 2-year-old with periorbital cellulitis
- ○ **D.** A 1-year-old with a fractured tibia

125. During the change of shift, the oncoming nurse notes a discrepancy in the number of percocette listed and the number present in the narcotic drawer. The nurse's first action should be to:

- ○ **A.** Notify the hospital pharmacist
- ○ **B.** Notify the nursing supervisor
- ○ **C.** Notify the Board of Nursing
- ○ **D.** Notify the director of nursing

126. Due to a high census, it has been necessary for a number of clients to be transferred to other units within the hospital. Which client should be transferred to the postpartum unit?

- ○ **A.** A 66-year-old female with gastroenteritis
- ○ **B.** A 40-year-old female with a hysterectomy
- ○ **C.** A 27-year-old male with severe depression
- ○ **D.** A 28-year-old male with ulcerative colitis

127. A client with glomerulonephritis is placed on a low-sodium diet. Which of the following snacks is suitable for the client with sodium restriction?

Quick Answer: 53
Detailed Answer: 67

   ○ **A.** Peanut butter cookies

   ○ **B.** Grilled cheese sandwich

   ○ **C.** Cottage cheese and fruit

   ○ **D.** Fresh peach

128. A home health nurse is making preparations for morning visits. Which one of the following clients should the nurse visit first?

Quick Answer: 53
Detailed Answer: 67

   ○ **A.** A client with a stroke with tube feedings

   ○ **B.** A client with congestive heart failure complaining of night-time dyspnea

   ○ **C.** A client with a thoracotomy six months ago

   ○ **D.** A client with Parkinson's disease

129. A client with cancer develops xerostomia. The nurse can help alleviate the discomfort the client is experiencing associated with xerostomia by:

Quick Answer: 53
Detailed Answer: 68

   ○ **A.** Offering hard candy

   ○ **B.** Administering analgesic medications

   ○ **C.** Splinting swollen joints

   ○ **D.** Providing saliva substitute

130. The nurse is making assignments for the day. The staff consists of an RN, an LPN, and a nursing assistant. Which client could the nursing assistant care for?

Quick Answer: 53
Detailed Answer: 68

   ○ **A.** A client with Alzheimer's disease

   ○ **B.** A client with pneumonia

   ○ **C.** A client with appendicitis

   ○ **D.** A client with thrombophlebitis

131. The nurse is caring for a client with cerebral palsy. The nurse should provide frequent rest periods because:

Quick Answer: 53
Detailed Answer: 68

   ○ **A.** Grimacing and writhing movements decrease with relaxation and rest.

   ○ **B.** Hypoactive deep tendon reflexes become more active with rest.

   ○ **C.** Stretch reflexes are increased with rest.

   ○ **D.** Fine motor movements are improved by rest.

132. The physician has ordered a culture for the client with suspected gonorrhea. The nurse should obtain a culture of:

- ○ **A.** Blood
- ○ **B.** Nasopharyngeal secretions
- ○ **C.** Stool
- ○ **D.** Genital secretions

133. Which of the following post-operative diets is most appropriate for the client who has had a hemorrhoidectomy?

- ○ **A.** High-fiber
- ○ **B.** Lactose free
- ○ **C.** Bland
- ○ **D.** Clear-liquid

134. The client delivered a 9-pound infant two days ago. An effective means of managing discomfort from an episiotomy is:

- ○ **A.** Medicated suppository
- ○ **B.** Taking showers
- ○ **C.** Sitz baths
- ○ **D.** Ice packs

135. The nurse is assessing the client recently returned from surgery. The nurse is aware that the best way to assess pain is to:

- ○ **A.** Take the blood pressure, pulse, and temperature
- ○ **B.** Ask the client to rate his pain on a scale of 0–5
- ○ **C.** Watch the client's facial expression
- ○ **D.** Ask the client if he is in pain

136. The client is admitted with chronic obstructive pulmonary disease. Blood gases reveal pH 7.36, CO_2 45, O_2 84, bicarb 28. The nurse would assess the client to be in:

- ○ **A.** Uncompensated acidosis
- ○ **B.** Compensated alkalosis
- ○ **C.** Compensated respiratory acidosis
- ○ **D.** Uncompensated metabolic acidosis

137. The schizophrenic client has become disruptive and requires seclusion. Which staff member can institute seclusion?

- ○ **A.** The security guard
- ○ **B.** The registered nurse
- ○ **C.** The licensed practical nurse
- ○ **D.** The nursing assistant

138. The physician has ordered sodium warfarin for the client with thrombophlebitis. The order should be entered to administer the medication at:

Quick Answer: **53**
Detailed Answer: **68**

- ○ **A.** 0900
- ○ **B.** 1200
- ○ **C.** 1700
- ○ **D.** 2100

139. A 25-year-old male is brought to the emergency room with a piece of metal in his eye. The first action the nurse should take is:

Quick Answer: **53**
Detailed Answer: **69**

- ○ **A.** Use a magnet to remove the object.
- ○ **B.** Rinse the eye thoroughly with saline.
- ○ **C.** Cover both eyes with paper cups.
- ○ **D.** Patch the affected eye.

140. To ensure safety while administering a nitroglycerine patch, the nurse should:

Quick Answer: **53**
Detailed Answer: **69**

- ○ **A.** Wear gloves while applying the patch
- ○ **B.** Shave the area where the patch will be applied.
- ○ **C.** Wash the area thoroughly with soap and rinse with hot water.
- ○ **D.** Apply the patch to the buttocks.

141. The client with Cirrhosis is scheduled for a pericentesis. Which instruction should be given to the client before the exam?

Quick Answer: **53**
Detailed Answer: **69**

- ○ **A.** "You will need to lay flat during the exam."
- ○ **B.** "You need to empty your bladder before the procedure."
- ○ **C.** "You will be asleep during the procedure."
- ○ **D.** "The doctor will inject a medication to treat your illness during the procedure."

142. The client is scheduled for a Tensilon test to check for Myasthenia Gravis. Which medication should be kept available during the test?

Quick Answer: **53**
Detailed Answer: **69**

- ○ **A.** Atropine sulfate
- ○ **B.** Furosemide
- ○ **C.** Prostigmin
- ○ **D.** Promethazine

143. The first exercise that should be performed by the client who had a mastectomy 1 day earlier is:

Quick Answer: **53**
Detailed Answer: **69**

- ○ **A.** Walking the hand up the wall
- ○ **B.** Sweeping the floor
- ○ **C.** Combing her hair
- ○ **D.** Squeezing a ball

144. Which woman is not a candidate for RhoGam?

Quick Answer: **53**
Detailed Answer: **69**

- ○ **A.** A gravida 4 para 3 that is Rh negative with an Rh-positive baby
- ○ **B.** A gravida 1 para 1 that is Rh negative with an Rh-positive baby
- ○ **C.** A gravida II para 0 that is Rh negative admitted after a stillbirth delivery
- ○ **D.** A gravida 4 para 2 that is Rh negative with an Rh-negative baby

145. Which laboratory test would be the least effective in making the diagnosis of a myocardial infarction?

Quick Answer: **53**
Detailed Answer: **69**

- ○ **A.** AST
- ○ **B.** Troponin
- ○ **C.** CK-MB
- ○ **D.** Myoglobin

146. The client with a myocardial infarction comes to the nurse's station stating that he is ready to go home because there is nothing wrong with him. Which defense mechanism is the client using?

Quick Answer: **53**
Detailed Answer: **69**

- ○ **A.** Rationalization
- ○ **B.** Denial
- ○ **C.** Projection
- ○ **D.** Conversion reaction

147. The client is receiving total parenteral nutrition (TPN). Which lab test should be evaluated while the client is receiving TPN?

Quick Answer: **53**
Detailed Answer: **69**

- ○ **A.** Hemoglobin
- ○ **B.** Creatinine
- ○ **C.** Blood glucose
- ○ **D.** White blood cell count

148. The client with diabetes is preparing for discharge. During discharge teaching, the nurse assesses the client's ability to care for himself. Which statement made by the client would indicate a need for follow-up after discharge?

- ○ **A.** "I live by myself."
- ○ **B.** "I have trouble seeing."
- ○ **C.** "I have a cat in the house with me."
- ○ **D.** "I usually drive myself to the doctor."

Quick Answer: **53**
Detailed Answer: **69**

149. The client with cirrhosis of the liver is receiving Lactulose. The nurse is aware that the rationale for the order for Lactulose is:

- ○ **A.** To lower the blood glucose level
- ○ **B.** To lower the uric acid level
- ○ **C.** To lower the ammonia level
- ○ **D.** To lower the creatinine level

Quick Answer: **53**
Detailed Answer: **70**

150. The client is receiving peritoneal dialysis. If the dialysate returns cloudy, the nurse should:

- ○ **A.** Document the finding
- ○ **B.** Send a specimen to the lab
- ○ **C.** Strain the urine
- ○ **D.** Obtain a complete blood count

Quick Answer: **53**
Detailed Answer: **70**

151. The nurse employed in the emergency room is responsible for triage of four clients injured in a motor vehicle accident. Which of the following clients should receive priority in care?

- ○ **A.** A 10-year-old with lacerations of the face
- ○ **B.** A 15-year-old with sternal bruises
- ○ **C.** A 34-year-old with a fractured femur
- ○ **D.** A 50-year-old with dislocation of the elbow

Quick Answer: **53**
Detailed Answer: **70**

152. Which of the following roommates would be most suitable for the client with myasthenia gravis?

- ○ **A.** A client with hypothyroidism
- ○ **B.** A client with Crohn's disease
- ○ **C.** A client with pylonephritis
- ○ **D.** A client with bronchitis

Quick Answer: **53**
Detailed Answer: **70**

153. The nurse is observing a graduate nurse as she assesses the central venous pressure. Which observation would indicate that the graduate needs further teaching?

Quick Answer: **53**
Detailed Answer: **70**

   ○ **A.** The graduate places the client in a supine position to read the manometer.

   ○ **B.** The graduate turns the stop-cock to the off position from the IV fluid to the client.

   ○ **C.** The graduate instructs the client to perform the Valsalva maneuver during the CVP reading.

   ○ **D.** The graduate notes the level at the top of the meniscus.

154. The nurse is working with another nurse and a patient care assistant. Which of the following clients should be assigned to the registered nurse?

Quick Answer: **53**
Detailed Answer: **70**

   ○ **A.** A client 2 days post-appendectomy

   ○ **B.** A client 1 week post-thyroidectomy

   ○ **C.** A client 3 days post-splenectomy

   ○ **D.** A client 2 days post-thoracotomy

155. Which of the following roommates would be best for the client newly admitted with gastric resection?

Quick Answer: **53**
Detailed Answer: **70**

   ○ **A.** A client with Crohn's disease

   ○ **B.** A client with pneumonia

   ○ **C.** A client with gastritis

   ○ **D.** A client with phlebitis

156. The nurse is preparing a client for mammography. To prepare the client for a mammogram, the nurse should tell the client:

Quick Answer: **53**
Detailed Answer: **70**

   ○ **A.** To restrict her fat intake for 1 week before the test

   ○ **B.** To omit creams, powders, or deodorants before the exam

   ○ **C.** That mammography replaces the need for self-breast exams

   ○ **D.** That mammography requires a higher dose of radiation than x-rays

157. Which action by the novice nurse indicates a need for further teaching?

Quick Answer: **53**
Detailed Answer: **70**

   ○ **A.** The nurse fails to wear gloves to remove a dressing.

   ○ **B.** The nurse applies an oxygen saturation monitor to the ear lobe.

   ○ **C.** The nurse elevates the head of the bed to check the blood pressure.

   ○ **D.** The nurse places the extremity in a dependent position to acquire a peripheral blood sample.

158. The graduate nurse is assigned to care for the client on ventilator support, pending organ donation. Which goal should receive priority?

Quick Answer: 53
Detailed Answer: 70

   ○ **A.** Maintaining the client's systolic blood pressure at 70mmHg or greater

   ○ **B.** Maintaining the client's urinary output greater than 300cc per hour

   ○ **C.** Maintaining the client's body temperature of greater than 33°F rectal

   ○ **D.** Maintaining the client's hematocrit at less than 30%

159. The nurse is assigned to care for an infant with physiologic jaundice. Which action by the nurse would facilitate elimination of the bilirubin?

Quick Answer: 53
Detailed Answer: 71

   ○ **A.** Increasing the infant's fluid intake

   ○ **B.** Maintaining the infant's body temperature at 98.6°F

   ○ **C.** Minimizing tactile stimulation

   ○ **D.** Decreasing caloric intake

160. A home health nurse is planning for her daily visits. Which client should the home health nurse visit first?

Quick Answer: 53
Detailed Answer: 71

   ○ **A.** A client with AIDS being treated with Foscarnet

   ○ **B.** A client with a fractured femur in a long leg cast

   ○ **C.** A client with laryngeal cancer with a laryngectomy

   ○ **D.** A client with diabetic ulcers to the left foot

161. The charge nurse overhears the patient care assistant speaking harshly to the client with dementia. The charge nurse should:

Quick Answer: 53
Detailed Answer: 71

   ○ **A.** Change the nursing assistant's assignment

   ○ **B.** Explore the interaction with the nursing assistant

   ○ **C.** Discuss the matter with the client's family

   ○ **D.** Initiate a group session with the nursing assistant

162. The nurse notes the patient care assistant looking through the personal items of the client with cancer. Which action should be taken by the registered nurse?

Quick Answer: 53
Detailed Answer: 71

   ○ **A.** Notify the police department as a robbery

   ○ **B.** Report this behavior to the charge nurse

   ○ **C.** Monitor the situation and note whether any items are missing

   ○ **D.** Ignore the situation until items are reported missing

163. Which client can best be assigned to the newly licensed nurse?

- ○ **A.** The client receiving chemotherapy
- ○ **B.** The client post–coronary bypass
- ○ **C.** The client with a TURP
- ○ **D.** The client with diverticulitis

Quick Answer: **53**
Detailed Answer: **71**

164. The nurse has an order for medication to be administered intrathecally. The nurse is aware that medications will be administered by which method?

- ○ **A.** Intravenously
- ○ **B.** Rectally
- ○ **C.** Intramuscularly
- ○ **D.** Into the cerebrospinal fluid

Quick Answer: **53**
Detailed Answer: **71**

165. The client is admitted to the unit after a cholescystectomy. Montgomery straps are utilized with this client. The nurse is aware that Montgomery straps are utilized on this client because:

- ○ **A.** The client is at risk for evisceration.
- ○ **B.** The client will require frequent dressing changes.
- ○ **C.** The straps provide support for drains that are inserted into the incision.
- ○ **D.** No sutures or clips are used to secure the incision.

Quick Answer: **53**
Detailed Answer: **71**

166. A client with pancreatitis has been transferred to the intensive care unit. Which order would the nurse anticipate?

- ○ **A.** Blood pressure every 15 minutes
- ○ **B.** Insertion of a Levine tube
- ○ **C.** Cardiac monitoring
- ○ **D.** Dressing changes two times per day

Quick Answer: **53**
Detailed Answer: **71**

167. The nurse is caring for a client with a diagnosis of hepatitis who is experiencing pruritis. Which would be the most appropriate nursing intervention?

- ○ **A.** Suggest that the client take warm showers two times per day
- ○ **B.** Add baby oil to the client's bath water
- ○ **C.** Apply powder to the client's skin
- ○ **D.** Suggest a hot-water rinse after bathing

Quick Answer: **53**
Detailed Answer: **72**

168. The nurse recognizes that which of the following would be most appropriate to wear when providing direct care to a client with a cough?

- ○ **A.** Mask
- ○ **B.** Gown
- ○ **C.** Gloves
- ○ **D.** Shoe covers

Quick Answer: **53**
Detailed Answer: **72**

169. A client visits the clinic after the death of a parent. Which statement made by the client's sister signifies abnormal grieving?

- ○ **A.** "My sister still has episodes of crying, and it's been three months since Daddy died."
- ○ **B.** "Sally seems to have forgotten the bad things that Daddy did in his lifetime."
- ○ **C.** "She really had a hard time after Daddy's funeral. She said that she had a sense of longing."
- ○ **D.** "She has not been saddened at all by Daddy's death. She acts like nothing has happened."

Quick Answer: **53**
Detailed Answer: **72**

170. The nurse is obtaining a history on an 80-year-old client. Which statement made by the client might indicate a potential for fluid and electrolyte imbalance?

- ○ **A.** "My skin is always so dry."
- ○ **B.** "I often use laxatives."
- ○ **C.** "I have always liked to drink a lot of ice tea."
- ○ **D.** "I sometimes have a problem with dribbling urine."

Quick Answer: **53**
Detailed Answer: **72**

171. A client is admitted to the acute care unit. Initial laboratory values reveal serum sodium of 170meq/L. What behavior changes would be most common for this client?

- ○ **A.** Anger
- ○ **B.** Mania
- ○ **C.** Depression
- ○ **D.** Psychosis

Quick Answer: **53**
Detailed Answer: **72**

172. When assessing a client for risk of hyperphosphatemia, which piece of information is most important for the nurse to obtain?

- ○ **A.** A history of radiation treatment in the neck region
- ○ **B.** Any history of recent orthopedic surgery
- ○ **C.** A history of minimal physical activity
- ○ **D.** A history of the client's food intake

Quick Answer: **53**
Detailed Answer: **72**

173. The nurse on the 3–11 shift is assessing the chart of a client with an abdominal aneurysm scheduled for surgery in the morning and finds that the consent form has been signed, but the client is unclear about the surgery and possible complications. Which is the most appropriate action?

- ○ **A.** Call the surgeon and ask him or her to see the client to clarify the information
- ○ **B.** Explain the procedure and complications to the client
- ○ **C.** Check in the physician's progress notes to see if understanding has been documented
- ○ **D.** Check with the client's family to see if they understand the procedure fully

174. The nurse is preparing a client for surgery. Which item is most important to remove before sending the client to surgery?

- ○ **A.** Hearing aid
- ○ **B.** Contact lenses
- ○ **C.** Wedding ring
- ○ **D.** Artificial eye

175. A client is 2 days post-operative colon resection. After a coughing episode, the client's wound eviscerates. Which nursing action is most appropriate?

- ○ **A.** Reinsert the protruding organ and cover with 4×4s
- ○ **B.** Cover the wound with a sterile 4×4 and ABD dressing
- ○ **C.** Cover the wound with a sterile saline-soaked dressing
- ○ **D.** Apply an abdominal binder and manual pressure to the wound

176. The nurse is caring for a client with a malignancy. The classification of the primary tumor is Tis. The nurse should plan care for a tumor:

- ○ **A.** That cannot be assessed
- ○ **B.** That is in situ
- ○ **C.** With increasing lymph node involvement
- ○ **D.** With distant metastasis

177. A client with cancer is to undergo an intravenous pyelogram. The nurse should:

Quick Answer: **53**
Detailed Answer: **73**

- ○ **A.** Force fluids 24 hours before the procedure
- ○ **B.** Ask the client to void immediately before the study
- ○ **C.** Hold medication that affects the central nervous system for 12 hours pre- and post-test
- ○ **D.** Cover the client's reproductive organs with an x-ray shield.

178. A client arrives in the emergency room with a possible fractured femur. The nurse should anticipate an order for:

Quick Answer: **53**
Detailed Answer: **73**

- ○ **A.** Trendelenburg position
- ○ **B.** Ice to the entire extremity
- ○ **C.** Buck's traction
- ○ **D.** An abduction pillow

179. The nurse is performing an assessment on a client with possible pernicious anemia. Which data would support this diagnosis?

Quick Answer: **53**
Detailed Answer: **73**

- ○ **A.** A weight loss of 10 pounds in 2 weeks
- ○ **B.** Complaints of numbness and tingling in the extremities
- ○ **C.** A red, beefy tongue
- ○ **D.** A hemoglobin level of 12.0gm/dL

180. A client with suspected renal disease is to undergo a renal biopsy. The nurse plans to include which statement in the teaching session?

Quick Answer: **53**
Detailed Answer: **73**

- ○ **A.** "You will be sitting for the examination procedure."
- ○ **B.** "Portions of the procedure will cause pain or discomfort."
- ○ **C.** "You will be asleep during the procedure."
- ○ **D.** "You will not be able to drink fluids for 24 hours following the study."

181. The nurse is caring for a client scheduled for a surgical repair of a sacular abdominal aortic aneurysm. Which assessment is most crucial during the preoperative period?

Quick Answer: **53**
Detailed Answer: **73**

- ○ **A.** Assessment of the client's level of anxiety
- ○ **B.** Evaluation of the client's exercise tolerance
- ○ **C.** Identification of peripheral pulses
- ○ **D.** Assessment of bowel sounds and activity

182. A client in the cardiac step-down unit requires suctioning for excess mucous secretions. The dysrhythmia most commonly seen during suctioning is:

Quick Answer: **53**
Detailed Answer: **73**

- ○ **A.** Bradycardia
- ○ **B.** Tachycardia
- ○ **C.** Premature ventricular beats
- ○ **D.** Heart block

183. The nurse is performing discharge instruction to a client with an implantable defibrillator. What discharge instruction is essential?

Quick Answer: **53**
Detailed Answer: **73**

- ○ **A.** "You cannot eat food prepared in a microwave."
- ○ **B.** "You should avoid moving the shoulder on the side of the pacemaker site for 6 weeks."
- ○ **C.** "You should use your cell phone on your right side."
- ○ **D.** "You will not be able to fly on a commercial airliner with the defibrillator in place."

184. Six hours after birth, the infant is found to have an area of swelling over the right parietal area that does not cross the suture line. The nurse should chart this finding as:

Quick Answer: **54**
Detailed Answer: **73**

- ○ **A.** A cephalhematoma
- ○ **B.** Molding
- ○ **C.** Subdural hematoma
- ○ **D.** Caput succedaneum

185. A removal of the left lower lobe of the lung is performed on a client with lung cancer. Which post-operative measure would usually be included in the plan?

Quick Answer: **54**
Detailed Answer: **74**

- ○ **A.** Closed chest drainage
- ○ **B.** A tracheostomy
- ○ **C.** A Swan Ganz Monitor
- ○ **D.** Percussion vibration and drainage

186. The nurse is caring for a client with laryngeal cancer. Which finding ascertained in the health history would not be common for this diagnosis?

Quick Answer: **54**
Detailed Answer: **74**

- ○ **A.** Foul breath
- ○ **B.** Dysphagia
- ○ **C.** Diarrhea
- ○ **D.** Chronic hiccups

187. The nurse is caring for a new mother. The mother asks why her baby has lost weight since he was born. The best explanation of the weight loss is:

Quick Answer: **54**
Detailed Answer: **74**

- ○ **A.** The baby is dehydrated.
- ○ **B.** The baby is hypoglycemic.
- ○ **C.** The baby is allergic to the formula the mother is giving him.
- ○ **D.** A loss of 10% is normal in the first week due to meconium stools.

188. The nurse is performing discharge teaching on a client with diverticulitis who has been placed on a low-roughage diet. Which food would have to be eliminated from this client's diet?

Quick Answer: **54**
Detailed Answer: **74**

- ○ **A.** Roasted chicken
- ○ **B.** Noodles
- ○ **C.** Cooked broccoli
- ○ **D.** Custard

189. A client has rectal cancer and is scheduled for an abdominal perineal resection. What should be the priority nursing care during the post-op period?

Quick Answer: **54**
Detailed Answer: **74**

- ○ **A.** Teaching how to irrigate the illeostomy
- ○ **B.** Stopping electrolyte loss in the incisional area
- ○ **C.** Encouraging a high-fiber diet
- ○ **D.** Facilitating perineal wound drainage

190. The nurse is assisting a client with diverticulosis to select appropriate foods. Which food should be avoided?

Quick Answer: **54**
Detailed Answer: **74**

- ○ **A.** Bran
- ○ **B.** Fresh peaches
- ○ **C.** Cucumber salad
- ○ **D.** Yeast rolls

191. A 6-month-old client is admitted with possible intussuception. Which question during the nursing history is least helpful in obtaining information regarding this diagnosis?

Quick Answer: **54**
Detailed Answer: **74**

- ○ **A.** "Tell me about his pain."
- ○ **B.** "What does his vomit look like?"
- ○ **C.** "Describe his usual diet."
- ○ **D.** "Have you noticed changes in his abdominal size?"

192. The nurse is caring for a client with epilepsy who is being treated with carbamazepine (Tegretol). Which laboratory value might indicate a serious side effect of this drug?

- ○ **A.** Uric acid of 5mg/dL
- ○ **B.** Hematocrit of 33%
- ○ **C.** WBC 2000 per cubic millimeter
- ○ **D.** Platelets 150,000 per cubic millimeter

Quick Answer: **54**
Detailed Answer: **74**

193. A client is admitted with a Ewing's sarcoma. Which symptoms would be expected due to this tumor's location?

- ○ **A.** Hemiplegia
- ○ **B.** Aphasia
- ○ **C.** Nausea
- ○ **D.** Bone pain

Quick Answer: **54**
Detailed Answer: **74**

194. A infant weighs 7 pounds at birth. The expected weight by 1 year should be:

- ○ **A.** 10 pounds
- ○ **B.** 12 pounds
- ○ **C.** 18 pounds
- ○ **D.** 21 pounds

Quick Answer: **54**
Detailed Answer: **74**

195. The nurse is making initial rounds on a client with a C5 fracture and crutchfield tongs. Which equipment should be kept at the bedside?

- ○ **A.** A pair of forceps
- ○ **B.** A torque wrench
- ○ **C.** A pair of wire cutters
- ○ **D.** A screwdriver

Quick Answer: **54**
Detailed Answer: **74**

196. The nurse is visiting a home health client with osteoporosis. The client has a new prescription for alendronate (Fosamax). Which instruction should be given to the client?

- ○ **A.** Rest in bed after taking the medication for at least 30 minutes.
- ○ **B.** Avoid rapid movements after taking the medication.
- ○ **C.** Take the medication with water only.
- ○ **D.** Allow at least 1 hour between taking the medicine and taking other medications.

Quick Answer: **54**
Detailed Answer: **74**

197. The nurse is working in the emergency room when a client arrives with severe burns of the left arm, hands, face, and neck. Which action should receive priority?

Quick Answer: **54**
Detailed Answer: **75**

- ○ **A.** Starting an IV
- ○ **B.** Applying oxygen
- ○ **C.** Obtaining blood gases
- ○ **D.** Medicating the client for pain

198. A 24-year-old female client is scheduled for surgery in the morning. Which of the following is the primary responsibility of the nurse?

Quick Answer: **54**
Detailed Answer: **75**

- ○ **A.** Taking the vital signs
- ○ **B.** Obtaining the permit
- ○ **C.** Explaining the procedure
- ○ **D.** Checking the lab work

199. A client with cancer is admitted to the oncology unit. Stat lab values reveal Hgb 12.6, WBC 6500, K+ 1.9, uric acid 7.0, Na+ 136, and platelets 178,000. The nurse evaluates that the client is experiencing which of the following?

Quick Answer: **54**
Detailed Answer: **75**

- ○ **A.** Hypernatremia
- ○ **B.** Hypokalemia
- ○ **C.** Myelosuppression
- ○ **D.** Leukocytosis

200. The nurse is caring for a client scheduled for removal of the pituitary gland. The nurse should be particularly alert for:

Quick Answer: **54**
Detailed Answer: **75**

- ○ **A.** Nasal congestion
- ○ **B.** Abdominal tenderness
- ○ **C.** Muscle tetany
- ○ **D.** Oliguria

201. A client has cancer of the liver. The nurse should be most concerned about which nursing diagnosis?

Quick Answer: **54**
Detailed Answer: **75**

- ○ **A.** Alteration in nutrition
- ○ **B.** Alteration in urinary elimination
- ○ **C.** Alteration in skin integrity
- ○ **D.** Ineffective coping

202. The nurse is caring for a client with ascites. Which is the best method to use for determining early ascites?

- ○ **A.** Inspection of the abdomen for enlargement
- ○ **B.** Bimanual palpation for hepatomegaly
- ○ **C.** Daily measurement of abdominal girth
- ○ **D.** Assessment for a fluid wave

203. The client arrives in the emergency department after a motor vehicle accident. Nursing assessment findings include BP 68/34, pulse rate 130, and respirations 18. Which is the client's most appropriate priority nursing diagnosis?

- ○ **A.** Alteration in cerebral tissue perfusion
- ○ **B.** Fluid volume deficit
- ○ **C.** Ineffective airway clearance
- ○ **D.** Alteration in sensory perception

204. The home health nurse is visiting a 15-year-old with sickle cell disease. Which information obtained on the visit would cause the most concern? The client:

- ○ **A.** Likes to play baseball
- ○ **B.** Drinks several carbonated drinks per day
- ○ **C.** Has two sisters with sickle cell trait
- ○ **D.** Is taking Tylenol to control pain

205. The nurse on oncology is caring for a client with a white blood count of 600. During evening visitation, a visitor brings a potted plant. What action should the nurse take?

- ○ **A.** Allow the client to keep the plant
- ○ **B.** Place the plant by the window
- ○ **C.** Water the plant for the client
- ○ **D.** Tell the family members to take the plant home

206. The nurse is caring for the client following a thyroidectomy when suddenly the client becomes nonresponsive and pale, with a BP of 60 systolic. The nurse's initial action should be to:

- ○ **A.** Lower the head of the bed
- ○ **B.** Increase the infusion of normal saline
- ○ **C.** Administer atropine IV
- ○ **D.** Obtain a crash cart

207. The client pulls out the chest tube and fails to report the occurrence to the nurse. When the nurse discovers the incidence, he should take which initial action?

Quick Answer: 54
Detailed Answer: 76

  ○ **A.** Order a chest x-ray

  ○ **B.** Reinsert the tube

  ○ **C.** Cover the insertion site with a Vaseline gauze

  ○ **D.** Call the doctor

208. A client being treated with sodium warfarin has an INR of 8.0. Which intervention would be most important to include in the nursing care plan?

Quick Answer: 54
Detailed Answer: 76

  ○ **A.** Assess for signs of abnormal bleeding

  ○ **B.** Anticipate an increase in the Coumadin dosage

  ○ **C.** Instruct the client regarding the drug therapy

  ○ **D.** Increase the frequency of neurological assessments

209. Which snack selection by a client with osteoporosis indicates that the client understands the dietary management of the disease?

Quick Answer: 54
Detailed Answer: 76

  ○ **A.** A granola bar

  ○ **B.** A bran muffin

  ○ **C.** Yogurt

  ○ **D.** Raisins

210. The client with preeclampsia is admitted to the unit with an order for magnesium sulfate IV. Which action by the nurse indicates a lack of understanding of magnesium sulfate?

Quick Answer: 54
Detailed Answer: 76

  ○ **A.** The nurse places a sign over the bed not to check blood pressures in the left arm.

  ○ **B.** The nurse obtains an IV controller.

  ○ **C.** The nurse inserts a Foley catheter.

  ○ **D.** The nurse darkens the room.

211. The nurse is caring for a 12-year-old client with appendicitis. The client's mother is a Jehovah's Witness and refuses to sign the blood permit. What nursing action is most appropriate?

Quick Answer: 54
Detailed Answer: 76

  ○ **A.** Give the blood without permission

  ○ **B.** Encourage the mother to reconsider

  ○ **C.** Explain the consequences without treatment

  ○ **D.** Notify the physician of the mother's refusal

212. A client is admitted to the unit 2 hours after an injury with second-degree burns to the face, trunk, and head. The nurse would be most concerned with the client developing what?

- ○ **A.** Hypovolemia
- ○ **B.** Laryngeal edema
- ○ **C.** Hypernatremia
- ○ **D.** Hyperkalemia

Quick Answer: **54**
Detailed Answer: **76**

213. The nurse is evaluating nutritional outcomes for an elderly client with anorexia nervosa. Which data best indicates that the plan of care is effective?

- ○ **A.** The client selects a balanced diet from the menu.
- ○ **B.** The client's hematocrit improves.
- ○ **C.** The client's tissue turgor improves.
- ○ **D.** The client gains weight.

Quick Answer: **54**
Detailed Answer: **76**

214. The client is admitted following repair of a fractured tibia and cast application. Which nursing assessment should be reported to the doctor?

- ○ **A.** Pain beneath the cast
- ○ **B.** Warm toes
- ○ **C.** Pedal pulses weak and rapid
- ○ **D.** Paresthesia of the toes

Quick Answer: **54**
Detailed Answer: **76**

215. The client is having a cardiac catheterization. During the procedure, the client tells the nurse, "I'm feeling really hot." Which response would be best?

- ○ **A.** "You are having an allergic reaction. I will get an order for Benadryl."
- ○ **B.** "That feeling of warmth is normal when the dye is injected."
- ○ **C.** "That feeling of warmth indicates that the clots in the coronary vessels are dissolving."
- ○ **D.** "I will tell your doctor and let him explain to you the reason for the hot feeling that you are experiencing."

Quick Answer: **54**
Detailed Answer: **76**

216. Which action by the healthcare worker indicates a need for further teaching?

- ○ **A.** The nursing assistant wears gloves while giving the client a bath.
- ○ **B.** The nurse wears goggles while drawing blood from the client.
- ○ **C.** The doctor washes his hands before examining the client.
- ○ **D.** The nurse wears gloves to take the client's vital signs.

Quick Answer: **54**
Detailed Answer: **77**

217. The client is having electroconvulsive therapy for treatment of severe depression. Which of the following indicates that the client's ECT has been effective?

Quick Answer: 54
Detailed Answer: 77

   ○ **A.** The client loses consciousness.

   ○ **B.** The client vomits.

   ○ **C.** The client's ECG indicates tachycardia.

   ○ **D.** The client has a grand mal seizure.

218. The 5-year-old is being tested for enterobiasis (pinworms). To collect a specimen for assessment of pinworms, the nurse should teach the mother to:

Quick Answer: 54
Detailed Answer: 77

   ○ **A.** Place tape on the child's perianal area before putting the child to bed

   ○ **B.** Scrape the skin with a piece of cardboard and bring it to the clinic

   ○ **C.** Obtain a stool specimen in the afternoon

   ○ **D.** Bring a hair sample to the clinic for evaluation

219. The nurse is teaching the mother regarding treatment for enterobiasis. Which instruction should be given regarding the medication?

Quick Answer: 54
Detailed Answer: 77

   ○ **A.** Treatment is not recommended for children less than 10 years of age.

   ○ **B.** The entire family should be treated.

   ○ **C.** Medication therapy will continue for 1 year.

   ○ **D.** Intravenous antibiotic therapy will be ordered.

220. The registered nurse is making assignments for the day. Which client should not be assigned to the pregnant nurse?

Quick Answer: 54
Detailed Answer: 77

   ○ **A.** The client receiving linear accelerator radiation therapy for lung cancer

   ○ **B.** The client with a radium implant for cervical cancer

   ○ **C.** The client who has just been administered soluble brachytherapy for thyroid cancer

   ○ **D.** The client who returned from an intravenous pyelogram

221. Which client is at risk for opportunistic diseases such as pneumocystis pneumonia?

Quick Answer: 54
Detailed Answer: 77

   ○ **A.** The client with cancer who is being treated with chemotherapy

   ○ **B.** The client with Type I diabetes

   ○ **C.** The client with thyroid disease

   ○ **D.** The client with Addison's disease

222. The nurse caring for a client in the neonatal intensive care unit administers adult-strength Digitalis to the 3-pound infant. As a result of her actions, the baby suffers permanent heart and brain damage. The nurse can be charged with:

- ○ **A.** Negligence
- ○ **B.** Tort
- ○ **C.** Assault
- ○ **D.** Malpractice

223. Which assignment should not be performed by the registered nurse?

- ○ **A.** Inserting a Foley catheter
- ○ **B.** Inserting a nasogastric tube
- ○ **C.** Monitoring central venous pressure
- ○ **D.** Inserting sutures and clips in surgery

224. The client returns to the unit from surgery with a blood pressure of 90/50, pulse 132, respirations 30. Which action by the nurse should receive priority?

- ○ **A.** Document the finding.
- ○ **B.** Contact the physician.
- ○ **C.** Elevate the head of the bed.
- ○ **D.** Administer a pain medication.

225. Which nurse should be assigned to care for the postpartal client with preeclampsia?

- ○ **A.** The RN with 2 weeks of experience in postpartum
- ○ **B.** The RN with 3 years of experience in labor and delivery
- ○ **C.** The RN with 10 years of experience in surgery
- ○ **D.** The RN with 1 year of experience in the neonatal intensive care unit

226. Which medication is used to treat iron toxicity?

- ○ **A.** Narcan (naloxane)
- ○ **B.** Digibind (digoxin immune Fab)
- ○ **C.** Desferal (deferoxamine)
- ○ **D.** Zinecard (dexrazoxane)

227. The nurse is suspected of charting medication administration that he did not give. The nurse can be charged with:

- ○ **A.** Fraud
- ○ **B.** Malpractice
- ○ **C.** Negligence
- ○ **D.** Tort

228. The home health nurse is planning for the day's visits. Which client should be seen first?

    ○ **A.** The client with renal insufficiency

    ○ **B.** The client with Alzheimer's

    ○ **C.** The client with diabetes who has a decubitus ulcer

    ○ **D.** The client with multiple sclerosis who is being treated with IV cortisone

229. The emergency room is flooded with clients injured in a tornado. Which clients can be assigned to share a room in the emergency department during the disaster?

    ○ **A.** A schizophrenic client having visual and auditory hallucinations and the client with ulcerative colitis

    ○ **B.** The client who is six months pregnant with abdominal pain and the client with facial lacerations and a broken arm

    ○ **C.** A child whose pupils are fixed and dilated and his parents, and a client with a frontal head injury

    ○ **D.** The client who arrives with a large puncture wound to the abdomen and the client with chest pain

230. The nurse is caring for a 6-year-old client admitted with the diagnosis of conjunctivitis. Before administering eyedrops, the nurse should recognize that it is essential to consider which of the following?

    ○ **A.** The eye should be cleansed with warm water, removing any exudate, before instilling the eyedrops.

    ○ **B.** The child should be allowed to instill his own eyedrops.

    ○ **C.** Allow the mother to instill the eyedrops.

    ○ **D.** If the eye is clear from any redness or edema, the eyedrops should be held.

231. To assist with the prevention of urinary tract infections, the teenage girl should be taught to:

    ○ **A.** Drink citrus fruit juices

    ○ **B.** Avoid using tampons

    ○ **C.** Take showers instead of tub baths

    ○ **D.** Clean the perineum from front to back

232. A 2-year-old toddler is admitted to the hospital. Which of the following nursing interventions would you expect?

Quick Answer: **54**
Detailed Answer: **78**

- ○ **A.** Ask the parent/guardian to leave the room when assessments are being performed.
- ○ **B.** Ask the parent/guardian to take the child's favorite blanket home because anything from the outside should not be brought into the hospital.
- ○ **C.** Ask the parent/guardian to room-in with the child.
- ○ **D.** If the child is screaming, tell him this is inappropriate behavior.

233. Which instruction should be given to the client who is fitted for a behind-the-ear hearing aid?

Quick Answer: **54**
Detailed Answer: **78**

- ○ **A.** Remove the mold and clean every week.
- ○ **B.** Store the hearing aid in a warm place.
- ○ **C.** Clean the lint from the hearing aid with a toothpick.
- ○ **D.** Change the batteries weekly.

234. A priority nursing diagnosis for a child being admitted from surgery following a tonsillectomy is:

Quick Answer: **54**
Detailed Answer: **79**

- ○ **A.** Body image disturbance
- ○ **B.** Impaired verbal communication
- ○ **C.** Risk for aspiration
- ○ **D.** Pain

235. A client with bacterial pneumonia is admitted to the pediatric unit. What would the nurse expect the admitting assessment to reveal?

Quick Answer: **54**
Detailed Answer: **79**

- ○ **A.** High fever
- ○ **B.** Nonproductive cough
- ○ **C.** Rhinitis
- ○ **D.** Vomiting and diarrhea

236. The nurse is caring for a client admitted with acute laryngotracheobronchitis (LTB). Because of the possibility of complete obstruction of the airway, which of the following should the nurse have available?

Quick Answer: **54**
Detailed Answer: **79**

- ○ **A.** Intravenous access supplies
- ○ **B.** Emergency intubation equipment
- ○ **C.** Intravenous fluid-administration pump
- ○ **D.** Supplemental oxygen

237. A 5-year-old client with hyperthyroidism is admitted to the pediatric unit. What would the nurse expect the admitting assessment to reveal?

- ○ **A.** Bradycardia
- ○ **B.** Decreased appetite
- ○ **C.** Exophthalmos
- ○ **D.** Weight gain

238. The nurse is providing dietary instructions to the mother of an 8-year-old child diagnosed with celiac disease. Which of the following foods, if selected by the mother, would indicate her understanding of the dietary instructions?

- ○ **A.** Whole-wheat bread
- ○ **B.** Spaghetti
- ○ **C.** Hamburger on wheat bun with ketchup
- ○ **D.** Cheese omelet

239. The nurse is caring for a 9-year-old child admitted with asthma. Upon the morning rounds, the nurse finds an O$_2$ sat of 78%. Which of the following actions should the nurse take first?

- ○ **A.** Notify the physician
- ○ **B.** Do nothing; this is a normal O$_2$ sat for a 9-year-old
- ○ **C.** Apply oxygen
- ○ **D.** Assess the child's pulse

240. A gravida II para 0 is admitted to the labor and delivery unit. The doctor performs an amniotomy. Which observation would the nurse expect to make immediately after the amniotomy?

- ○ **A.** Fetal heart tones 160 beats per minute
- ○ **B.** A moderate amount of clear fluid
- ○ **C.** A small amount of greenish fluid
- ○ **D.** A small segment of the umbilical cord

241. The client is admitted to the unit. A vaginal exam reveals that she is 3cm dilated. Which of the following statements would the nurse expect her to make?

- ○ **A.** "I can't decide what to name the baby."
- ○ **B.** "It feels good to push with each contraction."
- ○ **C.** "Don't touch me. I'm trying to concentrate."
- ○ **D.** "When can I get my epidural?"

242. The client is having fetal heart rates of 100–110 beats per minute during the contractions. The first action the nurse should take is to:

- ○ **A.** Apply an internal monitor
- ○ **B.** Turn the client to her side
- ○ **C.** Get the client up and walk her in the hall
- ○ **D.** Move the client to the delivery room

Quick Answer: **54**
Detailed Answer: **79**

243. In evaluating the effectiveness of IV Pitocin for a client with secondary dystocia, the nurse should expect:

- ○ **A.** A rapid delivery
- ○ **B.** Cervical effacement
- ○ **C.** Infrequent contractions
- ○ **D.** Progressive cervical dilation

Quick Answer: **54**
Detailed Answer: **80**

244. A vaginal exam reveals a breech presentation in a newly admitted client. The nurse should take which of the following actions at this time?

- ○ **A.** Prepare the client for a caesarean section
- ○ **B.** Apply the fetal heart monitor
- ○ **C.** Place the client in the Trendelenburg position
- ○ **D.** Perform an ultrasound exam

Quick Answer: **54**
Detailed Answer: **80**

245. The nurse is caring for a client admitted to labor and delivery. The nurse is aware that the infant is in distress if she notes:

- ○ **A.** Contractions every three minutes
- ○ **B.** Absent variability
- ○ **C.** Fetal heart tone accelerations with movement
- ○ **D.** Fetal heart tone 120–130bpm

Quick Answer: **54**
Detailed Answer: **80**

246. The following are all nursing diagnoses appropriate for a gravida 4 para 3 in labor. Which one would be most appropriate for the client as she completes the latent phase of labor?

- ○ **A.** Impaired gas exchange related to hyperventilation
- ○ **B.** Alteration in placental perfusion related to maternal position
- ○ **C.** Impaired physical mobility related to fetal-monitoring equipment
- ○ **D.** Potential fluid volume deficit related to decreased fluid intake

Quick Answer: **54**
Detailed Answer: **80**

247. As the client reaches 8cm dilation, the nurse notes a pattern on the fetal monitor that shows a drop in the fetal heart rate of 30bpm beginning at the peak of the contraction and ending at the end of the contraction. The FHR baseline is 165–175bpm with variability of 0–2bpm. What is the most likely explanation of this pattern?

    ○ **A.** The baby is asleep.

    ○ **B.** The umbilical cord is compressed.

    ○ **C.** There is a vagal response.

    ○ **D.** There is uteroplacental insufficiency.

Quick Answer: **54**
Detailed Answer: **80**

248. The nurse notes variable decelerations on the fetal monitor strip. The most appropriate initial action would be to:

    ○ **A.** Notify her doctor

    ○ **B.** Increase the rate of IV fluid

    ○ **C.** Reposition the client

    ○ **D.** Readjust the monitor

Quick Answer: **54**
Detailed Answer: **80**

249. Which of the following is a characteristic of a reassuring fetal heart rate pattern?

    ○ **A.** A fetal heart rate of 180bpm

    ○ **B.** A baseline variability of 35bpm

    ○ **C.** A fetal heart rate of 90 at the baseline

    ○ **D.** Acceleration of FHR with fetal movements

Quick Answer: **54**
Detailed Answer: **80**

250. The nurse asks the client with an epidural anesthesia to void every hour during labor. The rationale for this intervention is:

    ○ **A.** The bladder fills more rapidly because of the medication used for the epidural.

    ○ **B.** Her level of consciousness is altered.

    ○ **C.** The sensation of the bladder filling is diminished or lost.

    ○ **D.** She is embarrassed to ask for the bedpan that frequently.

Quick Answer: **54**
Detailed Answer: **80**

Quick Check Answer Key

1.	B	31.	B	61.	D
2.	A	32.	A	62.	C
3.	C	33.	C	63.	D
4.	B	34.	B	64.	B
5.	B	35.	D	65.	A
6.	B	36.	A	66.	A
7.	B	37.	D	67.	C
8.	C	38.	C	68.	D
9.	D	39.	B	69.	A
10.	A	40.	A	70.	B
11.	D	41.	B	71.	C
12.	C	42.	B	72.	A
13.	A	43.	B	73.	C
14.	C	44.	B	74.	A
15.	A	45.	D	75.	C
16.	C	46.	C	76.	C
17.	A	47.	C	77.	D
18.	C	48.	A	78.	D
19.	B	49.	A	79.	C
20.	D	50.	C	80.	B
21.	B	51.	B	81.	A
22.	C	52.	B	82.	C
23.	A	53.	A	83.	B
24.	A	54.	A	84.	A
25.	B	55.	C	85.	A
26.	A	56.	D	86.	A
27.	B	57.	A	87.	D
28.	A	58.	C	88.	C
29.	A	59.	A	89.	C
30.	B	60.	D	90.	C

91. D	122. D	153. C
92. D	123. A	154. D
93. B	124. B	155. D
94. D	125. B	156. B
95. A	126. B	157. A
96. C	127. D	158. A
97. B	128. B	159. A
98. B	129. D	160. C
99. D	130. A	161. B
100. C	131. A	162. B
101. A	132. D	163. D
102. D	133. D	164. D
103. B	134. C	165. B
104. A	135. B	166. B
105. B	136. C	167. B
106. A	137. B	168. A
107. B	138. C	169. D
108. A	139. C	170. B
109. A	140. A	171. B
110. C	141. B	172. A
111. D	142. A	173. A
112. B	143. D	174. B
113. B	144. D	175. C
114. B	145. A	176. B
115. A	146. B	177. B
116. D	147. C	178. C
117. D	148. B	179. C
118. A	149. C	180. B
119. D	150. B	181. C
120. C	151. B	182. A
121. A	152. A	183. C

184. A	**207.** C	**230.** A
185. A	**208.** A	**231.** D
186. C	**209.** C	**232.** C
187. D	**210.** A	**233.** B
188. C	**211.** D	**234.** C
189. D	**212.** B	**235.** A
190. C	**213.** D	**236.** B
191. C	**214.** D	**237.** C
192. C	**215.** B	**238.** D
193. D	**216.** D	**239.** C
194. D	**217.** D	**240.** B
195. B	**218.** A	**241.** D
196. C	**219.** B	**242.** B
197. B	**220.** B	**243.** D
198. A	**221.** A	**244.** B
199. B	**222.** D	**245.** B
200. A	**223.** D	**246.** D
201. A	**224.** B	**247.** D
202. C	**225.** B	**248.** C
203. B	**226.** C	**249.** D
204. A	**227.** A	**250.** C
205. D	**228.** D	
206. B	**229.** B	

Answers and Rationales

1. **Answer B is correct.** The client with passive-aggressive personality disorder often has underlying hostility that is exhibited as acting-out behavior. Answers A, C, and D are incorrect. Although these individuals might have a high IQ, it cannot be said that they have superior intelligence. They also do not necessarily have dependence on others or an inability to share feelings.

2. **Answer A is correct.** Clients with antisocial personality disorder must have limits set on their behavior because they are artful in manipulating others. Answer B is not correct because they do express feelings and remorse. Answers C and D are incorrect because it is unnecessary to minimize interactions with others or encourage them to act out rage more than they already do.

3. **Answer C is correct.** To prevent the client from inducing vomiting after eating, the client should be observed for 1–2 hours after meals. Allowing privacy as stated in answer A will only give the client time to vomit. Praising the client for eating all of a meal does not correct the psychological aspects of the disease; thus, answer B is incorrect. Encouraging the client to choose favorite foods might increase stress and the chance of choosing foods that are low in calories and fats so D is not correct.

4. **Answer B is correct.** The 4-year-old is more prone to accidental poisoning because children at this age are much more mobile. Answers A, C, and D are incorrect because the 6-month-old is still too small to be extremely mobile, the 12-year-old has begun to understand risk, and the 13-year-old is also aware that injuries can occur and is less likely to become injured than the 4-year-old.

5. **Answer B is correct.** Parallel play is play that is demonstrated by two children playing side by side but not together. The play in answers A and C is participative play because the children are playing together. The play in answer D is solitary play because the mother is not playing with Mary.

6. **Answer B is correct.** The first action that the nurse should take when beginning to examine the infant is to listen to the heart and lungs. If the nurse elicits the Babinski reflex, palpates the abdomen, or looks in the child's ear first, the child will begin to cry and it will be difficult to obtain an objective finding while listening to the heart and lungs. Therefore, answers A, C, and D are incorrect.

7. **Answer B is correct.** A 2-year-old is expected only to use magical thinking, such as believing that a toy bear is a real bear. Answers A, C, and D are not expected until the child is much older. Abstract thinking, conservation of matter, and the ability to look at things from the perspective of others are not skills for small children.

8. **Answer C is correct.** Children at 24 months can verbalize their needs. Answers A and B are incorrect because children at 24 months understand yes and no, but they do not understand the meaning of all words. Answer D is incorrect; asking "why?" comes later in development.

9. **Answer D is correct.** Urokinase is a thrombolytic used to destroy a clot following a myocardial infraction. If the client exhibits overt signs of bleeding, the nurse should stop the medication, call the doctor immediately, and prepare the antidote, which is Amicar. Answer B is not correct because simply stopping the urokinase is not enough. In answer A, vitamin K is not the antidote for urokinase, and reducing the urokinase, as stated in answer B, is not enough.

10. **Answer A is correct.** The client taking calcium preparations will frequently develop constipation. Answers B, C, and D do not apply.

11. **Answer C is correct.** C indicates a lack of understanding of the correct method of administering heparin. A, B, and D indicate understanding and are, therefore, incorrect answers.

12. **Answer C is correct.** If the finger cannot be used, the next best place to apply the oxygen monitor is the earlobe. It can also be placed on the forehead, but the choices in answers A, B, and D will not provide the needed readings.

13. **Answer A is correct.** The client is exhibiting a widened pulse pressure, tachycardia, and tachypnea. The next action after obtaining these vital signs is to notify the doctor for additional orders. Rechecking the vital signs, as in answer B, is wasting time. The doctor may order arterial blood gases and an ECG.

14. **Answer C is correct.** The client with a femoral popliteal bypass graft should avoid activities that can occlude the femoral artery graft. Sitting in the straight chair and wearing tight clothes are prohibited for this reason. Resting in a supine position, resting in a recliner, or sleeping in right Sim's are allowed, as stated in answers A, B, and D.

15. **Answer A is correct.** The best time to apply antithrombolytic stockings is in the morning before rising. If the doctor orders them later in the day, the client should return to bed, wait 30 minutes, and apply the stockings. Answers B, C, and D are incorrect because there is likely to be more peripheral edema if the client is standing or has just taken a bath; before retiring in the evening is wrong because late in the evening, more peripheral edema will be present.

16. **Answer C is correct.** The client admitted 1 hour ago with shortness of breath should be seen first because this client might require oxygen therapy. The client in answer A with an oxygen saturation of 99% is stable. Answer B is incorrect because this client will have some inflammatory process after surgery, so a temperature of 100.2°F is not unusual. The client in answer D is stable and can be seen later.

17. **Answer A is correct.** The best roommate for the post-surgical client is the client with hypothyroidism. This client is sleepy and has no infectious process. Answers B, C, and D are incorrect because the client with a diabetic ulcer, ulcerative colitis, or pneumonia can transmit infection to the post-surgical client.

18. **Answer C is correct.** The client taking an anticoagulant should not take aspirin because it will further increase bleeding. He should return to have a Protime drawn for bleeding time, report a rash, and use an electric razor. Therefore, answers A, B, and D are incorrect.

19. **Answer B is correct.** Because the aorta is clamped during surgery, the blood supply to the kidneys is impaired. This can result in renal damage. A urinary output of 20mL is oliguria. In answer A, the pedal pulses that are thready and regular are within normal limits. For answer C, it is desirable for the client's blood pressure to be slightly low after surgical repair of an aneurysm. The oxygen saturation of 97% in answer D is within normal limits and, therefore, incorrect.

20. **Answer D is correct.** When assisting the client with bowel and bladder training, the least helpful factor is the sexual function. Dietary history, mobility, and fluid intake are important factors; these must be taken into consideration because they relate to constipation, urinary function, and the ability to use the urinal or bedpan. Therefore, answers A, B, and C are incorrect.

21. **Answer B is correct.** To correctly measure the client for crutches, the nurse should measure approximately 3 inches under the axilla. Answer A allows for too much distance under the arm. The elbows should be flexed approximately 35°, not 10°, as stated in answer C. The crutches should be approximately 6 inches from the side of the foot, not 20 inches, as stated in answer D.

22. **Answer C is correct.** The temporal lobe is responsible for taste, smell, and hearing. The occipital lobe is responsible for vision. The frontal lobe is responsible for judgment, foresight, and behavior. The parietal lobe is responsible for ideation, sensory functions, and language. Therefore, answers A, B, and D are incorrect.

23. **Answer A is correct.** Damage to the hypothalamus can result in an elevated temperature because this portion of the brain helps to regulate body temperature. Answers B, C, and D are incorrect because there is no data to support the possibility of an infection, a cooling blanket might not be required, and the frontal lobe is not responsible for regulation of the body temperature.

24. **Answer A is correct.** A low-protein diet is required because protein breaks down into nitrogenous waste and causes an increased workload on the kidneys. Answers B, C, and D are incorrect.

25. **Answer B is correct.** To safely administer heparin, the nurse should obtain an infusion controller. Too rapid infusion of heparin can result in hemorrhage. Answers A, C, and D are incorrect. It is not necessary to have a buretrol, an infusion filter, or a three-way stop-cock.

26. **Answer A is correct.** If the blood pressure cuff is too small, the result will be a blood pressure that is a false elevation. Answers B, C, and D are incorrect. If the blood pressure cuff is too large, a false low will result. Answers C and D have basically the same meaning.

27. **Answer B is correct.** The child with nephotic syndrome will exhibit extreme edema. Elevating the scrotum on a small pillow will help with the edema. Applying ice is contraindicated; heat will increase the edema. Administering a diuretic might be ordered, but it will not directly help the scrotal edema. Therefore, answers A, C, and D are incorrect.

28. **Answer A is correct.** The elevated white blood cell count should be reported because this indicates infection. A bruit will be heard if the client has an aneurysm, and a negative Babinski is normal in the adult, as are pupils that are equal and reactive to light and accommodation; thus, answers B, C, and D are incorrect.

29. **Answer A is correct.** If the nurse cannot elicit the patella reflex (knee jerk), the client should be asked to pull against the palms. This helps the client to relax the legs and makes it easier to get an objective reading. Answers B, C, and D will not help with the test.

30. **Answer B is correct.** If the doctor orders 0.4mgm IM and the drug is available in 0.8/1mL, the nurse should make the calculation: ?mL = 1mL / 0.8mgm; × .4mg / 1 = 0.5m:. Answers A, C, and D are incorrect.

31. **Answer B is correct.** The pulmonary artery pressure will measure the pressure during systole, diastole, and the mean pressure in the pulmonary artery. It will not measure the pressure in the left ventricle, the pressure in the pulmonary veins, or the pressure in the right ventricle. Therefore, answers A, C, and D are incorrect.

32. **Answer A is correct.** The normal central venous pressure is 5–10cm of water. A reading of 2cm is low and should be reported. Answers B, C, and D indicate that the nurse believes that the reading is too high and is incorrect.

33. **Answer C is correct.** The treatment for ventricular tachycardia is lidocaine. A precordial thump is sometimes successful in slowing the rate, but this should be done only if a defibrillator is available. In answer A, atropine sulfate will speed the rate further; in answer B, checking the potassium is indicated but is not the priority; and in answer D, defibrillation is used for pulseless ventricular tachycardia or ventricular fibrillation. Also, defibrillation should begin at 200 joules and be increased to 360 joules.

34. **Answer B is correct.** The client should be asked to perform the Valsalva maneuver while the chest tube is being removed. This prevents changes in pressure until an occlusive dressing can be applied. Answers A and C are not recommended, and sneezing is difficult to perform on command.

35. **Answer D is correct.** The potassium level of 2.5meq/L is extremely low. The normal is 3.5–5.5meq/L. Lasix (furosemide) is a nonpotassium sparing diuretic, so answer A is incorrect. The nurse cannot alter the doctor's order, as stated in answer B, and answer C will not help with this situation.

36. **Answer A is correct.** An occult blood test should be done periodically to detect any intestinal bleeding on the client with Coumadin therapy. Answers B, C, and D are not directly related to the question.

37. **Answer D is correct.** After administering any subcutaneous anticoagulant, the nurse should check the site for bleeding. Answers A and C are incorrect because aspirating and massaging the site are not done. Checking the pulse is not necessary, as in answer B.

38. **Answer C is correct.** Acupuncture uses needles, and because HIV is transmitted by blood and body fluids, the nurse should question this treatment. Answer A describes acupressure, and answers B and D describe massage therapy with the use of oils.

39. **Answer B is correct.** The fifth vital sign is pain. Nurses should assess and record pain just as they would temperature, respirations, pulse, and blood pressure. Answers A, C, and D are included in the charting but are not considered to be the fifth vital sign and are, therefore, incorrect.

40. **Answer A is correct.** Narcan is the antidote for the opioid analgesics. Toradol (answer B) is a nonopoid analgesic; aspirin (answer C) is an analgesic, anticoagulant, and antipyretic; and atropine (answer D) is an anticholengergic.

41. **Answer B is correct.** The client is concerned about overdosing himself. The machine will deliver a set amount as ordered and allow the client to self-administer a small amount of medication. PCA pumps usually are set to lock out the amount of medication that the client can give himself at 5- to 15-minute intervals. Answer A does not address the client's concerns, answer C is incorrect, and answer D does not address the client's concerns.

42. **Answer B is correct.** Skin irritation can occur if the TENS unit is used for prolonged periods of time. To prevent skin irritations, the client should change the location of the electrodes often. Electrocution is not a risk because it uses a battery pack; thus, answer A is incorrect. Answer C is incorrect because the unit should not be used on sensitive areas of the body. Answer D is incorrect because no creams are to be used with the device.

43. **Answer B is correct.** An advanced directive allows the client to make known his wishes regarding care if he becomes unable to act on his own. Much confusion regarding life-saving measures can occur if the client does not have an advanced directive. Answers A, C, and D are incorrect because the nurse doesn't need to know about funeral plans and cannot make decisions for the client, and active euthanasia is illegal in most states in the United States.

44. **Answer B is correct.** To decrease the potential for soreness of the nipples, the client should be taught to break the suction before removing the baby from the breast. Answer A is incorrect because feeding the baby during the first 48 hours after delivery will provide colostrum but will not help the soreness of the nipples. Answers C and D are incorrect because applying hot, moist soaks several times per day might cause burning of the breast and cause further drying. Wearing a support bra will help with engorgement but will not help the nipples.

45. **Answer D is correct.** Facial grimace is an indication of pain. The blood pressure in answer A is within normal limits. The client's inability to concentrate and dilated pupils, as stated in answers B and C, may be related to the anesthesia that he received during surgery.

46. **Answer C is correct.** Epidural anesthesia involves injecting an anesthetic into the epidural space. If the anesthetic rises above the respiratory center, the client will have impaired breathing; thus, monitoring for respiratory depression is necessary. Answer A, seizure activity, is not likely after an epidural. Answer B, postural hypertension, is not likely. Answer D, hematuria, is not related to epidural anesthesia.

47. **Answer C is correct.** Pain is a late sign of oral cancer. Answers A, B, and D are incorrect because a feeling of warmth, odor, and a flat ulcer in the mouth are all early occurrences of oral cancer.

48. **Answer A is correct.** The best diagnostic tool for cancer is the biopsy. Other assessment includes checking the lymph nodes. Answers B, C, and D will not confirm a diagnosis of oral cancer.

49. **Answer A is correct.** Maintaining a patient's airway is paramount in the post-operative period. This is the priority of nursing care. Answers B, C, and D are applicable but are not the priority.

50. **Answer C is correct.** *H. pylori* bacteria has been linked to peptic ulcers. Answers A, B, and D are not typically cultured within the stomach, duodenum, or esophagus, and are not related to the development of peptic ulcers.

51. **Answer B is correct.** Individuals with ulcers within the duodenum typically complain of pain occurring 2–3 hours after a meal, as well as at night. The pain is usually relieved by eating. The pain associated with gastric ulcers, answer A, occurs 30 minutes after eating. Answer C is too vague and does not distinguish the type of ulcer. Answer D is associated with a stress ulcer.

52. **Answer B is correct.** A barium enema is contraindicated in the client with diverticulitis because it can cause bowel perforation. Answers A, C, and D are appropriate diagnostic studies for the client with suspected diverticulitis.

53. **Answer A is correct.** Clients with celiac disease should refrain from eating foods containing gluten. Foods with gluten include wheat barley, oats, and rye. The other foods are allowed.

54. **Answer A is correct.** The nurse should reinforce the need for a diet balanced in all nutrients and fiber. Foods that often cause diarrhea and bloating associated with irritable bowel syndrome include fried foods, caffeinated beverages, alcohol, and spicy foods. Therefore, answers B, C, and D are incorrect.

55. **Answer C is correct.** Fluid volume deficit can lead to metabolic acidosis and electrolyte loss. The other nursing diagnoses in answers A, B, and D might be applicable but are of lesser priority.

56. **Answer D is correct.** Alcohol will cause extreme nausea if consumed with Flagyl. Answer A is incorrect because the full course of treatment should be taken. The medication should be taken with a full 8 oz. of water, with meals, and the client should avoid direct sunlight because he will most likely be photosensitive; therefore, answers A, B, and C are incorrect.

57. **Answer A is correct.** Before beginning feedings, an x-ray is often obtained to check for placement. Aspirating stomach content and checking the pH for acidity is the best method of checking for placement. Other methods include placing the end in water and checking for bubbling, and injecting air and listening over the epigastric area. Answers B and C are not correct. Answer D is incorrect because warming in the microwave is contraindicated.

58. **Answer C is correct.** Antacids should be administered with other medications. If antacids are taken with many medications, they render the other medications inactive. All other answers are incorrect.

59. **Answer A is correct.** The client with a colostomy can swim and carry on activities as before the colostomy. Answers B and C are incorrect, and answer D shows a lack of empathy.

60. **Answer D is correct.** The use of a sitz bath will help with the pain and swelling associated with a hemorroidectomy. The client should eat foods high in fiber, so answer A is incorrect. Ice packs, as stated in answer B, are ordered immediately after surgery only. Answer C is incorrect because taking a laxative daily can result in diarrhea.

61. **Answer D is correct.** Low hemoglobin and hematocrit might indicate intestinal bleeding. Answers A, B, and C are incorrect, because they do not require immediate action.

62. **Answer C is correct.** The new diabetic has a knowledge deficit. Answers A, B, and D are not supported within the stem and so are incorrect.

63. **Answer D Is correct.** Peptic ulcers are not always related to stress but are a component of the disease. Answers A and B are incorrect because peptic ulcers are not caused by overeating or continued exposure to stress. Answer C is incorrect because peptic ulcers are related to but not directly caused by stress.

64. **Answer B is correct.** Many medications can irritate the stomach and contribute to abdominal pain. For answer A, not all interactions between medications will cause abdominal pain. Although this might provide an opportunity for teaching, this is not the best time to teach. Therefore, answer C is incorrect. Answer D is incorrect because medication may not be the cause of the pain.

65. **Answer A is correct.** The nurse should inspect first, then auscultate, and finally palpate. If the nurse palpates first the assessment might be unreliable. Therefore, answers B, C, and D are incorrect.

66. **Answer A is correct.** The hospital will certainly honor the wishes of family members even if the patient has signed a donor card. Answer B is incorrect, answer C is not empathetic to the family and is untrue, and answer D is not good nursing etiquette and, therefore, is incorrect.

67. **Answer C is correct.** The nurse should explore the cause for the lack of motivation. The client might be anemic and lack energy, or the client might be depressed. Alternating staff, as stated in answer A, will prevent a bond from being formed with the nurse. Answer B is not enough, and answer D is not necessary.

68. **Answer D is correct.** The nurse who has had the chickenpox has immunity to the illness and will not transmit chickenpox to the client. Answer A is incorrect because there could be no need to reassign the nurse. Answer B is incorrect because the nurse should be assessed before coming to the conclusion that she cannot spread the infection to the client. Answer C is incorrect because there is still a risk, even though chickenpox has formed scabs.

69. **Answer A is correct.** The nurse should not take the blood pressure on the affected side. Also, venopunctures and IVs should not be used in the affected area. Answers B, C, and D are all indicated for caring for the client. The arm should be elevated to decrease edema. It is best to position the client on the unaffected side and perform a dextrostix on the unaffected side.

70. **Answer B is correct.** Gentamycin is an aminoglycocide. These drugs are toxic to the auditory nerve and the kidneys. The hematocrit is not of significant consideration in this client; therefore, answer A is incorrect. Answer C is incorrect because we would expect the white blood cell count to be elevated in this client because gentamycin is an antibiotic. Answer D is incorrect because the erythrocyte count is also particularly significant to check.

71. **Answer C is correct.** The most definitive diagnostic tool for HIV is the Western Blot. The white blood cell count, as stated in answer A, is not the best indicator, but a white blood cell count of less than 3,500 requires investigation. The ELISA test, answer B, is a screening exam. Answer D is not specific enough.

72. **Answer A is correct.** The "bull's eye" rash is indicative of Lyme's disease, a disease spread by ticks. The signs and symptoms include elevated temperature, headache, nausea, and the rash. Although answers B and D are important, the question asked which question would be *best*. Answer C has no significance.

73. **Answer C is correct.** The client that needs the least-skilled nursing care is the client with the thyroidectomy 4 days ago. Answers A, B, and D are incorrect because the other clients are less stable and require a registered nurse.

74. **Answer A is correct.** Hyphema is blood in the anterior chamber of the eye and around the eye. The client should have the head of the bed elevated and ice applied. Answers B, C, and D are incorrect and do not treat the problem.

75. **Answer C is correct.** $FeSO_4$ or iron should be given with ascorbic acid (vitamin C). This helps with the absorption. It should not be given with meals or milk because this decreases the absorption; thus, answers A and B are incorrect. Giving it undiluted, as stated in answer D, is not good because it tastes bad.

76. **Answer C is correct.** The best protector for the client with an ileostomy to use is stomahesive. Answer A is not correct because the bag will not seal if the client uses Karaya powder. Answer B is incorrect because there is no need to irrigate an ileostomy. Neosporin, answer D, is not used to protect the skin because it is an antibiotic.

77. **Answer D is correct.** Vitamin K is given after delivery because the newborn's intestinal tract is sterile and lacks vitamin K needed for clotting. Answer A is incorrect because vitamin K is not directly given to stop hemorrhage. Answers B and C are incorrect because vitamin K does not prevent infection or replace electrolytes.

78. **Answer D is correct.** The vital signs should be taken before any chemotherapy agent. If it is an IV infusion of chemotherapy, the nurse should check the IV site as well. Answers B and C are incorrect because it is not necessary to check the electrolytes or blood gasses.

79. **Answer C is correct.** Before chemotherapy, an antiemetic should be given because most chemotherapy agents cause nausea. It is not necessary to give a bolus of IV fluids, medicate for pain, or allow the client to eat; therefore, answers A, B, and D are incorrect.

80. **Answer B is correct.** Pitocin is used to cause the uterus to contract and decrease bleeding. A uterus deviated to the left, as stated in answer A, indicates a full bladder. It is not desirable to have a boggy uterus, making answer C incorrect. This lack of muscle tone will increase bleeding. Answer D is incorrect because Pitocin does not affect the position of the uterus.

81. **Answer A is correct.** Household contacts should take INH approximately 6 months. Answers B, C, and D are incorrect because they indicate either too short or too long of a time to take the medication.

82. **Answer C is correct.** Viokase is a pancreatic enzyme that is used to facilitate digestion. It should be given with meals and snacks, and it works well in foods such as applesauce. Answers A, B, and D are incorrect.

83. **Answer B is correct.** Trough levels are the lowest blood levels and should be done 30 minutes before the third IV dose or 30 minutes before the fourth IM dose. Answers A, C, and D are incorrect.

84. **Answer A is correct.** Regular insulin should be drawn up before the NPH. They can be given together, so there is no need for two injections, making answer D incorrect. Answer B is obviously incorrect, and answer C is incorrect because it certainly does matter which is drawn first: Contamination of NPH into regular insulin will result in a hypoglycemic reaction at unexpected times.

85. **Answer A is correct.** Clients having dye procedures should be assessed for allergies to iodine or shellfish. Answers B and D are incorrect because there is no need for the client to be assessed for reactions to blood or eggs. Because an IV cholangiogram is done to detect gallbladder disease, there is no need to ask about answer C.

86. **Answer A is correct.** Methergine is a drug that causes uterine contractions. It is used for postpartal bleeding that is not controlled by Pitocin. Answers B, C, and D are incorrect: Stadol is an analgesic; magnesium sulfate is used for preeclampsia; and phenergan is an antiemetic.

87. **Answer D is correct.** Cyclosporin is an immunosuppressant, and the client with a liver transplant will be on immunosuppressants for the rest of his life. Answers A, B, and C, then, are incorrect.

88. **Answer C is correct.** Histamine blockers are frequently ordered for clients who are hospitalized for prolonged periods and who are in a stressful situation. They are not used to treat discomfort, correct electrolytes, or treat nausea; therefore, answers A, B, and D are incorrect.

89. **Answer C is correct.** The time of onset for regular insulin is 30–60 minutes. Answers A, B, and D are incorrect because they are not the correct times.

90. **Answer C is correct.** The client should be taught to eat his meals even if he is not hungry, to prevent a hypoglycemic reaction. Answers A, B, and D are incorrect because they indicate knowledge of the nurse's teaching.

91. **Answer D is correct.** Taking antibiotics and oral contraceptives together decreases the effectiveness of the oral contraceptives. Answers A, B, and C are not necessarily true.

92. **Answer D is correct.** Taking corticosteroids in the morning mimics the body's natural release of cortisol. Answer A is not necessarily true, and answers B and C are not true.

93. **Answer B is correct.** Rifampin can change the color of the urine and body fluid. Teaching the client about these changes is best because he might think this is a complication. Answer A is not necessary, answer C is not true, and answer D is not true because this medication should be taken regularly during the course of the treatment.

94. **Answer D is correct.** Cytoxan can cause hemorrhagic cystitis, so the client should drink at least eight glasses of water a day. Answers A and B are not necessary and, so, are incorrect. Nausea often occurs with chemotherapy, so answer C is incorrect.

95. **Answer A is correct.** Crystals in the solution are not normal and should not be administered to the client. Discard the bad solution immediately. Answer B is incorrect because warming the solution will not help. Answer C is incorrect, and answer D requires a doctor's order.

96. **Answer C is correct.** Theodur is a bronchodilator, and a side effect of bronchodilators is tachycardia, so checking the pulse is important. Extreme tachycardia should be reported to the doctor. Answers A, B, and D are not necessary.

97. **Answer B is correct.** The diagnosis of meningitis at age 6 months correlates to a diagnosis of cerebral palsy. Cerebral palsy, a neurological disorder, is often associated with birth trauma or infections of the brain or spinal column. Answers A, C and D are not related to the question.

98. **Answer B is correct.** Children at 18 months of age like push-pull toys. Children at approximately 3 years of age begin to dress themselves and build a tower of eight blocks. At age four, children can copy a horizontal or vertical line. Therefore, answers A, C, and D are incorrect.

99. **Answer D is correct.** A complication of a tonsillectomy is bleeding, and constant swallowing may indicate bleeding. Decreased appetite is expected after a tonsillectomy, as is a low-grade temperature; thus, answers A and B are incorrect. In answer C, chest congestion is not normal but is not associated with the tonsillectomy.

100. **Answer C is correct.** Hyperplasia of the gums is associated with Dilantin therapy. Answer A is not related to the therapy; answer B is a side effect; and answer D is not related to the question.

101. **Answer A is correct.** If the client eats foods high in tyramine, he might experience malignant hypertension. Tyramine is found in cheese, sour cream, Chianti wine, sherry, beer, pickled herring, liver, canned figs, raisins, bananas, avocados, chocolate, soy sauce, fava beans, and yeast. These episodes are treated with Regitine, an alpha-adrenergic blocking agent. Answers B, C, and D are not related to the question.

102. **Answer D is correct.** Quinidine can cause widened Q-T intervals and heart block. Other signs of myocardial toxicity are notched P waves and widened QRS complexes. The most common side effects are diarrhea, nausea, and vomiting. The client might experience tinnitus, vertigo, headache, visual disturbances, and confusion. Answers A, B, and C are not related to the use of quinidine.

103. **Answer B is correct.** Lidocaine is used to treat ventricular tachycardia. This medication slowly exerts an antiarrhythmic effect by increasing the electric stimulation threshold of the ventricles without depressing the force of ventricular contractions. It is not used for atrial arrhythmias; thus, answer A is incorrect. Answers C and D are incorrect because it slows the heart rate, so it is not used for heart block or brachycardia.

104. **Answer A is correct.** Sites for the application of nitroglycerin should be rotated, to prevent skin irritation. It can be applied to the back and upper arms, not to the lower extremities, making answer B incorrect. Answer C is incorrect because nitroglycerine should not be rubbed into the skin, and answer D is incorrect because the medication should be covered with a prepared dressing made of a thin paper substance, not gauze.

105. **Answer B is correct.** A persistent cough might be related to an adverse reaction to Captoten. Answers A and D are incorrect because tinnitus and diarrhea are not associated with the medication. Muscle weakness might occur when beginning the treatment but is not an adverse effect; thus, answer C is incorrect.

106. **Answer A is correct.** Lasix should be given approximately 1mL per minute to prevent hypotension. Answers B, C, and D are incorrect because it is not necessary to be given in an IV piggyback, with saline, or through a filter.

107. **Answer B is correct.** The antidote for heparin is protamine sulfate. Cyanocobalamine is B12, Streptokinase is a thrombolytic, and sodium warfarin is an anticoagulant. Therefore, answers A, C, and D are incorrect.

108. **Answer A is correct.** The pregnant nurse should not be assigned to any client with radioactivity present. The client receiving linear accelerator therapy is not radioactive because he travels to the radium department for therapy, and the radiation stays in the department. The client in answer B does pose a risk to the pregnant nurse. The client in answer C is radioactive in very small doses. For approximately 72 hours, the client should dispose of urine and feces in special containers and use plastic spoons and forks. The client in answer D is also radioactive in small amounts, especially upon return from the procedure.

109. **Answer A is correct.** The client with Cushing's disease has adrenocortical hyper-secretion. This increase in the level of cortisone causes the client to be immune suppressed. In answer B, the client with diabetes poses no risk to other clients. The client in answer C has an increase in growth hormone and poses no risk to himself or others. The client in answer D has hyperthyroidism or myxedema, and poses no risk to others or himself.

110. **Answer C is correct.** Assault is defined as striking or touching the client inappropriately, so a nurse assistant striking a client could be charged with assault. Answer A, negligence, is failing to perform care for the client. Answer B, a tort, is a wrongful act committed on the client or their belongings. Answer D, malpractice, is failure to perform an act that the nurse assistant knows should be done, or the act of doing something wrong that results in harm to the client.

111. **Answer D is correct.** The licensed practical nurse cannot start a blood transfusion, but can assist the registered nurse with identifying the client and taking vital signs. Answers A, B, and C are duties that the licensed practical nurse can perform.

112. **Answer B is correct.** The vital signs are abnormal and should be reported to the doctor immediately. Answer A, continuing to monitor the vital signs, can result in deterioration of the client's condition. Answer C, asking the client how he feels, would supply only subjective data. Involving the LPN, in Answer D, is not the best solution to help this client because he is unstable.

113. **Answer B is correct.** Thalasemia is a genetic disorder that causes the red blood cells to have a shorter life span. Frequent blood transfusions are necessary to provide oxygen to the tissues. Answer A is incorrect because fluid therapy will not help; answer C is incorrect because oxygen therapy will also not help; and answer D is incorrect because iron should be given sparingly because these clients do not use iron stores adequately.

114. **Answer B is correct.** Cystic fibrosis is a disease of the exocrine glands. The child with cystic fibrosis will be salty. A sweat test result of 60meq/L and higher is considered positive. Answers A, C, and D are incorrect because these test results are within the normal range and are not reported on the sweat test.

115. **Answer A is correct.** A meningomylocele is an opening in the spine. The nurse should keep the defect covered with a sterile saline gauze until the defect can be repaired. Answer B is incorrect because the child should be placed in the prone position. Answer C is incorrect because feeding the child slowly is not necessary. Answer D is not correct because this is not the priority of care.

116. **Answer D is correct.** Absent femoral pulses indicates coarctation of the aorta. This defect causes strong bounding pulses and elevated blood pressure in the upper body, and low blood pressure in the lower extremities. Answers A, B, and C are incorrect because they are normal findings in the newborn.

117. **Answer D is correct.** Clostrium dificille is primarily spread through the GI tract, resulting from poor hand washing and contamination with stool containing clostridium dificille. Answers A, B, and C are incorrect because the mode of transmission is not by sputum, through the urinary tract, or by unsterile surgical equipment.

118. **Answer A is correct.** The first client to be seen is the one who recently returned from surgery. The other clients in answers B, C, and D are more stable and can be seen later.

119. **Answer D is correct.** Cyanocolamine is a B12 medication that is used for pernicious anemia, and a reticulocyte count of 1% indicates that it is having the desired effect. Answers A, B, and C are white blood cells and have nothing to do with this medication.

120. **Answer C is correct.** The client taking antabuse should not eat or drink anything containing alcohol or vinegar. The other foods in answers A, B, and D are allowed.

121. **Answer A is correct.** The client with unilateral neglect will neglect one side of the body. Answers B, C, and D are not associated with unilateral neglect.

122. **Answer D is correct.** Because the client is immune suppressed, foods should be served in sealed containers, to avoid food contaminants. Answer B is incorrect because of possible infection from visitors. Answer A is not necessary, but the utensils should be cleaned thoroughly and rinsed in hot water. Answer C might be a good idea, but alcohol can be drying and can cause the skin to break down.

123. **Answer A is correct.** Identifying oneself as a nurse without a license defrauds the public and can be prosecuted. A tort is a wrongful act; malpractice is failing to act appropriately as a nurse or acting in a way that harm comes to the client; and negligence is failing to perform care. Therefore, answers B, C, and D are incorrect.

124. **Answer B is correct.** The client with the appendectomy is the most stable of these clients and can be assigned to a nursing assistant. The client with bronchiolitis has an alteration in the airway; the client with periorbital cellulitis has an infection; and the client with a fracture might be an abused child. Therefore, answers A, C, and D are incorrect.

125. **Answer B is correct.** The first action the nurse should take is to report the finding to the nurse supervisor and follow the chain of command. If it is found that the pharmacy is in error, it should be notified, as stated in answer A. Answers C and D, notifying the director of nursing and the Board of Nursing, might be necessary if theft is found, but not as a first step; thus, these are incorrect for this question.

126. **Answer B is correct.** The best client to transport to the postpartum unit is the 40-year-old female with a hysterectomy. The nurses on the postpartum unit will be aware of normal amounts of bleeding and will be equipped to care for this client. The clients in answers A and D will be best cared for on a medical-surgical unit. The client with depression in answer C should be transported to the psychiatric unit.

127. **Answer D is correct.** The fresh peach is the lowest in sodium of these choices. Answers A, B, and C have much higher amounts of sodium.

128. **Answer B is correct.** The client with congestive heart failure who is complaining of nighttime dyspnea should be seen because airway is number one in nursing care. In answers A, C, and D, the clients are more stable. A brain attack in answer A is the new terminology for a stroke.

129. **Answer D is correct.** Xerostomia is dry mouth, and offering the client a saliva substitute will help the most. Eating hard candy in answer A can further irritate the mucosa and cut the tongue and lips. Administering an analgesic might not be necessary; thus, answer B is incorrect. Splinting swollen joints, in answer C, is not associated with xerostomia.

130. **Answer A is correct.** The client with Alzheimer's disease is the most stable of these clients and can be assigned to the nursing assistant, who can perform duties such as feeding and assisting the client with activities of daily living. The clients in answers B, C, and D are less stable and should be attended by a registered nurse.

131. **Answer A is correct.** Frequent rest periods help to relax tense muscles and preserve energy. Answers B, C, and D are incorrect because they are untrue statements about cerebral palsy.

132. **Answer D is correct.** A culture for gonorrhea is taken from the genital secretions. The culture is placed in a warm environment, where it can grow nisseria gonorrhea. Answers A, B, and C are incorrect because these cultures do not test for gonorrhea.

133. **Answer D is correct.** After surgery, the client will be placed on a clear-liquid diet and progressed to a regular diet. Stool softeners will be included in the plan of care, to avoid constipation. Later, a high-fiber diet, in answer A, is encouraged, but this is not the first diet after surgery. Answers B and C are not diets for this type of surgery.

134. **Answer C is correct.** A sitz bath will help with swelling and improve healing. Ice packs, in answer D, can be used immediately after delivery, but answers A and B are not used in this instance.

135. **Answer B is correct.** The best way to evaluate pain levels is to ask the client to rate his pain on a scale. In answer A, the blood pressure, pulse, and temperature can alter for other reasons than pain. Answers C and D are not as effective in determining pain levels.

136. **Answer C is correct.** The client is experiencing compensated metabolic acidosis. The pH is within the normal range but is lower than 7.40, so it is on the acidic side. The CO_2 level is elevated, the oxygen level is below normal, and the bicarb level is slightly elevated. In respiratory disorders, the pH will be the inverse of the CO_2 and bicarb levels. This means that if the pH is low, the CO_2 and bicarb levels will be elevated. Answers A, B, and D are incorrect because they do not fall into the range of symptoms.

137. **Answer B is correct.** The registered nurse is the only one of these who can legally put the client in seclusion. The only other healthcare worker who is allowed to initiate seclusion is the doctor; therefore, answers A, C, and D are incorrect.

138. **Answer C is correct.** Sodium warfarin is administered in the late afternoon, at approximately 1700 hours. This allows for accurate bleeding times to be drawn in the morning. Therefore, answers A, B, and D are incorrect.

139. **Answer C is correct.** Covering both eyes prevents consensual movement of the affected eye. Answer A is incorrect because the nurse should not attempt to remove the object from the eye because this might cause trauma. Rinsing the eye, as stated in answer B, might be ordered by the doctor, but this is not the first step for the nurse. Answer D is not correct because often when one eye moves, the other also moves.

140. **Answer A is correct.** To protect herself, the nurse should wear gloves when applying a nitroglycerine patch or cream. Answer B is incorrect because shaving the shin might abrade the area. Answer C is incorrect because washing with hot water will vasodilate and increase absorption. The patches should be applied to areas above the waist, making answer D incorrect.

141. **Answer B is correct.** The client scheduled for a pericentesis should be told to empty the bladder, to prevent the risk of puncturing the bladder when the needle is inserted. A pericentesis is done to remove fluid from the peritoneal cavity. The client will be positioned sitting up or leaning over an overbed table, making answer A incorrect. The client is usually awake during the procedure, and medications are not commonly instilled during the procedure; thus answers C and D are incorrect.

142. **Answer A is correct.** Atropine sulfate is the antidote for Tensilon and is given to treat cholenergic crises. Furosemide (answer B) is a diuretic; Prostigmin (answer C) is the treatment for myasthenia gravis; and Promethazine (answer D) is an antiemetic, antianxiety medication. Thus, answers B, C, and D are incorrect.

143. **Answer D is correct.** The first exercise that should be done by the client with a mastectomy is squeezing the ball. Answers A, B, and C are incorrect as the first step; they are implemented later.

144. **Answer D is correct.** The mothers in answers A, B, and C all require RhoGam and, thus, are incorrect. Answer D is the only mother who does not require a RhoGam injection.

145. **Answer A is correct.** Answer A, AST, is not specific for myocardial infarction. Troponin, CK-MB, and Myoglobin, in answers B, C, and D, are more specific, although myoglobin is also elevated in burns and trauma to muscles.

146. **Answer B is correct.** The client who says he has nothing wrong is in denial about his myocardial infarction. Rationalization is making excuses for what happened, projection is projecting feeling or thoughts onto others, and conversion reaction is converting a psychological trauma into a physical illness; thus, answers A, C, and D are incorrect.

147. **Answer C is correct.** When the client is receiving TPN, the blood glucose level should be drawn. TPN is a solution that contains large amounts of glucose. Answers A, B, and D are not directly related to the question and are incorrect.

148. **Answer B is correct.** A client with diabetes who has trouble seeing would require follow-up after discharge. The lack of visual acuity for the client preparing and injecting insulin might require help. Answers A, C, and D will not prevent the client from being able to care for himself and, thus, are incorrect.

149. **Answer C is correct.** Lactulose is administered to the client with cirrhosis to lower ammonia levels. Answers A, B, and D are incorrect because they do not have an effect on the other lab values.

150. **Answer B is correct.** If the dialysate returns cloudy, infection might be present and must be evaluated. Documenting the finding, as stated in answer A, as not enough; straining the urine, in answer C, is incorrect; and dialysate, in answer D, is not urine at all. However, the physician might order a white blood cell count.

151. **Answer B is correct.** The teenager with sternal bruising might be experiencing airway and oxygenation problems and, thus, should be seen first. In answer A, the 10 year old with lacerations has superficial bleeding. The client in answer C with a fractured femur should be immobilized but can be seen after the client with sternal bruising. The client in answer D with the dislocated elbow can be seen later as well.

152. **Answer A is correct.** The most suitable roommate for the client with myasthenia gravis is the client with hypothyroidism because he is quiet. The client with Crohn's disease in answer B will be up to the bathroom frequently; the client with pylonephritis in answer C has a kidney infection and will be up to urinate frequently. The client in answer D with bronchitis will be coughing and will disturb any roommate.

153. **Answer C is correct.** The client should not be instructed to do the Valsalva maneuver during central venous pressure reading. If the nurse tells the client to perform the Valsalva maneuver, he needs further teaching. Answers A, B, and D are incorrect because they indicate that the nurse understands the correct way to check the CVP.

154. **Answer D is correct.** The most critical client should be assigned to the registered nurse; in this case, that is the client 2 days post-thoracotomy. The clients in answers A and B are ready for discharge, and the client in answer C who had a splenectomy 3 days ago is stable enough to be assigned to a PN.

155. **Answer D is correct.** The most suitable roommate for the client with gastric reaction is the client with phlebitis because the client with phlebitis will not transmit any infection to the surgical client. Crohn's disease clients, in answer A, have frequent stools and might transmit infections. The client in answer B with pneumonia is coughing and will disturb the gastric client. The client with gastritis, in answer C, is vomiting and has diarrhea, which also will disturb the gastric client.

156. **Answer B is correct.** The client having a mammogram should be instructed to omit deodorants or powders beforehand because these could cause a false positive reading. Answer A is incorrect because there is no need to restrict fat. Answer C is incorrect because doing a mammogram does not replace the need for self-breast exams. Answer D is incorrect because a mammogram does not require a higher dose of radiation than an x-ray.

157. **Answer A is correct.** The nurse who fails to wear gloves to remove a contaminated dressing needs further instruction. Answers B, C, and D are incorrect because these answers indicate understanding by the nurse.

158. **Answer A is correct.** When the cadaver client is being prepared to donate an organ, the systolic blood pressure should be maintained at 70mmHg or greater, to ensure a blood supply to the donor organ. Answers B, C, and D are incorrect because these actions are not necessary for the donated organ to remain viable.

159. **Answer A is correct.** Bilirubin is excreted through the kidneys, thus the need for increased fluids. Maintaining the body temperature is important but will not assist in eliminating bilirubin; therefore, answer B is incorrect. Answers C and D are incorrect because they do not relate to the question.

160. **Answer C is correct.** The client with laryngeal cancer has a potential airway alteration and should be seen first. The clients in answers A, B, and D are not in immediate danger and can be seen later in the day.

161. **Answer B is correct.** The best action for the nurse to take is to explore the interaction with the nursing assistant. This will allow for clarification of the situation. Changing the assignment in answer A might need to be done, but talking to the nursing assistant is the first step. Answer C is incorrect because discussing the incident with the family is not necessary at this time; it might cause more problems than it solves. Answer C is not a first step, even though initiating a group session might be a plan for the future.

162. **Answer B is correct.** The best action at this time is to report the incident to the charge nurse. Further action might be needed, but it will be done by the charge nurse. Answers A, C, and D are incorrect because notifying the police is overreacting at this time, and monitoring or ignoring the situation is an inadequate response.

163. **Answer D is correct.** The best client to assign to the newly licensed nurse is the most stable client; in this case, it is the client with diverticulitis. The client receiving chemotherapy and the client with a coronary bypass both need nurses experienced in these areas, so answers A and B are incorrect. Answer C is incorrect because the client with a transurethral prostatectomy might bleed, so this client should be assigned to a nurse who knows how much bleeding is within normal limits.

164. **Answer D is correct.** Intrathecal medications are administered into the cerebrospinal fluid. This method of administering medications is reserved for the client metastases, the client with chronic pain, or the client with cerebrospinal infections. Answers A, B, and C are incorrect because intravenous, rectal, and intramuscular injections are entirely different procedures.

165. **Answer B is correct.** Montgomery straps are used to secure dressings that require frequent dressing changes because the client with a cholecystectomy usually has a large amount of draining on the dressing. Montgomery straps are also used for clients who are allergic to several types of tape. This client is not at higher risk of evisceration than other clients, so answer A is incorrect. Montgomery straps are not used to secure the drains, so answer C is incorrect. Sutures or clips are used to secure the wound of the client who has had gallbladder surgery, so answer D is incorrect.

166. **Answer B is correct.** The client with pancreatitis frequently has nausea and vomiting. Lavage is often used to decompress the stomach and rest the bowel, so the insertion of a Levine tube should be anticipated. Answers A and C are incorrect because blood pressures are not required every 15 minutes, and cardiac monitoring might be needed, but this is individualized to the client. Answer D is incorrect because there are no dressings to change on this client.

167. **Answer B is correct.** Oils can be applied to help with the dry skin and to decrease itching, so adding baby oil to bath water is soothing to the skin. Answer A is incorrect because two baths per day is too frequent and can cause more dryness. Answer C is incorrect because powder is also drying. Rinsing with hot water, as stated in answer D, dries out the skin as well.

168. **Answer A is correct.** If the nurse is exposed to the client with a cough, the best item to wear is a mask. If the answer had included a mask, gloves, and a gown, all would be appropriate, but in this case, only one item is listed; therefore, answers B and C are incorrect. Shoe covers are not necessary, so answer D is incorrect.

169. **Answer D is correct.** Abnormal grieving is exhibited by a lack of feeling sad; if the client's sister appears not to grieve, it might be abnormal grieving. She thinks the client might be suppressing feelings of grief. Answers A, B, and C are all normal expressions of grief and, therefore, incorrect.

170. **Answer B is correct.** Frequent use of laxatives can lead to diarrhea and electrolyte loss. Answers A, C, and D are not of particular significance in this case and, therefore, are incorrect.

171. **Answer B is correct.** The client with serum sodium of 170meq/L has hypernatremia and might exhibit manic behavior. Answers A, C, and D are not associated with hypernatremia and are, therefore, incorrect.

172. **Answer A is correct.** Radiation to the neck might have damaged the parathyroid glands, which are located on the thyroid gland, interferes with calcium and phosphorus regulation. Answer B has no significance to this case; answers C and D are more related to calcium only, not to phosphorus regulation.

173. **Answer A is correct.** It is the responsibility of the physician to explain and clarify the procedure to the client, so the nurse should call the surgeon to explain to the client. Answers B, C, and D are incorrect because they are not within the nurse's responsibility.

174. **Answer B is correct.** It is most important to remove the contact lenses because leaving them in can lead to corneal drying, particularly with contact lenses that are not extended-wear lenses. Leaving in the hearing aid or artificial eye will not harm the client. Leaving the wedding ring on is also allowed; usually, the ring is covered with tape. Therefore, answers A, C, and D are incorrect.

175. **Answer C is correct.** If the client eviscerates, the abdominal content should be covered with a sterile saline-soaked dressing. Reinserting the content should not be the action and will require that the client return to surgery; thus, answer A is incorrect. Answers B and D are incorrect because they not appropriate to this case.

176. **Answer B is correct.** Cancer in situ means that the cancer is still localized to the primary site. *T* stands for "tumor" and the *IS* for "in situ." Cancer is graded in terms of tumor, grade, node involvement, and mestatasis. Answers A, C, and D pertain to these other classifications.

177. **Answer B is correct.** A full bladder or bowel can obscure the visualization of the kidney ureters and urethra. Answer A is incorrect because there is no need to force fluids before the test. Answer C is incorrect because there is no need to withhold medication for 12 hours before the test. Answer D is incorrect because the client's reproductive organs should not be covered.

178. **Answer C is correct.** The client with a fractured femur will be placed in Buck's traction to realign the leg and to decrease spasms and pain. The Trendelenburg position is the wrong position for this client, so answer A is incorrect. Ice might be ordered after repair, but not for the entire extremity, so answer B is incorrect. An abduction pillow is ordered after a total hip replacement, not for a fractured femur; therefore, answer D is incorrect.

179. **Answer C is correct.** A red, beefy tongue is characteristic of the client with pernicious anemia. Answer A, a weight loss of 10 pounds in 2 weeks, is abnormal but is not seen in pernicious anemia. Numbness and tingling, in answer B, can be associated with anemia but are not particular to pernicious anemia. This is more likely associated with peripheral vascular diseases involving vasculature. In answer D, the hemoglobin is normal and does not support the diagnosis.

180. **Answer B is correct.** Portions of the exam are painful, especially when the sample is being withdrawn, so this should be included in the session with the client. Answer A is incorrect because the client will be positioned prone, not in a sitting position, for the exam. Anesthesia is not commonly given before this test, making answer C incorrect. Answer D is incorrect because the client can eat and drink following the test.

181. **Answer C is correct.** The assessment that is most crucial to the client is the identification of peripheral pulses because the aorta is clamped during surgery. This decreases blood circulation to the kidneys and lower extremities. The nurse must also assess for the return of circulation to the lower extremities. Answer A is of lesser concern, answer B is not advised at this time, and answer D is of lesser concern than answer A.

182. **Answer A is correct.** Suctioning can cause a vagal response, lowering the heart rate and causing bradycardia. Answers B, C and D can occur as well, but they are less likely.

183. **Answer C is correct.** The client with an internal defibrillator should learn to use any battery-operated machinery on the opposite side. He should also take his pulse rate and report dizziness or fainting. Answers A, B, and D are incorrect because the client can eat food prepared in the microwave, move his shoulder on the affected side, and fly in an airplane.

184. **Answer A is correct.** A swelling over the right parietal area is a cephalhematoma, an area of bleeding outside the cranium. This type of hematoma does not cross the suture line. Answer B, molding, is overlapping of the bones of the cranium and, thus, incorrect. In answer C, a subdural hematoma, or intracranial bleeding, is ominous and can be seen only on a CAT scan or x-ray. A caput succedaneum, in answer D, crosses the suture line and is edema.

185. **Answer A is correct.** The client with a lung resection will have chest tubes and a drainage-collection device. He probably will not have a tracheostomy or Swanz Ganz monitoring, and he will not have an order for percussion, vibration, or drainage. Therefore, answers B, C, and D are incorrect.

186. **Answer C is correct.** The client with mouth and throat cancer will have all the findings in answers A, B, and D except the correct answer of diarrhea.

187. **Answer D is correct.** A loss of 10% is normal due to meconium stool and water loss. There is no evidence to indicate dehydration, hypoglycemia, or allergy to the infant formula; thus, answers A, B, and C are incorrect.

188. **Answer C is correct.** The client with diverticulitis should avoid eating foods that are gas forming and that increase abdominal discomfort, such as cooked broccoli. Foods such as those listed in answers A, B, and D are allowed.

189. **Answer D is correct.** The client with a perineal resection will have a perineal incision. Drains will be used to facilitate wound drainage. This will help prevent infection of the surgical site. The client will not have an illeostomy, as in answer A; he will have some electrolyte loss, but treatment is not focused on preventing the loss, so answer B is incorrect. A high-fiber diet, in answer C, is not ordered at this time.

190. **Answer C is correct.** The client with diverticulitis should avoid foods with seeds. The foods in answers A, B, and D are allowed; in fact, bran cereal and fruit will help prevent constipation.

191. **Answer C is correct.** The least-helpful questions are those describing his usual diet. Answers A, B, and D are useful in determining the extent of disease process and, thus, are incorrect.

192. **Answer C is correct.** Tegretol can suppress the bone marrow and decrease the white blood cell count; thus, a lab value of WBC 2,000 per cubic millimeter indicates side effects of the drug. Answers A and D are within normal limits, and answer B is a lower limit of normal; therefore answers A, B, and D are incorrect.

193. **Answer D is correct.** Sarcoma is a type of bone cancer; therefore, bone pain would be expected. Answers A, B, and C are not specific to this type of cancer and are incorrect.

194. **Answer D is correct.** A birth weight of 7 pounds would indicate 21 pounds in 1 year, or triple his birth weight. Answers A, B, and C therefore are incorrect.

195. **Answer B is correct.** A torque wrench is kept at the bedside to tighten and loosen the screws of crutchfield tongs. This wrench controls the amount of pressure that is placed on the screws. A pair of forceps, wire cutters, and a screwdriver, in answers A, C, and D, would not be used and, thus, are incorrect. Wire cutters should be kept with the client who has wired jaws.

196. **Answer C is correct.** Fosamax should be taken with water only. The client should also remain upright for at least 30 minutes after taking the medication. Answers A, B, and D are not applicable to taking Fosamax and, thus, are incorrect.

197. **Answer B is correct.** The client with burns to the neck needs airway assessment and supplemental oxygen, so applying oxygen is the priority. The next action should be to start an IV and medicate for pain, making answers A and C incorrect. Answer D, obtaining blood gases is of less priority.

198. **Answer A is correct.** The primary responsibility of the nurse is to take the vital signs before any surgery. The actions in answers B, C, and D are the responsibility of the doctor and, therefore, are incorrect for this question.

199. **Answer B is correct.** The only lab result that is abnormal is the potassium. A potassium level of 1.9 indicates hypokalemia. The findings in answers A, C, and D are not revealed in the stem.

200. **Answer A is correct.** Removal of the pituitary gland is usually done by a transphenoidal approach, through the nose. Nasal congestion further interferes with the airway. Answers B, C, and D are not correct because they are not directly associated with the pituitary gland.

201. **Answer A is correct.** Cancer of the liver frequently leads to severe nausea and vomiting, thus the need for altering nutritional needs. The problems in answers B, C, and D are of lesser concern and, thus, are incorrect in this instance.

202. **Answer C is correct.** Daily measuring of the abdominal girth is the best method of determining early ascites. Measuring with a paper tape measure and marking the measured area is the most objective method of estimating ascites. Inspection and checking for fluid waves, in answers A and D, are more subjective and, thus, are incorrect for this question. Palpation of the liver, in answer B, will not tell the amount of ascites.

203. **Answer B is correct.** The vital signs indicate hypovolemic shock or fluid volume deficit. In answers A, C, and D, cerebral tissue perfusion, airway clearance, and sensory perception alterations are not symptoms and, therefore, are incorrect.

204. **Answer A is correct.** The client with sickle cell is likely to experience symptoms of hypoxia if he becomes dehydrated or lacks oxygen. Extreme exercise, especially in warm weather, can exacerbate the condition, so the fact that the client plays baseball should be of great concern to the visiting nurse. Answers B, C, and D are not factors for concern with sickle cell disease.

205. **Answer D is correct.** The client with neutropenia should not have potted or cut flowers in the room. Cancer patients are extremely susceptible to bacterial infections. Answers A, B, and C will not help to prevent bacterial invasions and, therefore, are incorrect.

206. **Answer B is correct.** Clients who have not had surgery to the face or neck would benefit from lowering the head of the bed, as in answer A. However, in this situation lowering the client's head could further interfere with the airway. Therefore, the best answer is answer B, increasing the infusion and placing the client in supine position. Answers C and D are not necessary at this time.

207. **Answer C is correct.** If the client pulls the chest tube out of the chest, the nurse should first cover the insertion site with an occlusive dressing, such as a Vaseline gauze. Then the nurse should call the doctor, who will order a chest x-ray and possibly reinsert the tube. Answers A, B, and D are not the first priority in this case.

208. **Answer A is correct.** An INR of 8 indicates that the blood is too thin. The normal INR is 2.0–3.0, so answer B is incorrect because the doctor will not increase the dosage of coumadin. Answer C is incorrect because now is not the time to instruct the client about the therapy. Answer D is not correct because there is no need to increase the neurological assessment.

209. **Answer C is correct.** The food indicating the client's understanding of dietary management of osteoporosis is the yogurt, with approximately 400mg of calcium. The other foods are good choices, but not as good as the yogurt; therefore, answers A, B, and D are incorrect.

210. **Answer A is correct.** There is no need to avoid taking the blood pressure in the left arm. Answers B, C, and D are all actions that should be taken for the client receiving magnesium sulfate for preeclampsia.

211. **Answer D is correct.** If the client's mother refuses the blood transfusion, the doctor should be notified. Because the client is a minor, the court might order treatment. Answer A is incorrect because the mother is the legal guardian and can refuse the blood transfusion to be given to her daughter. Answers B and C are incorrect because it is not the primary responsibility of the nurse to encourage the mother to consent or explain the consequences.

212. **Answer B is correct.** The nurse should be most concerned with laryngeal edema because of the area of burn. Answer A is of secondary priority. Hyponatremia and hypokalemia are also of concern but are not the primary concern; thus, answers C and D are incorrect.

213. **Answer D is correct.** The client with anorexia shows the most improvement by weight gain. Selecting a balanced diet is useless if the client does not eat the diet, so answer A is incorrect. The hematocrit, in answer B, might improve by several means, such as blood transfusion, but that does not indicate improvement in the anorexic condition, so B is incorrect. The tissue turgor indicates fluid, not improvement of anorexia, so answer C is incorrect.

214. **Answer D is correct.** Paresthesia of the toes is not normal and can indicate compartment syndrome. At this time, pain beneath the cast is normal and, thus, would not be reported as a concern. The client's toes should be warm to the touch, and pulses should be present. Answers A, B, and C, then, are incorrect.

215. **Answer B is correct.** The best response from the nurse is to let the client know that it is normal to have a warm sensation when dye is injected for this procedure. Answers A, C, and D indicate that the nurse believes that the hot feeling is abnormal and, so, are incorrect.

216. **Answer D is correct.** It is not necessary to wear gloves when taking the vital signs of the client, thus indicating further teaching for the nursing assistant. If the client has an active infection with methicillin-resistant staphylococcus aureus, gloves should be worn, but this is not indicated in this instance. The actions in answers A, B, and C are incorrect because they are indicative of infection control not mentioned in the question.

217. **Answer D is correct.** During ECT, the client will have a grand mal seizure. This indicates completion of the electroconvulsive therapy. Answers A, B, and C are incorrect because they do not indicate that the ECT has been completed.

218. **Answer A is correct.** An infection with pinworms begins when the eggs are ingested or inhaled. The eggs hatch in the upper intestine and mature in 2–8 weeks. The females then mate and migrate out the anus, where they lay up to 17,000 eggs, causing intense itching. The mother should be told to use a flashlight to examine the rectal area about 2–3 hours after the child is asleep. Placing clear tape on a tongue blade will allow the eggs to adhere to the tape. The specimen should then be evaluated in a lab. There is no need to scrape the skin, collect a stool specimen, or bring a sample of hair; therefore, answers B, C, and D are incorrect.

219. **Answer B is correct.** Erterobiasis, or pinworms, is treated with Vermox (mebendazole) or Antiminth (pyrantel pamoate). The entire family should be treated, to ensure that no eggs remain. Because a single treatment is usually sufficient, there is usually good compliance. The family should then be tested again in 2 weeks, to ensure that no eggs remain. Answers A, C, and D are inappropriate for this treatment and, therefore, incorrect.

220. **Answer B is correct.** The pregnant nurse should not be assigned to any client with radioactivity present, and the client with a radium implant poses the most risk to the pregnant nurse. The clients in answers A, C, and D are not radioactive; therefore, these answers are incorrect.

221. **Answer A is correct.** The client with cancer being treated with chemotherapy is immune suppressed and is at risk for opportunistic diseases such as pneumocystis. Answers B, C, and D are incorrect because these clients are not at a higher risk for opportunistic diseases than other clients.

222. **Answer D is correct.** Injecting an infant with an adult dose of Digitalis is considered malpractice, or failing to perform or performing an act that causes harm to the client. In answer A, negligence is failing to perform care for the client and, thus, is incorrect. In answer B, a tort is a wrongful act committed on the client or his belongings but, in this case, was accidental. Assault, in answer C, is not pertinent to this incident.

223. **Answer D is correct.** The registered nurse cannot insert sutures or clips unless specially trained to do so, as in the case of a nurse practitioner skilled to perform this task. The registered nurse can insert a Foley catheter, insert a nasogastric tube, and monitor central venous pressure.

224. **Answer B is correct.** The vital signs are abnormal and should be reported to the doctor immediately. A, B, and D are incorrect actions.

225. **Answer B is correct.** The nurse in answer B has the most experience in knowing possible complications involving preeclampsia. The nurse in answer A is a new nurse to the unit, and the nurses in answers C and D have no experience with the postpartum client.

226. **Answer C is correct.** Desferal is used to treat iron toxicity. Answers A, B, and D are incorrect because they are antidotes for other drugs: Narcan is used to treat narcotic overdose; Digibind is used to treat dioxin toxicity; and Zinecard is used to treat doxorubicin toxicity.

227. **Answer A is correct.** If the nurse charts information that he did not perform, she can be charged with fraud. Answer B is incorrect because malpractice is harm that results to the client due to an erroneous action taken by the nurse. Answer C is incorrect because negligence is failure to perform a duty that the nurse knows should be performed. Answer D is incorrect because a tort is a wrongful act to the client or his belongings.

228. **Answer D is correct.** The client who should receive priority is the client with multiple sclerosis and who is being treated with IV cortisone. This client is at highest risk for complications. Answers A, B, and C are incorrect because these clients are more stable and can be seen later.

229. **Answer B is correct.** Out of all of these clients, it is best to place the pregnant client and the client with a broken arm and facial lacerations in the same room. These two clients probably do not need immediate attention and are least likely to disturb each other. The clients in answers A, C, and D need to be placed in separate rooms because their conditions are more serious, they might need immediate attention, and they are more likely to disturb other patients.

230. **Answer A is correct.** Before instilling eyedrops, the nurse should cleanse the area with warm water. A 6-year-old child is not developmentally ready to instill his own eyedrops, so answer B is incorrect. The mother cannot be allowed to administer the eye drops in the hospital setting so answer C incorrect. Although the eye might appear to be clear, the nurse should instill the eyedrops, as ordered (answer D).

231. **Answer D is correct.** To prevent urinary tract infections, the girl should clean the perineum from front to back to prevent e. coli contamination. Answer A is incorrect because drinking citrus juices will not prevent UTIs. Answers B and C are incorrect because UTI's are not associated with the use of tampons or with tub baths.

232. **Answer C is correct.** The nurse should encourage rooming in, to promote parent-child attachment. It is okay for the parents to be in the room for assessment of the child, so answer A is incorrect. Allowing the child to have items that are familiar to him is allowed and encouraged; thus, answer B is incorrect. Answer D is incorrect and shows a lack of empathy for the child's distress; it is an inappropriate response from the nurse.

233. **Answer B is correct.** The hearing aid should be stored in a warm, dry place and should be cleaned daily. A toothpick is inappropriate to clean the aid because it might break off in the hearing aide. Changing the batteries weekly is not necessary; therefore, answers A, C, and D are incorrect.

234. **Answer C is correct.** Always remember your ABC's (airway, breathing, circulation) when selecting an answer. Although answers B and D might be appropriate for this child, answer C should have the highest priority. Answer A does not apply for a child who has undergone a tonsillectomy.

235. **Answer A is correct.** If the child has bacterial pneumonia, a high fever is usually present. Bacterial pneumonia usually presents with a productive cough, so answer B is incorrect. Rhinitis, as stated in answer C, is often seen with viral pneumonia and is incorrect for this case. Vomiting and diarrhea are usually not seen with pneumonia; thus, answer D is incorrect.

236. **Answer B is correct.** For a child with LTB and the possibility of complete obstruction of the airway, emergency intubation equipment should always be kept at the bedside. Intravenous supplies and fluid will not treat an obstruction, nor will supplemental oxygen; therefore, answers A, C, and D are incorrect.

237. **Answer C is correct.** Exophthalmos (protrusion of eyeballs) often occurs with hyperthyroidism. The client with hyperthyroidism will often exhibit tachycardia, increased appetite, and weight loss. Answers A, B, and D are not associated with hyperthyroidism.

238. **Answer D is correct.** The child with celiac disease should be on a gluten-free diet. Answer D is the only choice of foods that do not contain gluten. Therefore, answers A, B, and C are incorrect.

239. **Answer C is correct.** Remember the ABC's (airway, breathing, circulation) when answering this question. Before notifying the physician or assessing the child's pulse, oxygen should be applied to increase the child's oxygen saturation. The normal oxygen saturation for a child is 92%–100%. Answer A is important but not the priority, answer B is inappropriate, and answer D is also not the priority.

240. **Answer B is correct.** Normal amniotic fluid is straw colored and odorless, so this is the observation the nurse should expect. An amniotomy is artificial rupture of membranes, causing a straw-colored fluid to appear in the vaginal area. Fetal heart tones of 160 indicate tachycardia, and this is not the observation to watch for. Greenish fluid is indicative of meconium, not amniotic fluid. If the nurse notes the umbilical cord, the client is experiencing a prolapsed cord. This would need to be reported immediately. For this question, answers A, C, and D are incorrect.

241. **Answer D is correct.** The client is usually given epidural anesthesia at approximately three centimeters dilation. Answer A is vague, answer B would indicate the end of the first stage of labor, and answer C indicates the transition phase, not the latent phase of labor.

242. **Answer B is correct.** The normal fetal heart rate is 120–160bpm. A heart rate of 100–110bpm is bradycardia. The first action would be to turn the client to the left side and apply oxygen. Answer A is not indicated at this time. Answer C is not the best action for clients experiencing bradycardia. There is no data to indicate the need to move the client to the delivery room at this time, so answer D is incorrect as well.

243. **Answer D is correct.** The expected effect of Pitocin is progressive cervical dilation. Pitocin causes more intense contractions, which can increase the pain; thus, answer A is incorrect. Answers B and C are incorrect because cervical effacement is caused by pressure on the presenting part and there are not infrequent contractions.

244. **Answer B is correct.** Applying a fetal heart monitor is the appropriate action at this time. Preparing for a caesarean section is premature; placing the client in Trendelenburg is also not an indicated action, and an ultrasound is not needed based on the finding. Therefore, answer B is the best answer, and answers A, C, and D are incorrect.

245. **Answer B is correct.** Absent variability is not normal and could indicate a neurological problem. Answers A, C, and D are normal findings.

246. **Answer D is correct.** Clients admitted in labor are told not to eat during labor, to avoid nausea and vomiting. Ice chips might be allowed, although this amount of fluid might not be sufficient to prevent fluid volume deficit. In answer A, impaired gas exchange related to hyperventilation would be indicated during the transition phase, not the early phase of labor. Answers B and C are not correct because clients during labor are allowed to change position as she desires.

247. **Answer D is correct.** This information indicates a late deceleration. This type of deceleration is caused by uteroplacental insufficiency, or lack of oxygen. Answer A is incorrect because there is no data to support the conclusion that the baby is asleep; answer B results in a variable deceleration; and answer C is indicative of an early deceleration.

248. **Answer C is correct.** The initial action by the nurse observing a variable deceleration should be to turn the client to the side, preferably the left side. Administering oxygen is also indicated. Answer A is not called for at this time. Answer B is incorrect because it is not needed, and answer D is incorrect because there is no data to indicate that the monitor has been applied incorrectly.

249. **Answer D is correct.** Answers A, B, and C indicate ominous findings on the fetal heart monitor and so are incorrect in this instance. Accelerations with movement are normal, so answer D is the reassuring pattern.

250. **Answer C is correct.** Epidural anesthesia decreases the urge to void and sensation of a full bladder. A full bladder decreases the progression of labor. Answers A, B, and D are incorrect because the bladder does not fill more rapidly due to the epidural, the client is not in a trancelike state, and the client's level of consciousness is not altered, and there is no evidence that the client is too embarrassed to ask for a bedpan.

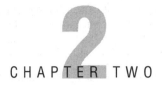

CHAPTER TWO

Practice Exam 2 and Rationales

1. The nurse is caring for a client with systemic lupus erythematosis (SLE). The major complication associated with systemic lupus erythematosis is:

   ○ **A.** Nephritis

   ○ **B.** Cardiomegaly

   ○ **C.** Desquamation

   ○ **D.** Meningitis

2. A client with benign prostatic hypertrophy has been started on Proscar (finasteride). The nurse's discharge teaching should include:

   ○ **A.** Telling the client's wife not to touch the tablets

   ○ **B.** Explaining that the medication should be taken with meals

   ○ **C.** Telling the client that symptoms will improve in 1–2 weeks

   ○ **D.** Instructing the client to take the medication at bedtime, to prevent nocturia

3. A 5-year-old child is hospitalized for correction of congenital hip dysplasia. During the assessment of the child, the nurse can expect to find the presence of:

   ○ **A.** Scarf sign

   ○ **B.** Harlequin sign

   ○ **C.** Cullen's sign

   ○ **D.** Trendelenburg sign

4. Which diet is associated with an increased risk of colorectal cancer?

   ○ **A.** Low protein, complex carbohydrates

   ○ **B.** High protein, simple carbohydrates

   ○ **C.** High fat, refined carbohydrates

   ○ **D.** Low carbohydrates, complex proteins

5. The nurse is caring for an infant following a cleft lip repair. While comforting the infant, the nurse should avoid:

Quick Answer: **131**
Detailed Answer: **134**

- ○ **A.** Holding the infant
- ○ **B.** Offering a pacifier
- ○ **C.** Providing a mobile
- ○ **D.** Offering sterile water

6. The physician has diagnosed a client with cirrhosis characterized by asterixis. If the nurse assesses the client with asterixis, he can expect to find:

Quick Answer: **131**
Detailed Answer: **134**

- ○ **A.** Irregular movement of the wrist
- ○ **B.** Enlargement of the breasts
- ○ **C.** Dilated veins around the umbilicus
- ○ **D.** Redness of the palmar surfaces

7. The physician has ordered Amoxil (amoxicillin) 500mg capsules for a client with esophageal varices. The nurse can best care for the client's needs by:

Quick Answer: **131**
Detailed Answer: **134**

- ○ **A.** Giving the medication as ordered
- ○ **B.** Providing extra water with the medication
- ○ **C.** Giving the medication with an antacid
- ○ **D.** Requesting an alternate form of the medication

8. A client with an inguinal hernia asks the nurse why he should have surgery when he has had a hernia for years. The nurse understands that surgery is recommended to:

Quick Answer: **131**
Detailed Answer: **134**

- ○ **A.** Prevent strangulation of the bowel
- ○ **B.** Prevent malabsorptive disorders
- ○ **C.** Decrease secretion of bile salts
- ○ **D.** Increase intestinal motility

9. The nurse is providing dietary instructions for a client with iron-deficiency anemia. Which food is a poor source of iron?

Quick Answer: **131**
Detailed Answer: **135**

- ○ **A.** Tomatoes
- ○ **B.** Legumes
- ○ **C.** Dried fruits
- ○ **D.** Nuts

10. A client is admitted with suspected acute pancreatitis. Which lab finding confirms the diagnosis?

Quick Answer: **131**
Detailed Answer: **135**

- ○ **A.** Blood glucose of 260mg/dL
- ○ **B.** White cell count of 21,000cu/mm
- ○ **C.** Platelet count of 250,000cu/mm
- ○ **D.** Serum amylase level of 600 units/dL

11. The nurse is teaching a client with Parkinson's disease ways to prevent curvatures of the spine associated with the disease. To prevent spinal flexion, the nurse should tell the client to:

Quick Answer: **131**
Detailed Answer: **135**

- ○ **A.** Periodically lie prone without a neck pillow
- ○ **B.** Sleep only in dorsal recumbent position
- ○ **C.** Rest in supine position with his head elevated
- ○ **D.** Sleep on either side, but keep his back straight

12. The physician has ordered Dilantin (phenytoin) 100mg intravenously for a client with generalized tonic clonic seizures. The nurse should administer the medication:

Quick Answer: **131**
Detailed Answer: **135**

- ○ **A.** Rapidly with an IV push
- ○ **B.** With IV dextrose
- ○ **C.** Slowly over 2–3 minutes
- ○ **D.** Through a small vein

13. The nurse is planning dietary changes for a client following an episode of acute pancreatitis. Which diet is suitable for the client?

Quick Answer: **131**
Detailed Answer: **135**

- ○ **A.** Low calorie, low carbohydrate
- ○ **B.** High calorie, low fat
- ○ **C.** High protein, high fat
- ○ **D.** Low protein, high carbohydrate

14. A client is admitted with a diagnosis of polycythemia vera. The nurse should closely monitor the client for:

Quick Answer: **131**
Detailed Answer: **135**

- ○ **A.** Increased blood pressure
- ○ **B.** Decreased respirations
- ○ **C.** Increased urinary output
- ○ **D.** Decreased oxygen saturation

15. A client with hypothyroidism frequently complains of feeling cold. The nurse should tell the client that she will be more comfortable if she:

Quick Answer: **131**
Detailed Answer: **135**

- ○ **A.** Uses an electric blanket at night
- ○ **B.** Dresses in extra layers of clothing
- ○ **C.** Applies a heating pad to her feet
- ○ **D.** Takes a hot bath morning and evening

16. The nurse caring for a client with a closed head injury obtains an intracranial pressure (ICP) reading of 17mmHg. The nurse recognizes that:

Quick Answer: **131**
Detailed Answer: **135**

- ○ **A.** The ICP is elevated and the doctor should be notified.
- ○ **B.** The ICP is normal; therefore, no further action is needed.
- ○ **C.** The ICP is low and the client needs additional IV fluids.
- ○ **D.** The ICP reading is not as reliable as the Glascow coma scale.

17. A client has been hospitalized with a diagnosis of laryngeal cancer. Which factor is most significant in the development of laryngeal cancer?

Quick Answer: **131**
Detailed Answer: **136**

- ○ **A.** A family history of laryngeal cancer
- ○ **B.** Chronic inhalation of noxious fumes
- ○ **C.** Frequent straining of the vocal cords
- ○ **D.** A history of frequent alcohol and tobacco use

18. The nurse is completing an assessment history of a client with pernicious anemia. Which complaint differentiates pernicious anemia from other types of anemia?

Quick Answer: **131**
Detailed Answer: **136**

- ○ **A.** Difficulty in breathing after exertion
- ○ **B.** Numbness and tingling in the extremities
- ○ **C.** A faster than usual heart rate
- ○ **D.** Feelings of lightheadedness

19. A client with rheumatoid arthritis is beginning to develop flexion contractures of the knees. The nurse should tell the client to:

Quick Answer: **131**
Detailed Answer: **136**

- ○ **A.** Lie prone and let her feet hang over the mattress edge
- ○ **B.** Lie supine, with her feet rotated inward
- ○ **C.** Lie on her right side and point her toes downward
- ○ **D.** Lie on her left side and allow her feet to remain in a neutral position

20. The chart of a client with schizophrenia states that the client has echolalia. The nurse can expect the client to:

- ○ **A.** Speak using words that rhyme
- ○ **B.** Repeat words or phrases used by others
- ○ **C.** Include irrelevant details in conversation
- ○ **D.** Make up new words with new meanings

21. The mother of a 1-year-old with sickle cell anemia wants to know why the condition didn't show up in the nursery. The nurse's response is based on the knowledge that:

- ○ **A.** There is no test to measure abnormal hemoglobin in newborns.
- ○ **B.** Infants do not have insensible fluid loss before a year of age.
- ○ **C.** Infants rarely have infections that would cause them to have a sickling crises.
- ○ **D.** The presence of fetal hemoglobin protects the infant.

22. Which early morning activity helps to reduce the symptoms associated with rheumatoid arthritis?

- ○ **A.** Brushing the teeth
- ○ **B.** Drinking a glass of juice
- ○ **C.** Holding a cup of coffee
- ○ **D.** Brushing the hair

23. A client with B negative blood requires a blood transfusion during surgery. If no B negative blood is available, the client should be transfused with:

- ○ **A.** A positive blood
- ○ **B.** B positive blood
- ○ **C.** O negative blood
- ○ **D.** AB negative blood

24. The nurse notes that a post-operative client's respirations have dropped from 14 to 6 breaths per minute. The nurse administers Narcan (naloxone) per standing order. Following administration of the medication, the nurse should assess the client for:

- ○ **A.** Pupillary changes
- ○ **B.** Projectile vomiting
- ○ **C.** Wheezing respirations
- ○ **D.** Sudden, intense pain

25. A newborn weighed 7 pounds at birth. At 6 months of age, the infant could be expected to weigh:

Quick Answer: **131**
Detailed Answer: **136**

- ○ **A.** 14 pounds
- ○ **B.** 18 pounds
- ○ **C.** 25 pounds
- ○ **D.** 30 pounds

26. A client with nontropical sprue has an exacerbation of symptoms. Which meal selection is responsible for the recurrence of the client's symptoms?

Quick Answer: **131**
Detailed Answer: **136**

- ○ **A.** Tossed salad with oil and vinegar dressing
- ○ **B.** Baked potato with sour cream and chives
- ○ **C.** Cream of tomato soup and crackers
- ○ **D.** Mixed fruit and yogurt

27. A client with congestive heart failure has been receiving digoxia (Laxoxin). Which finding indicates that the medication is having a desired effect?

Quick Answer: **131**
Detailed Answer: **137**

- ○ **A.** Increased urinary output
- ○ **B.** Stabilized weight
- ○ **C.** Improved appetite
- ○ **D.** Increased pedal edema

28. Which play activity is best suited to the gross motor skills of the toddler?

Quick Answer: **131**
Detailed Answer: **137**

- ○ **A.** Coloring book and crayons
- ○ **B.** Ball
- ○ **C.** Building cubes
- ○ **D.** Swing set

29. A client in labor admits to using alcohol throughout the pregnancy. The most recent use was the day before. Based on the client's history, the nurse should give priority to assessing the newborn for:

Quick Answer: **131**
Detailed Answer: **137**

- ○ **A.** Respiratory depression
- ○ **B.** Wide-set eyes
- ○ **C.** Jitteriness
- ○ **D.** Low-set ears

30. The physician has ordered Basalgel (aluminum carbonate gel) for a client with recurrent indigestion. The nurse should teach the client common side effects of the medication, which include:

Quick Answer: **131**
Detailed Answer: **137**

- ○ **A.** Constipation
- ○ **B.** Urinary retention
- ○ **C.** Diarrhea
- ○ **D.** Confusion

31. A client is admitted with suspected abdominal aortic aneurysm (AAA). A common complaint of the client with an abdominal aortic aneurysm is:

Quick Answer: **131**
Detailed Answer: **137**

- ○ **A.** Loss of sensation in the lower extremities
- ○ **B.** Back pain that lessens when standing
- ○ **C.** Decreased urinary output
- ○ **D.** Pulsations in the periumbilical area

32. The nurse is caring for a client hospitalized with nephotic syndrome. Based on the client's treatment, the nurse should:

Quick Answer: **131**
Detailed Answer: **137**

- ○ **A.** Limit the number of visitors
- ○ **B.** Provide a low-protein diet
- ○ **C.** Discuss the possibility of dialysis
- ○ **D.** Offer the client additional fluids

33. A client is admitted with acute adrenal crisis. During the intake assessment, the nurse can expect to find that the client has:

Quick Answer: **131**
Detailed Answer: **137**

- ○ **A.** Low blood pressure
- ○ **B.** A slow, regular pulse
- ○ **C.** Warm, flushed skin
- ○ **D.** Increased urination

34. A 5-month-old infant is admitted to the ER with a temperature of 103.6°F and irritability. The mother states that the child has been listless for the past several hours and that he had a seizure on the way to the hospital. A lumbar puncture confirms a diagnosis of bacterial meningitis. The nurse should assess the infant for:

Quick Answer: **131**
Detailed Answer: **137**

- ○ **A.** Periorbital edema
- ○ **B.** Tenseness of the anterior fontanel
- ○ **C.** Positive Babinski reflex
- ○ **D.** Negative scarf sign

35. A client with AIDS is admitted with a diagnosis of pneumocystis carinii pneumonia. Shortly after his admission, he becomes confused and disoriented. He attempts to pull out his IV and refuses to wear an O_2 mask. Based upon his mental status, the priority nursing diagnosis is:

Quick Answer: **131**
Detailed Answer: **137**

- ○ **A.** Social isolation
- ○ **B.** Risk for injury
- ○ **C.** Ineffective coping
- ○ **D.** Anxiety

88   Chapter 2

36. The doctor has ordered Ampicillin 100mg every 6 hours IV push for an infant weighing 7kg. The suggested dose for infants is 25–50mg/kg/day in equally divided doses. The nurse should:

- ○ **A.** Give the medication as ordered
- ○ **B.** Give half the amount ordered
- ○ **C.** Give the ordered amount q 12 hrs.
- ○ **D.** Check the order with the doctor

Quick Answer: **131**
Detailed Answer: **137**

37. An elderly client is hospitalized for a transurethral prostatectomy. Which finding should be reported to the doctor immediately?

- ○ **A.** Hourly urinary output of 40–50cc
- ○ **B.** Bright red urine with many clots
- ○ **C.** Dark red urine with few clots
- ○ **D.** Requests for pain med q 4 hrs.

Quick Answer: **131**
Detailed Answer: **138**

38. Which statement by the parent of a child with sickle cell anemia indicates an understanding of the disease?

- ○ **A.** "The pain he has is due to the presence of too many red blood cells."
- ○ **B.** "He will be able to go snow-skiing with his friends as long as he stays warm."
- ○ **C.** "He will need extra fluids in summer to prevent dehydration."
- ○ **D.** "There is very little chance that his brother will have sickle cell."

Quick Answer: **131**
Detailed Answer: **138**

39. A toddler with otitis media has just completed antibiotic therapy. A recheck appointment should be made to:

- ○ **A.** Determine whether the ear infection has affected her hearing
- ○ **B.** Make sure that she has taken all the antibiotic
- ○ **C.** Document that the infection has completely cleared
- ○ **D.** Obtain a new prescription, in case the infection recurs

Quick Answer: **131**
Detailed Answer: **138**

40. A 9-year-old is admitted with suspected rheumatic fever. Which finding is suggestive of Sydenham's chorea?

- ○ **A.** Irregular movements of the extremities and facial grimacing
- ○ **B.** Painless swellings over the extensor surfaces of the joints
- ○ **C.** Faint areas of red demarcation over the back and abdomen
- ○ **D.** Swelling, inflammation, and effusion of the joints

Quick Answer: **131**
Detailed Answer: **138**

41. A child with croup is placed in a cool, high-humidity tent connected to room air. The primary purpose of the tent is to:

- ○ **A.** Prevent insensible water loss
- ○ **B.** Provide a moist environment with oxygen at 30%
- ○ **C.** Prevent dehydration and reduce fever
- ○ **D.** Liquefy secretions and relieve laryngeal spasm

Quick Answer: **131**
Detailed Answer: **138**

42. The nurse is suctioning the tracheostomy of an adult client. The recommended pressure setting for performing tracheostomy suctioning on the adult client is:

- ○ **A.** 40–60mmHg
- ○ **B.** 60–80mmHg
- ○ **C.** 80–120mmHg
- ○ **D.** 120–140mmHg

Quick Answer: **131**
Detailed Answer: **138**

43. A client is admitted with a diagnosis of myxedema. An initial assessment of the client would reveal the symptoms of:

- ○ **A.** Slow pulse rate, weight loss, diarrhea, and cardiac failure
- ○ **B.** Weight gain, lethargy, slowed speech, and decreased respiratory rate
- ○ **C.** Rapid pulse, constipation, and bulging eyes
- ○ **D.** Decreased body temperature, weight loss, and increased respirations

Quick Answer: **131**
Detailed Answer: **138**

44. Which statement describes the contagious stage of varicella?

- ○ **A.** The contagious stage is 1 day before the onset of the rash until the appearance of vesicles.
- ○ **B.** The contagious stage lasts during the vesicular and crusting stages of the lesions.
- ○ **C.** The contagious stage is from the onset of the rash until the rash disappears.
- ○ **D.** The contagious stage is 1 day before the onset of the rash until all the lesions are crusted.

Quick Answer: **131**
Detailed Answer: **138**

45. The nurse is reviewing the results of a sweat test taken from a child with cystic fibrosis. Which finding supports the client's diagnosis?

- ○ **A.** A sweat potassium concentration less than 40mEq/L
- ○ **B.** A sweat chloride concentration greater than 60mEq/L
- ○ **C.** A sweat potassium concentration greater than 40mEq/L
- ○ **D.** A sweat chloride concentration less than 40mEq/L

Quick Answer: **131**
Detailed Answer: **138**

46. A client in labor has an order for Demerol (meperidine) 75 mg. IM to be administered 10 minutes before delivery. The nurse should:

Quick Answer: **131**
Detailed Answer: **138**

○ **A.** Wait until the client is placed on the delivery table and administer the medication

○ **B.** Question the order

○ **C.** Give the medication IM during the delivery to prevent pain from the episiotomy

○ **D.** Give the medication as ordered

47. Which of the following statements describes Piaget's stage of concrete operations?

Quick Answer: **131**
Detailed Answer: **139**

○ **A.** Reflex activity proceeds to imitative behavior.

○ **B.** The ability to see another's point of view increases.

○ **C.** Thought processes become more logical and coherent.

○ **D.** The ability to think abstractly leads to logical conclusion.

48. A client admitted to the psychiatric unit claims to be the Pope and insists that he will not be kept away from his subjects. The most likely explanation for the client's delusion is:

Quick Answer: **131**
Detailed Answer: **139**

○ **A.** A reaction formation

○ **B.** A stressful event

○ **C.** Low self-esteem

○ **D.** Overwhelming anxiety

49. Which of the following statements reflects Kohlberg's theory of the moral development of the preschool-age child?

Quick Answer: **131**
Detailed Answer: **139**

○ **A.** Obeying adults is seen as correct behavior.

○ **B.** Showing respect for parents is seen as important.

○ **C.** Pleasing others is viewed as good behavior.

○ **D.** Behavior is determined by consequences.

50. The nurse is caring for an 8-year-old following a routine tonsillectomy. Which finding should be reported immediately?

Quick Answer: **131**
Detailed Answer: **139**

○ **A.** Reluctance to swallow

○ **B.** Drooling of blood-tinged saliva

○ **C.** An axillary temperature of 99°F

○ **D.** Respiratory stridor

51. The nurse is admitting a client with a suspected duodenal ulcer. The client will most likely report that his abdominal discomfort decreases when he:

Quick Answer: **131**
Detailed Answer: **139**

   ○ **A.** Avoids eating
   ○ **B.** Rests in a recumbent position
   ○ **C.** Eats a meal or snack
   ○ **D.** Sits upright after eating

52. The nurse is assessing a newborn in the well-baby nursery. Which finding should alert the nurse to the possibility of a cardiac anomaly?

Quick Answer: **131**
Detailed Answer: **139**

   ○ **A.** Diminished femoral pulses
   ○ **B.** Harlequin's sign
   ○ **C.** Circumoral pallor
   ○ **D.** Acrocyanosis

53. A 2-year-old is hospitalized with a diagnosis of Kawasaki's disease. A severe complication of Kawasaki's disease is:

Quick Answer: **131**
Detailed Answer: **139**

   ○ **A.** The development of Brushfield spots
   ○ **B.** The eruption of Hutchinson's teeth
   ○ **C.** The development of coxa plana
   ○ **D.** The creation of a giant aneurysm

54. The charge nurse is formulating a discharge teaching plan for a client with mild preeclampsia. The nurse should give priority to:

Quick Answer: **131**
Detailed Answer: **139**

   ○ **A.** Teaching the client to report a nosebleed
   ○ **B.** Instructing the client to maintain strict bed rest
   ○ **C.** Telling the client to notify the doctor of pedal edema
   ○ **D.** Advising the client to avoid sodium sources in the diet

55. The nurse is preparing to discharge a client who is taking an MAOI. The nurse should instruct the client to:

Quick Answer: **131**
Detailed Answer: **139**

   ○ **A.** Wear protective clothing and sunglasses when outside
   ○ **B.** Avoid over-the-counter cold and hayfever preparations
   ○ **C.** Drink at least eight glasses of water a day
   ○ **D.** Increase his intake of high-quality protein

56. Which of the following meal selections is appropriate for the client with celiac disease?

Quick Answer: **131**
Detailed Answer: **139**

   ○ **A.** Toast, jam, and apple juice
   ○ **B.** Peanut butter cookies and milk
   ○ **C.** Rice Krispies bar and milk
   ○ **D.** Cheese pizza and Kool-Aid

57. A client with hyperthyroidism is taking lithium carbonate to inhibit thyroid hormone release. Which complaint by the client should alert the nurse to a problem with the client's medication?

- ○ **A.** The client complains of blurred vision.
- ○ **B.** The client complains of increased thirst and increased urination.
- ○ **C.** The client complains of increased weight gain over the past year.
- ○ **D.** The client complains of rhinorrhea.

Quick Answer: **131**
Detailed Answer: **139**

58. The physician has ordered intravenous fluid with potassium for a client admitted with gastroenteritis and dehydration. Before adding potassium to the intravenous fluid, the nurse should:

- ○ **A.** Assess the urinary output
- ○ **B.** Obtain arterial blood gases
- ○ **C.** Perform a dextrostick
- ○ **D.** Obtain a stool culture

Quick Answer: **131**
Detailed Answer: **140**

59. A 2-month-old infant has just received her first Tetramune injection. The nurse should tell the mother that the immunization:

- ○ **A.** Will need to be repeated when the child is 4 years of age
- ○ **B.** Is given to determine whether the child is susceptible to pertussis
- ○ **C.** Is one of a series of injections that protects against diphtheria, pertussis, tetanus and H.influenza b
- ○ **D.** Is a one-time injection that protects against measles, mumps, rubella and varicella

Quick Answer: **131**
Detailed Answer: **140**

60. A client with Addison's disease has been receiving glucocorticoid therapy. Which finding indicates a need for dosage adjustment?

- ○ **A.** Dryness of the skin and mucus membranes
- ○ **B.** Dizziness when rising to a standing position
- ○ **C.** A weight gain of 6 pounds in the past week
- ○ **D.** Difficulty in remaining asleep

Quick Answer: **131**
Detailed Answer: **140**

61. The nurse is caring for an obstetrical client in early labor. After the rupture of membranes, the nurse should give priority to:

- ○ **A.** Applying an internal monitor
- ○ **B.** Assessing fetal heart tones
- ○ **C.** Assisting with epidural anesthesia
- ○ **D.** Inserting a Foley catheter

62. The physician has prescribed Synthroid (levothyroxine) for a client with myxedema. Which statement indicates that the client understands the nurse's teaching regarding the medication?

- ○ **A.** "I will take the medication each morning after breakfast."
- ○ **B.** "I will check my heart rate before taking the medication."
- ○ **C.** "I will report visual disturbances to my doctor."
- ○ **D.** "I will stop the medication if I develop gastric upset."

63. The nurse is caring for a client with a radium implant for the treatment of cervical cancer. While caring for the client with a radioactive implant, the nurse should:

- ○ **A.** Provide emotional support by spending additional time with the client
- ○ **B.** Stand at the foot of the bed when talking to the client
- ○ **C.** Avoid handling items used by the client
- ○ **D.** Wear a badge to monitor the amount of time spent in the client's room

64. The nurse is caring for a client hospitalized with bipolar disorder, manic phase who is taking lithium. Which of the following snacks would be best for the client with mania?

- ○ **A.** Potato chips
- ○ **B.** Diet cola
- ○ **C.** Apple
- ○ **D.** Milkshake

65. The physician has prescribed imipramine (ToFranil) for a client with depression. The nurse should continue to monitor the client's affect because the maximal effects of tricyclic antidepressant medication do not occur for:

- ○ **A.** 48–72 hours
- ○ **B.** 5–7 days
- ○ **C.** 2–4 weeks
- ○ **D.** 3–6 months

66. An elderly client with glaucoma has been prescribed Timoptic eyedrops. Timoptic should be used with caution in clients with a history of:

Quick Answer: **131**
Detailed Answer: **140**

- ○ **A.** Diabetes
- ○ **B.** Gastric ulcers
- ○ **C.** Emphysema
- ○ **D.** Pancreatitis

67. A 2-year-old is hospitalized with suspected intussusception. Which finding is associated with intussusception?

Quick Answer: **131**
Detailed Answer: **140**

- ○ **A.** "Currant jelly" stools
- ○ **B.** Projectile vomiting
- ○ **C.** "Ribbonlike" stools
- ○ **D.** Palpable mass over the flank

68. Which of the following findings would be expected in the infant with biliary atresia?

Quick Answer: **131**
Detailed Answer: **141**

- ○ **A.** Rapid weight gain and hepatomegaly
- ○ **B.** Dark stools and poor weight gain
- ○ **C.** Abdominal distention and poor weight gain
- ○ **D.** Abdominal distention and rapid weight gain

69. A client is being treated for cancer with linear acceleration radiation. The physician has marked the radiation site with a blue marking pen. The nurse should:

Quick Answer: **131**
Detailed Answer: **141**

- ○ **A.** Remove the unsightly markings with acetone or alcohol
- ○ **B.** Cover the radiation site with loose gauze dressing
- ○ **C.** Sprinkle baby powder over the radiated area
- ○ **D.** Refrain from using soap or lotion on the marked area

70. The blood alcohol concentration of a client admitted following a motor vehicle accident is 460mg/dL. The nurse should give priority to monitoring the client for:

Quick Answer: **131**
Detailed Answer: **141**

- ○ **A.** Loss of coordination
- ○ **B.** Respiratory depression
- ○ **C.** Visual hallucinations
- ○ **D.** Tachycardia

71. The nurse is caring for a client with acromegaly. Following a transphenoidal hypophysectomy, the nurse should:

   ○ **A.** Monitor the client's blood sugar

   ○ **B.** Suction the mouth and pharynx every hour

   ○ **C.** Place the client in low Trendelenburg position

   ○ **D.** Encourage the client to cough

Quick Answer: **131**
Detailed Answer: **141**

72. A client newly diagnosed with diabetes is started on Precose (acarbose). The nurse should tell the client that the medication should be taken:

   ○ **A.** 1 hour before meals

   ○ **B.** 30 minutes after meals

   ○ **C.** With the first bite of a meal

   ○ **D.** Daily at bedtime

Quick Answer: **131**
Detailed Answer: **141**

73. A client with a deep decubitus ulcer is receiving therapy in the hyperbaric oxygen chamber. Before therapy, the nurse should:

   ○ **A.** Apply a lanolin-based lotion to the skin

   ○ **B.** Wash the skin with water and pat dry

   ○ **C.** Cover the area with a petroleum gauze

   ○ **D.** Apply an occlusive dressing to the site

Quick Answer: **131**
Detailed Answer: **141**

74. The physician has ordered DDAVP (desmopressin acetate) for a client with diabetes insipidus. Which finding indicates that the medication is having its intended effect?

   ○ **A.** The client's appetite has improved.

   ○ **B.** The client's morning blood sugar was 120mg/dL.

   ○ **C.** The client's urinary output has decreased.

   ○ **D.** The client's activity level has increased.

Quick Answer: **131**
Detailed Answer: **141**

75. A client with pregnancy-induced hypertension is scheduled for a C-section. Before surgery, the nurse should keep the client:

   ○ **A.** On her right side

   ○ **B.** Supine with a small pillow

   ○ **C.** On her left side

   ○ **D.** In knee chest position

Quick Answer: **131**
Detailed Answer: **141**

76. The physician has prescribed Coumadin (sodium warfarin) for a client having transient ischemic attacks. Which laboratory test measures the therapeutic level of Coumadin?

Quick Answer: **131**
Detailed Answer: **141**

- ○ **A.** Prothrombin time
- ○ **B.** Clot retraction time
- ○ **C.** Partial thromboplastin time
- ○ **D.** Bleeding time

77. An adolescent client with cystic acne has a prescription for Accutane (isotretinoin). Which lab work is needed before beginning the medication?

Quick Answer: **131**
Detailed Answer: **141**

- ○ **A.** Complete blood count
- ○ **B.** Clean-catch urinalysis
- ○ **C.** Liver profile
- ○ **D.** Thyroid function test

78. Twenty-four hours after an uncomplicated labor and delivery, a client's WBC is 12,000cu/mm. The elevation in the client's WBC is most likely an indication of:

Quick Answer: **131**
Detailed Answer: **142**

- ○ **A.** A normal response to the birth process
- ○ **B.** An acute bacterial infection
- ○ **C.** A sexually transmitted virus
- ○ **D.** Dehydration from being NPO during labor

79. The home health nurse is visiting a client who plans to deliver her baby at home. Which statement by the client indicates an understanding regarding screening for phenylketonuria (PKU)?

Quick Answer: **131**
Detailed Answer: **142**

- ○ **A.** "I will need to take the baby to the clinic within 24 hours of delivery to have blood drawn."
- ○ **B.** "I will need to schedule a home visit for PKU screening when the baby is 3 days old."
- ○ **C.** "I will remind the midwife to save a specimen of cord blood for the PKU test."
- ○ **D.** "I will have the PKU test done when I take her for her first immunizations."

80. The physician has ordered intubation and mechanical ventilation for a client with periods of apnea following a closed head injury. Arterial blood gases reveal a pH of 7.47, PCO_2 of 28, and HCO_3 of 23. These findings indicate that the client has:

    ○ **A.** Respiratory acidosis

    ○ **B.** Respiratory alkalosis

    ○ **C.** Metabolic acidosis

    ○ **D.** Metabolic alkalosis

Quick Answer: **131**
Detailed Answer: **142**

81. A client is diagnosed with emphysema and cor pulmonale. Which findings are characteristic of cor pulmonale?

    ○ **A.** Hypoxia, shortness of breath, and exertional fatigue

    ○ **B.** Weight loss, increased RBC, and fever

    ○ **C.** Rales, edema, and enlarged spleen

    ○ **D.** Edema of the lower extremities and distended neck veins

Quick Answer: **131**
Detailed Answer: **142**

82. A client with a laryngectomy returns from surgery with a nasogastric tube in place. The primary reason for placement of the nasogastric tube is to:

    ○ **A.** Prevent swelling and dysphagia

    ○ **B.** Decompress the stomach

    ○ **C.** Prevent contamination of the suture line

    ○ **D.** Promote healing of the oral mucosa

Quick Answer: **131**
Detailed Answer: **142**

83. The physician orders the removal of an in-dwelling catheter the second postoperative day for a client with a prostatectomy. The client complains of pain and dribbling of urine the first time he voids. The nurse should tell the client that:

    ○ **A.** Using warm compresses over the bladder will lessen the discomfort.

    ○ **B.** Perineal exercises will be started in a few days to help relieve his symptoms.

    ○ **C.** If the symptoms don't improve, the catheter will have to be reinserted.

    ○ **D.** His complaints are common and will improve over the next few days.

Quick Answer: **131**
Detailed Answer: **142**

84. A client with a right lobectomy is being transported from the intensive care unit to a medical unit. The nurse understands that the client's chest drainage system:

    ○ **A.** Can be disconnected from suction if the chest tube is clamped

    ○ **B.** Can be disconnected from suction, but the chest tube should remain unclamped

    ○ **C.** Must remain connected by means of a portable suction

    ○ **D.** Must be kept even with the client's shoulders during the transport

Quick Answer: **131**
Detailed Answer: **142**

85. A nurse is caring for a client with a myocardial infarction. The nurse recognizes that the most common complication in the client following a myocardial infarction is:

- ○ **A.** Right ventricular hypertrophy
- ○ **B.** Cardiac dysrhythmia
- ○ **C.** Left ventricular hypertrophy
- ○ **D.** Hyperkalemia

Quick Answer: **131**
Detailed Answer: **142**

86. A client develops a temperature of 102°F following coronary artery bypass surgery. The nurse should notify the physician immediately because elevations in temperature:

- ○ **A.** Increase cardiac output
- ○ **B.** Indicate cardiac tamponade
- ○ **C.** Decrease cardiac output
- ○ **D.** Indicate graft rejection

Quick Answer: **131**
Detailed Answer: **142**

87. The chart indicates that a client has expressive aphasia following a stroke. The nurse understands that the client will have difficulty with:

- ○ **A.** Speaking and writing
- ○ **B.** Comprehending spoken words
- ○ **C.** Carrying out purposeful motor activity
- ○ **D.** Recognizing and using an object correctly

Quick Answer: **131**
Detailed Answer: **143**

88. A client receiving Parnate (tranylcypromine) is admitted in a hypertensive crisis. Which food is most likely to produce a hypertensive crisis when taken with the medication?

- ○ **A.** Processed cheese
- ○ **B.** Cottage cheese
- ○ **C.** Cream cheese
- ○ **D.** Cheddar cheese

Quick Answer: **131**
Detailed Answer: **143**

89. To prevent deformities of the knee joints in a client with an exacerbation of rheumatoid arthritis, the nurse should:

- ○ **A.** Tell the client to remain on bed rest until swelling subsides
- ○ **B.** Discourage passive range of motion because it will cause further swelling
- ○ **C.** Encourage motion of the joint within the limits of pain
- ○ **D.** Tell the client she will need joint immobilization for 2–3 weeks

Quick Answer: **131**
Detailed Answer: **143**

90. The nurse is assessing a trauma client in the emergency room when she notes a penetrating abdominal wound with exposed viscera. The nurse should:

- ○ **A.** Apply a clean dressing to protect the wound
- ○ **B.** Cover the exposed visera with a sterile saline gauze
- ○ **C.** Gently replace the abdominal contents
- ○ **D.** Cover the area with a petroleum gauze

91. A client is admitted to the emergency room with multiple injuries. What is the proper sequence for managing the client?

- ○ **A.** Assess for head injuries, control hemorrhage, establish an airway, prevent hypovolemic shock
- ○ **B.** Control hemorrhage, prevent hypovolemic shock, establish an airway, assess for head injuries
- ○ **C.** Establish an airway, control hemorrhage, prevent hypovolemic shock, assess for head injuries
- ○ **D.** Prevent hypovolemic shock, assess for head injuries, establish an airway, control hemorrhage

92. The nurse is teaching the mother of a child with attention deficit disorder regarding the use of Ritalin (methylphenidate). The nurse recognizes that the mother understands her teaching when she states the importance of:

- ○ **A.** Offering high-calorie snacks
- ○ **B.** Watching for signs of infection
- ○ **C.** Observing for signs of oversedation
- ○ **D.** Using a sunscreen with an SPF of 30

93. A home health nurse has several elderly clients in her case load. Which of the following clients is most likely to be a victim of elder abuse?

- ○ **A.** A 76-year-old female with Alzheimer's disease
- ○ **B.** A 70-year-old male with diabetes mellitus
- ○ **C.** A 64-year-old female with a hip replacement
- ○ **D.** A 72-year-old male with Parkinson's disease

94. A camp nurse is applying sunscreen to a group of children enrolled in swim classes. Chemical sunscreens are most effective when applied:

- ○ **A.** Just before sun exposure
- ○ **B.** 5 minutes before sun exposure
- ○ **C.** 15 minutes before sun exposure
- ○ **D.** 30 minutes before sun exposure

95. The physician has made a diagnosis of "shaken child" syndrome for a 13-month-old who was brought to the emergency room after a reported fall from his highchair. Which finding supports the diagnosis of "shaken child" syndrome?

- ○ **A.** Fracture of the clavicle
- ○ **B.** Periorbital bruising
- ○ **C.** Retinal hemorrhages
- ○ **D.** Fracture of the humerus

96. A post-operative client has an order for Demerol (meperidine) 75mg and Phenergan (promethazine) 25mg IM every 3–4 hours as needed for pain. The combination of the two medications produces a/an:

- ○ **A.** Agonist effect
- ○ **B.** Synergistic effect
- ○ **C.** Antagonist effect
- ○ **D.** Excitatory effect

97. Which obstetrical client is most likely to have an infant with respiratory distress syndrome?

- ○ **A.** A 28-year-old with a history of alcohol use during the pregnancy
- ○ **B.** A 24-year-old with a history of diabetes mellitus
- ○ **C.** A 30-year-old with a history of smoking during the pregnancy
- ○ **D.** A 32-year-old with a history of pregnancy-induced hypertension

98. A client with a C4 spinal cord injury has been placed in traction with cervical tongs. Nursing care should include:

- ○ **A.** Releasing the traction for 5 minutes each shift
- ○ **B.** Loosening the pins if the client complains of headache
- ○ **C.** Elevating the head of the bed 90°
- ○ **D.** Performing sterile pin care as ordered

99. The nurse is assessing a client following a coronary artery bypass graft (CABG). The nurse should give priority to reporting:

- ○ **A.** Chest drainage of 150mL in the past hour
- ○ **B.** Confusion and restlessness
- ○ **C.** Pallor and coolness of skin
- ○ **D.** Urinary output of 40mL per hour

100. Before administering a client's morning dose of Lanoxin (digoxin), the nurse checks the apical pulse rate and finds a rate of 54. The appropriate nursing intervention is to:

- ○ **A.** Record the pulse rate and administer the medication
- ○ **B.** Administer the medication and monitor the heart rate
- ○ **C.** Withhold the medication and notify the doctor
- ○ **D.** Withhold the medication until the heart rate increases

101. What information should the nurse give a new mother regarding the introduction of solid foods for her infant?

- ○ **A.** Solid foods should not be given until the extrusion reflex disappears at 8–10 months of age.
- ○ **B.** Solid foods should be introduced one at a time, with 4- to 7-day intervals.
- ○ **C.** Solid foods can be mixed in a bottle or infant feeder, to make feeding easier.
- ○ **D.** Solid foods should begin with fruits and vegetables.

102. When performing Leopold maneuvers on a client at 32 weeks gestation, the nurse would expect to find:

- ○ **A.** No fetal movement
- ○ **B.** Minimal fetal movement
- ○ **C.** Moderate fetal movement
- ○ **D.** Active fetal movement

103. A client with a history of phenylketonuria (PKU) is seen in the local family planning clinic. While completing the intake history, the nurse provides information for a healthy pregnancy. Which statement indicates that the client needs further teaching?

- ○ **A.** "I can use artificial sweeteners to keep me from gaining too much weight when I get pregnant."
- ○ **B.** "I need to go back on a low-phenylalanine diet before I get pregnant."
- ○ **C.** "Fresh fruits and raw vegetables will make good between-meal snacks for me."
- ○ **D.** "My baby could be mentally retarded if I don't stick to a diet eliminating phenylalanine."

104. The nurse is teaching the mother of an infant with galactosemia. Which information should be included in the nurse's teaching?

Quick Answer: **132**
Detailed Answer: **144**

- ○ **A.** Check food and drug labels for the presence of lactose.
- ○ **B.** Foods containing galactose can be gradually added.
- ○ **C.** Future children will not be affected.
- ○ **D.** Sources of galactose are essential for growth.

105. Which finding is associated with Tay Sachs disease?

Quick Answer: **132**
Detailed Answer: **144**

- ○ **A.** Pallor of the conjunctiva
- ○ **B.** Cherry-red spots on the macula
- ○ **C.** Blue-tinged sclera
- ○ **D.** White flecks in the iris

106. A client with schizophrenia is started on Zyprexa (olanzapine). Three weeks later, the client develops severe muscle rigidity and elevated temperature. The nurse should give priority to:

Quick Answer: **132**
Detailed Answer: **144**

- ○ **A.** Withholding all morning medications
- ○ **B.** Ordering a CBC and CPK
- ○ **C.** Administering prescribed anti-Parkinsonian medication
- ○ **D.** Transferring the client to a medical unit

107. A client with human immunodeficiency syndrome has gastrointestinal symptoms, including diarrhea. The nurse should teach the client to avoid:

Quick Answer: **132**
Detailed Answer: **144**

- ○ **A.** Calcium-rich foods
- ○ **B.** Canned or frozen vegetables
- ○ **C.** Processed meat
- ○ **D.** Raw fruits and vegetables

108. A 4-year-old is admitted with acute leukemia. It will be most important to monitor the child for:

Quick Answer: **132**
Detailed Answer: **145**

- ○ **A.** Abdominal pain and anorexia
- ○ **B.** Fatigue and bruising
- ○ **C.** Bleeding and pallor
- ○ **D.** Petechiae and mucosal ulcers

109. A 5-month-old is diagnosed with atopic dermatitis. Nursing interventions will focus on:

Quick Answer: **132**
Detailed Answer: **145**

- ○ **A.** Preventing infection
- ○ **B.** Administering antipyretics
- ○ **C.** Keeping the skin free of moisture
- ○ **D.** Limiting oral fluid intake

110. A client on a mechanical ventilator begins to fight the ventilator. Which medication will be ordered for the client?

Quick Answer: **132**
Detailed Answer: **145**

- ○ **A.** Sublimaze (fentanyl)
- ○ **B.** Pavulon (pancuronium bromide)
- ○ **C.** Versed (midazolam)
- ○ **D.** Atarax (hydroxyzine)

111. A client with a history of diverticulitis complains of abdominal pain, fever, and diarrhea. Which food is responsible for the client's symptoms?

Quick Answer: **132**
Detailed Answer: **145**

- ○ **A.** Mashed potatoes
- ○ **B.** Steamed carrots
- ○ **C.** Baked fish
- ○ **D.** Whole-grain cereal

112. The home health nurse is visiting a client with Paget's disease. An important part of preventive care for the client with Paget's disease is:

Quick Answer: **132**
Detailed Answer: **145**

- ○ **A.** Keeping the environment free of clutter
- ○ **B.** Advising the client to see the dentist regularly
- ○ **C.** Encouraging the client to take the influenza vaccine
- ○ **D.** Telling the client to take a daily multivitamin

113. The physician has scheduled a Whipple procedure for a client with pancreatic cancer. The nurse recognizes that the client's cancer is located in:

Quick Answer: **132**
Detailed Answer: **145**

- ○ **A.** The tail of the pancreas
- ○ **B.** The head of the pancreas
- ○ **C.** The body of the pancreas
- ○ **D.** The entire pancreas

114. A child with cystic fibrosis is being treated with inhalation therapy with Pulmozyme (dornase alfa). A side effect of the medication is:

Quick Answer: **132**
Detailed Answer: **145**

- ○ **A.** Weight gain
- ○ **B.** Hair loss
- ○ **C.** Sore throat
- ○ **D.** Brittle nails

115. Four days after delivery, a client develops complications of postpartal hemorrhage. The most common cause of late postpartal hemorrhage is:

Quick Answer: **132**
Detailed Answer: **145**

- ○ **A.** Uterine atony
- ○ **B.** Retained placental fragments
- ○ **C.** Cervical laceration
- ○ **D.** Perineal tears

116. On a home visit, the nurse finds four young children alone. The youngest of the children has bruises on the face and back and circular burns on the inner aspect of the right forearm. The nurse should:

Quick Answer: **132**
Detailed Answer: **145**

- ○ **A.** Contact child welfare services
- ○ **B.** Transport the child to the emergency room
- ○ **C.** Take the children to an abuse shelter
- ○ **D.** Stay with the children until an adult arrives

117. A client is diagnosed with post-traumatic stress disorder following a rape by an unknown assailant. The nurse should give priority to:

Quick Answer: **132**
Detailed Answer: **145**

- ○ **A.** Providing a supportive environment
- ○ **B.** Controlling the client's feelings of anger
- ○ **C.** Discussing the details of the attack
- ○ **D.** Administering a hypnotic for sleep

118. The doctor has ordered Percocet (oxycodone) for a client following abdominal surgery. The primary objective of nursing care for the client receiving an opiate analgesic is:

Quick Answer: **132**
Detailed Answer: **145**

- ○ **A.** Preventing addiction
- ○ **B.** Alleviating pain
- ○ **C.** Facilitating mobility
- ○ **D.** Preventing nausea

119. A client with emphysema is receiving intravenous aminophylline. Which aminophylline level is associated with signs of toxicity?

Quick Answer: **132**
Detailed Answer: **146**

- ○ **A.** 5 micrograms/mL
- ○ **B.** 10 micrograms/mL
- ○ **C.** 20 micrograms/mL
- ○ **D.** 25 micrograms/mL

120. Which finding is the best indication that a client with ineffective airway clearance needs suctioning?

Quick Answer: **132**
Detailed Answer: **146**

- ○ **A.** Oxygen saturation
- ○ **B.** Respiratory rate
- ○ **C.** Breath sounds
- ○ **D.** Arterial blood gases

121. A client with tuberculosis has a prescription for Myambutol (ethambutol HCl). The nurse should tell the client to notify the doctor immediately if he notices:

   ○ **A.** Gastric distress

   ○ **B.** Changes in hearing

   ○ **C.** Red discoloration of body fluids

   ○ **D.** Changes in color vision

Quick Answer: **132**
Detailed Answer: **146**

122. The primary cause of anemia in a client with chronic renal failure is:

   ○ **A.** Poor iron absorption

   ○ **B.** Destruction of red blood cells

   ○ **C.** Lack of intrinsic factor

   ○ **D.** Insufficient erythropoietin

Quick Answer: **132**
Detailed Answer: **146**

123. Which of the following nursing interventions has the highest priority for the client scheduled for an intravenous pyelogram?

   ○ **A.** Providing the client with a favorite meal for dinner

   ○ **B.** Asking if the client has allergies to shellfish

   ○ **C.** Encouraging fluids the evening before the test

   ○ **D.** Telling the client what to expect during the test

Quick Answer: **132**
Detailed Answer: **146**

124. A client has ataxia following a cerebral vascular accident. The nurse should:

   ○ **A.** Supervise the client's ambulation

   ○ **B.** Measure the client's intake and output

   ○ **C.** Request a consult for speech therapy

   ○ **D.** Provide the client with a magic slate

Quick Answer: **132**
Detailed Answer: **146**

125. The doctor has prescribed aspirin 325mg daily for a client with transient ischemic attacks. The nurse explains that aspirin was prescribed to:

   ○ **A.** Prevent headaches

   ○ **B.** Boost coagulation

   ○ **C.** Prevent cerebral anoxia

   ○ **D.** Decrease platelet aggregation

Quick Answer: **132**
Detailed Answer: **146**

126. The nurse is preparing to administer regular insulin by continuous IV infusion to a client with diabetic ketoacidosis. The nurse should:

- ○ **A.** Mix the insulin with Dextrose 5% in Water
- ○ **B.** Flush the IV tubing with the insulin solution and discard the first 50mL
- ○ **C.** Avoid using a pump or controller with the infusion
- ○ **D.** Mix the insulin with Ringer's lactate

Quick Answer: **132**
Detailed Answer: **146**

127. While reviewing the chart of a client with a history of hepatitis B, the nurse finds a serologic marker of HB8 AG. The nurse recognizes that the client:

- ○ **A.** Has chronic hepatitis B
- ○ **B.** Has recovered from hepatitis B infection
- ○ **C.** Has immunity to infection with hepatitis C
- ○ **D.** Has no chance of spreading the infection to others

Quick Answer: **132**
Detailed Answer: **146**

128. A client with tuberculosis who has been on combined therapy with rifampin and isoniazid asks the nurse how long he will have to take medication. The nurse should tell the client that:

- ○ **A.** Medication is rarely needed after 2 weeks.
- ○ **B.** He will need to take medication the rest of his life.
- ○ **C.** The course of therapy is usually 6 months.
- ○ **D.** He will be re-evaluated in 1 month to see if further medication is needed.

Quick Answer: **132**
Detailed Answer: **146**

129. Which developmental milestone puts the 4-month-old infant at greatest risk for injury?

- ○ **A.** Switching objects from one hand to another
- ○ **B.** Crawling
- ○ **C.** Standing
- ○ **D.** Rolling over

Quick Answer: **132**
Detailed Answer: **146**

130. A newborn is diagnosed with congenital syphilis. Classic signs of congenital syphilis are:

- ○ **A.** Red papular rash, desquamation, white strawberry tongue
- ○ **B.** Rhinitis, maculopapular rash, hepatosplenomegaly
- ○ **C.** Red edematous cheeks, maculopapular rash on the trunk and extremities
- ○ **D.** Epicanthal folds, low-set ears, protruding tongue

Quick Answer: **132**
Detailed Answer: **147**

131. Infants should be restrained in a car seat in a semi-reclined position facing the rear of the car until they weigh:

- ○ **A.** 10 pounds
- ○ **B.** 15 pounds
- ○ **C.** 20 pounds
- ○ **D.** 25 pounds

132. The nurse is caring for a client with irritable bowel syndrome. Irritable bowel syndrome is characterized by:

- ○ **A.** Development of pouches in the wall of the intestine
- ○ **B.** Alternating bouts of constipation and diarrhea
- ○ **C.** Swelling, thickening, and abscess formation
- ○ **D.** Hypocalcemia and iron-deficiency anemia

133. A client taking Dilantin (phenytoin) for tonic-clonic seizures is preparing for discharge. Which information should be included in the client's discharge care plan?

- ○ **A.** The medication can cause dental staining.
- ○ **B.** The client will need to avoid a high-carbohydrate diet.
- ○ **C.** The client will need a regularly scheduled blood work.
- ○ **D.** The medication can cause problems with drowsiness.

134. Assessment of a newborn male reveals that the infant has hypospadias. The nurse knows that:

- ○ **A.** The infant should not be circumcised.
- ○ **B.** Surgical correction will be done by 6 months of age.
- ○ **C.** Surgical correction is delayed until 6 years of age.
- ○ **D.** The infant should be circumcised to facilitate voiding.

135. The nurse is providing dietary teaching for a client with elevated cholesterol levels. Which cooking oil is *not* suggested for the client on a low-cholesterol diet?

- ○ **A.** Safflower oil
- ○ **B.** Sunflower oil
- ○ **C.** Coconut oil
- ○ **D.** Canola oil

136. A client is hospitalized with signs of transplant rejection following a recent renal transplant. Assessment of the client would be expected to reveal:

Quick Answer: **132**
Detailed Answer: **147**

- ○ **A.** A weight loss of 2 pounds in 1 day
- ○ **B.** A serum creatinine 1.25mg/dL
- ○ **C.** Urinary output of 50mL/hr
- ○ **D.** Rising blood pressure

137. A client is admitted with a blood alcohol level of 180mg/dL. The nurse recognizes that the alcohol in the client's system should be fully metabolized within:

Quick Answer: **132**
Detailed Answer: **147**

- ○ **A.** 3 hours
- ○ **B.** 5 hours
- ○ **C.** 7 hours
- ○ **D.** 9 hours

138. The nurse is caring for a client with stage III Alzheimer's disease. A characteristic of this stage is:

Quick Answer: **132**
Detailed Answer: **147**

- ○ **A.** Memory loss
- ○ **B.** Failing to recognize familiar objects
- ○ **C.** Wandering at night
- ○ **D.** Failing to communicate

139. The doctor has prescribed Cortone (cortisone) for a client with systemic lupus erythematosis. Which instruction should be given to the client?

Quick Answer: **132**
Detailed Answer: **147**

- ○ **A.** Take the medication 30 minutes before eating.
- ○ **B.** Report changes in appetite and weight.
- ○ **C.** Wear sunglasses to prevent cataracts.
- ○ **D.** Schedule a time to take the influenza vaccine.

140. The nurse is caring for a client with an above-the-knee amputation (AKA). To prevent contractures, the nurse should:

Quick Answer: **132**
Detailed Answer: **148**

- ○ **A.** Place the client in a prone position 15–30 minutes twice a day
- ○ **B.** Keep the foot of the bed elevated on shock blocks
- ○ **C.** Place trochanter rolls on either side of the affected leg
- ○ **D.** Keep the client's leg elevated on two pillows

141. The mother of a 6-month-old asks when her child will have all his baby teeth. The nurse knows that most children have all their primary teeth by age:

Quick Answer: **132**
Detailed Answer: **148**

- ○ **A.** 12 months
- ○ **B.** 18 months
- ○ **C.** 24 months
- ○ **D.** 30 months

142. A client with an esophageal tamponade develops symptoms of respiratory distress, including inspiratory stridor. The nurse should give priority to:

Quick Answer: **132**
Detailed Answer: **148**

- ○ **A.** Applying oxygen at 4L via nasal cannula
- ○ **B.** Removing the tube after deflating the balloons
- ○ **C.** Elevating the head of the bed to 45°
- ○ **D.** Increasing the pressure in the esophageal balloon

143. The nurse is assessing the heart sounds of a client with mitral stenosis following a history of rheumatic fever. To hear a mitral murmur, the nurse should place the stethoscope at:

Quick Answer: **132**
Detailed Answer: **148**

- ○ **A.** The third intercostal space right of the sternum
- ○ **B.** The third intercostal space left of the sternum
- ○ **C.** The fourth intercostal space beneath the sternum
- ○ **D.** The fourth intercostal space midclavicular line

144. While caring for a client with cervical cancer, the nurse notes that the radioactive implant is lying in the bed. The nurse should:

Quick Answer: **132**
Detailed Answer: **148**

- ○ **A.** Place the implant in a biohazard bag and return it to the lab
- ○ **B.** Give the client a pair of gloves and ask her to reinsert the implant
- ○ **C.** Use tongs to pick up the implant and return it to a lead-lined container
- ○ **D.** Discard the implant in the commode and double-flush

145. The nurse is preparing to discharge a client following a laparoscopic cholecystectomy. The nurse should:

Quick Answer: **132**
Detailed Answer: **148**

- ○ **A.** Tell the client to avoid a tub bath for 48 hours
- ○ **B.** Tell the client to expect clay-colored stools
- ○ **C.** Tell the client that she can expect lower abdominal pain for the next week
- ○ **D.** Tell the client to report pain in the back or shoulders

146. A high school student returns to school following a 3-week absence due to mononucleosis. The school nurse knows it will be important for the client:

Quick Answer: **132**
Detailed Answer: **148**

- ○ **A.** To drink additional fluids throughout the day
- ○ **B.** To avoid contact sports for 1–2 months
- ○ **C.** To have a snack twice a day to prevent hypoglycemia
- ○ **D.** To continue antibiotic therapy for 6 months

147. An adolescent with cystic fibrosis has an order for pancreatic enzyme replacement. The nurse knows that the medication should be given:

- ○ **A.** At bedtime
- ○ **B.** With meals and snacks
- ○ **C.** Twice daily
- ○ **D.** Daily in the morning

Quick Answer: **132**
Detailed Answer: **148**

148. The doctor has prescribed a diet high in vitamin B12 for a client with pernicious anemia. Which foods are good sources of B12?

- ○ **A.** Meat, eggs, dairy products
- ○ **B.** Peanut butter, raisins, molasses
- ○ **C.** Broccoli, cauliflower, cabbage
- ○ **D.** Shrimp, legumes, bran cereals

Quick Answer: **132**
Detailed Answer: **148**

149. A client with hypertension has begun an aerobic exercise program. The nurse should tell the client that the recommended exercise regimen should begin slowly and build up to:

- ○ **A.** 20–30 minutes three times a week
- ○ **B.** 45 minutes two times a week
- ○ **C.** 1 hour four times a week
- ○ **D.** 1 hour two times a week

Quick Answer: **132**
Detailed Answer: **149**

150. A home health nurse is visiting a client who is receiving diuretic therapy for congestive heart failure. Which medication places the client at risk for the development of hypokalemia?

- ○ **A.** Aldactone (spironolactone)
- ○ **B.** Demadex (torsemide)
- ○ **C.** Dyrenium (triamterene)
- ○ **D.** Midamor (amiloride hydrochloride)

Quick Answer: **132**
Detailed Answer: **149**

151. A client with breast cancer is returned to the room following a right total mastectomy. The nurse should:

- ○ **A.** Elevate the client's right arm on pillows
- ○ **B.** Place the client's right arm in a dependent sling
- ○ **C.** Keep the client's right arm on the bed beside her
- ○ **D.** Place the client's right arm across her body

Quick Answer: **132**
Detailed Answer: **149**

152. The physician has ordered nitroglycerin buccal tablets for a client with stable angina. The nurse knows that nitroglyerin:

Quick Answer: **132**
Detailed Answer: **149**

- ○ **A.** Slows contractions of the heart
- ○ **B.** Dilates coronary blood vessels
- ○ **C.** Increases the ventricular fill time
- ○ **D.** Strengthens contractions of the heart

153. A trauma client is admitted to the emergency room following a motor vehicle accident. Examination reveals that the left side of the chest moves inward when the client inhales. The finding is suggestive of:

Quick Answer: **132**
Detailed Answer: **149**

- ○ **A.** Pneumothorax
- ○ **B.** Mediastinal shift
- ○ **C.** Pulmonary contusion
- ○ **D.** Flail chest

154. A neurological consult has been ordered for a pediatric client with suspected absence seizures. The client with absence seizures can be expected to have:

Quick Answer: **132**
Detailed Answer: **140**

- ○ **A.** Short, abrupt muscle contractions
- ○ **B.** Quick, severe bilateral jerking movements
- ○ **C.** Abrupt loss of muscle tone
- ○ **D.** Brief lapse in consciousness

155. To decrease the likelihood of seizures and visual hallucinations in a client with alcohol withdrawal, the nurse should:

Quick Answer: **132**
Detailed Answer: **149**

- ○ **A.** Keep the room darkened by pulling the curtains
- ○ **B.** Keep the light over the bed on at all times
- ○ **C.** Keep the room quiet and dim the lights
- ○ **D.** Keep the television or radio turned on

156. A client with schizoaffective disorder is exhibiting Parkinsonian symptoms. Which medication is responsible for the development of Parkinsonian symptoms?

Quick Answer: **132**
Detailed Answer: **149**

- ○ **A.** Zyprexa (olanzapine)
- ○ **B.** Cogentin (benzatropine mesylate)
- ○ **C.** Benadryl (diphenhydramine)
- ○ **D.** Depakote (divalproex sodium)

157. Which activity is best suited to the 12-year-old with juvenile rheumatoid arthritis?

- ○ **A.** Playing video games
- ○ **B.** Swimming
- ○ **C.** Working crossword puzzles
- ○ **D.** Playing slow-pitch softball

158. The home health nurse is scheduled to visit four clients. Which client should she visit first?

- ○ **A.** A client with acquired immunodeficiency syndrome with a cough and reported temperature of 101°F
- ○ **B.** A client with peripheral vascular disease with an ulcer on the left lower leg
- ○ **C.** A client with diabetes mellitus who needs a diabetic control index drawn
- ○ **D.** A client with an autograft to burns of the chest and trunk

159. The glycosylated hemoglobin of a 40-year-old client with diabetes mellitus is 2.5%. The nurse understands that:

- ○ **A.** The client can have a higher-calorie diet.
- ○ **B.** The client has good control of her diabetes.
- ○ **C.** The client requires adjustment in her insulin dose.
- ○ **D.** The client has poor control of her diabetes.

160. A dexamethasone-suppression test has been ordered for a client with severe depression. The purpose of the dexamethasone suppression test is to:

- ○ **A.** Determine which social intervention will be best for the client
- ○ **B.** Help diagnose the seriousness of the client's clinical symptoms
- ○ **C.** Determine whether the client will benefit from electroconvulsive therapy
- ○ **D.** Reverse the depressive symptoms the client is experiencing

161. The physician has ordered Stadol (butorphanol) for a post-operative client. The nurse knows that the medication is having its intended effect if the client:

- ○ **A.** Is asleep 30 minutes after the injection
- ○ **B.** Asks for extra servings on his meal tray
- ○ **C.** Has an increased urinary output
- ○ **D.** States that he is feeling less nauseated

162. The mother of a child with cystic fibrosis tells the nurse that her child makes "snoring" sounds when breathing. The nurse is aware that many children with cystic fibrosis have:

- ○ **A.** Choanal atresia
- ○ **B.** Nasal polyps
- ○ **C.** Septal deviations
- ○ **D.** Enlarged adenoids

163. The nurse is caring for a client with full thickness burns to the lower half of the torso and lower extremities. During the emergent phase of injury, the primary nursing diagnosis would focus on:

- ○ **A.** Ineffective airway clearance
- ○ **B.** Impaired gas exchange
- ○ **C.** Fluid volume deficit
- ○ **D.** Pain

164. A client is hospitalized with hepatitis A. Which of the client's regular medications is contraindicated due to the current illness?

- ○ **A.** Prilosec (omeprazole)
- ○ **B.** Synthroid (levothyroxine)
- ○ **C.** Premarin (conjugated estrogens)
- ○ **D.** Lipitor (atorvastatin)

165. Which activity is suitable for a client who suffered an uncomplicated myocardial infarction (MI) 2 days ago?

- ○ **A.** Sitting in the bedside chair for 15 minutes three times a day
- ○ **B.** Remaining on strict bed rest with bedside commode privileges
- ○ **C.** Ambulating in the room and hall as tolerated
- ○ **D.** Sitting on the bedside for 5 minutes three times a day with assistance

166. The nurse has been teaching the role of diet in regulating blood pressure to a client with hypertension. Which meal selection indicates the client understands his new diet?

- ○ **A.** Cornflakes, whole milk, banana, and coffee
- ○ **B.** Scrambled eggs, bacon, toast, and coffee
- ○ **C.** Oatmeal, apple juice, dry toast, and coffee
- ○ **D.** Pancakes, ham, tomato juice, and coffee

167. An 18-month-old is being discharged following hypospadias repair. Which instruction should be included in the nurse's discharge teaching?

Quick Answer: **132**
Detailed Answer: **150**

- ○ **A.** The child should not play on his rocking horse.
- ○ **B.** Applying warm compresses will decrease pain.
- ○ **C.** Diapering should be avoided for 1–2 weeks.
- ○ **D.** The child will need a special diet to promote healing.

168. An obstetrical client calls the clinic with complaints of morning sickness. The nurse should tell the client to:

Quick Answer: **132**
Detailed Answer: **150**

- ○ **A.** Keep crackers at the bedside for eating before she arises
- ○ **B.** Drink a glass of whole milk before going to sleep at night
- ○ **C.** Skip breakfast but eat a larger lunch and dinner
- ○ **D.** Drink a glass of orange juice after adding a couple of teaspoons of sugar

169. The nurse is making assignments for the day. The staff consists of an RN, a novice RN, an LPN, and a nursing assistant. Which client should be assigned to the RN?

Quick Answer: **132**
Detailed Answer: **151**

- ○ **A.** A client with peptic ulcer disease
- ○ **B.** A client with skeletal traction for a fractured femur
- ○ **C.** A client with an abdominal cholecystectomy
- ○ **D.** A client with an esophageal tamponade

170. A child with Tetralogy of Fallot is scheduled for a modified Blalock Taussig procedure. The nurse understands that the surgery will:

Quick Answer: **132**
Detailed Answer: **151**

- ○ **A.** Reverse the direction of the blood flow
- ○ **B.** Allow better blood supply to the lungs
- ○ **C.** Relieve pressure on the ventricles
- ○ **D.** Prevent the need for further correction

171. The nurse has taken the blood pressure of a client hospitalized with methicillin-resistant staphylococcus aureus (MRSA). Which action by the nurse indicates an understanding regarding the care of clients with MRSA?

Quick Answer: **132**
Detailed Answer: **151**

- ○ **A.** The nurse leaves the stethoscope in the client's room for future use.
- ○ **B.** The nurse cleans the stethoscope with alcohol and returns it to the exam room.
- ○ **C.** The nurse uses the stethoscope to assess the blood pressure of other assigned clients.
- ○ **D.** The nurse cleans the stethoscope with water, dries it, and returns it to the nurse's station.

172. The physician has discussed the need for medication with the parents of an infant with congenital hypothyroidism. The nurse can reinforce the physician's teaching by telling the parents that:

- ○ **A.** The medication will be needed only during times of rapid growth.
- ○ **B.** The medication will be needed throughout the child's lifetime.
- ○ **C.** The medication schedule can be arranged to allow for drug holidays.
- ○ **D.** The medication is given one time daily every other day.

173. A client with diabetes mellitus has a prescription for Glucotrol XL (glipizide). The client should be instructed to take the medication:

- ○ **A.** At bedtime
- ○ **B.** With breakfast
- ○ **C.** Before lunch
- ○ **D.** After dinner

174. The nurse is caring for a client admitted with suspected myasthenia gravis. Which finding is usually associated with a diagnosis of myasthenia gravis?

- ○ **A.** Visual disturbances, including diplopia
- ○ **B.** Ascending paralysis and loss of motor function
- ○ **C.** Cogwheel rigidity and loss of coordination
- ○ **D.** Progressive weakness that is worse at the day's end

175. A preterm infant with sepsis is receiving Gentamycin (garamycin). Which physiological alteration places the preterm infant at increased risk for toxicity related to aminoglycoside therapy?

- ○ **A.** Lack of subcutaneous fat deposits
- ○ **B.** Immature central nervous system
- ○ **C.** Presence of fetal hemoglobin
- ○ **D.** Immaturity of the renal system

176. The nurse is teaching the parents of an infant with osteogenesis imperfecta. The nurse should tell the parents:

- ○ **A.** That the infant will need daily calcium supplements
- ○ **B.** That it is best to lift the infant by the buttocks when diapering
- ○ **C.** That the condition is a temporary one
- ○ **D.** That only the bones of the infant are affected by the disease

177. The home health nurse is visiting an elderly client following a hip replacement. Which finding requires further teaching?

- ○ **A.** The client shares her apartment with a cat.
- ○ **B.** The client has a grab bar near the commode.
- ○ **C.** The client usually sits on a soft, low sofa.
- ○ **D.** The client wears supportive shoes with nonskid soles.

178. Physician's orders for a client with acute pancreatitis include the following: strict NPO and nasogastric tube to low intermittent suction. The nurse recognizes that witholding oral intake will:

- ○ **A.** Reduce the secretion of pancreatic enzymes
- ○ **B.** Decrease the client's need for insulin
- ○ **C.** Prevent the secretion of gastric acid
- ○ **D.** Eliminate the need for pain medication

179. A client with diverticulitis is admitted with nausea, vomiting, and dehydration. Which finding suggests a complication of diverticulitis?

- ○ **A.** Pain in the left lower quadrant
- ○ **B.** Boardlike abdomen
- ○ **C.** Low-grade fever
- ○ **D.** Abdominal distention

180. The physician has ordered Vancocin (vancomycin) 500mg IV every 6 hours for a client with MRSA. The medication should be administered:

- ○ **A.** IV push
- ○ **B.** Over 15 minutes
- ○ **C.** Over 30 minutes
- ○ **D.** Over 60 minutes

181. The diagnostic work-up of a client hospitalized with complaints of progressive weakness and fatigue confirm a diagnosis of myasthenia gravis. The medication used to treat myasthenia gravis is:

- ○ **A.** Prostigmine (neostigmine)
- ○ **B.** Atropine (atropine sulfate)
- ○ **C.** Didronel (etidronate)
- ○ **D.** Tensilon (edrophonium)

182. A client with AIDS complains of a weight loss of 20 pounds in the past month. Which diet is suggested for the client with AIDS?

Quick Answer: **132**
Detailed Answer: **152**

- ○ **A.** High calorie, high protein, high fat
- ○ **B.** High calorie, high carbohydrate, low protein
- ○ **C.** High calorie, low carbohydrate, high fat
- ○ **D.** High calorie, high protein, low fat

183. The nurse is caring for a 4-year-old with cerebral palsy. Which nursing intervention will help ready the child for rehabilitative services?

Quick Answer: **132**
Detailed Answer: **152**

- ○ **A.** Patching one of the eyes to help strengthen the ocular muscles
- ○ **B.** Providing suckers and pinwheels to help strengthen tongue movement
- ○ **C.** Providing musical tapes to provide auditory training
- ○ **D.** Encouraging play with a video game to improve muscle coordination

184. A client is admitted with a diagnosis of duodenal ulcer. A common complaint of the client with a duodenal ulcer is:

Quick Answer: **132**
Detailed Answer: **152**

- ○ **A.** Epigastric pain that is relieved by eating
- ○ **B.** Weight loss
- ○ **C.** Epigastric pain that is worse after eating
- ○ **D.** Vomiting after eating

185. A client with otosderosis is scheduled for a stapedectomy. Which finding suggests a complication involving the seventh cranial nerve?

Quick Answer: **132**
Detailed Answer: **152**

- ○ **A.** Diminished hearing
- ○ **B.** Sensation of fullness in the ear
- ○ **C.** Inability to move the tongue side to side
- ○ **D.** Changes in facial sensation

186. At the 6-week check-up, the mother asks when she can expect the baby to sleep all night. The nurse should tell the mother that most infants begin to sleep all night by age:

Quick Answer: **132**
Detailed Answer: **152**

- ○ **A.** 1 month
- ○ **B.** 2 months
- ○ **C.** 3–4 months
- ○ **D.** 5–6 months

187. A client with emphysema has been receiving oxygen at 3L per minute by nasal cannula. The nurse knows that the goal of the client's oxygen therapy is achieved when the client's PaO_2 reading is:

- ○ **A.** 50–60mm Hg
- ○ **B.** 70–80mm Hg
- ○ **C.** 80–90mm Hg
- ○ **D.** 90–98mm Hg

Quick Answer: **133**
Detailed Answer: **152**

188. A client with diabetes insipidus is receiving DDAVP (desmopressin acetate). Which lab finding indicates that the medication is having its intended effect?

- ○ **A.** Blood glucose 92mg/dL
- ○ **B.** Urine specific gravity 1.020
- ○ **C.** White blood count of 7,500
- ○ **D.** Glycosylated hemoglobin 3.5mg/dL

Quick Answer: **133**
Detailed Answer: **152**

189. Which of the following pediatric clients is at greatest risk for latex allergy?

- ○ **A.** The child with a myelomeningocele
- ○ **B.** The child with epispadias
- ○ **C.** The child with coxa plana
- ○ **D.** The child with rheumatic fever

Quick Answer: **133**
Detailed Answer: **153**

190. The physician has ordered a serum aminophylline level for a client with chronic obstructive lung disease. The nurse knows that the therapeutic range for aminophylline is:

- ○ **A.** 1–3 micrograms/mL
- ○ **B.** 4–6 micrograms/mL
- ○ **C.** 7–9 micrograms/mL
- ○ **D.** 10–20 micrograms/mL

Quick Answer: **133**
Detailed Answer: **153**

191. The nurse is developing a plan of care for a client with acromegaly. Which nursing diagnosis should receive priority?

- ○ **A.** Alteration in body image related to change in facial features
- ○ **B.** Risk for immobility related to joint pain
- ○ **C.** Risk for ineffective airway clearance related to obstruction of airway by tongue
- ○ **D.** Sexual dysfunction related to altered hormone secretion

Quick Answer: **133**
Detailed Answer: **153**

192. A client with acute respiratory distress syndrome (ARDS) is placed on mechanical ventilation. To increase ventilation and perfusion to all areas of the lungs, the nurse should:

- ○ **A.** Tell the client to inhale deeply during the inspiratory cycle
- ○ **B.** Increase the positive end expiratory pressure (PEEP)
- ○ **C.** Turn the client every hour
- ○ **D.** Administer medication to prevent the client from fighting the ventilator

193. The nurse is teaching the mother of a child with cystic fibrosis how to do chest percussion. The nurse should tell the mother to:

- ○ **A.** Use the heel of her hand during percussion
- ○ **B.** Change the child's position every 20 minutes during percussion sessions
- ○ **C.** Do percussion after the child eats and at bedtime
- ○ **D.** Use cupped hands during percussion

194. A client with Addison's disease asks the nurse what he needs to know to manage his condition. The nurse should give priority to:

- ○ **A.** Emphasizing the need for strict adherence to his medication regimen
- ○ **B.** Teaching the client to avoid lotions and skin preparations containing alcohol
- ○ **C.** Explaining the need to avoid extremes of temperature
- ○ **D.** Assisting the client to choose a diet that contains adequate protein, fat, and carbohydrates

195. The nurse is caring for a client following the removal of a central line catheter when the client suddenly develops dyspnea and complains of substernal chest pain. The client is noticeably confused and fearful. Based on the client's symptoms, the nurse should suspect which complication of central line use?

- ○ **A.** Myocardial infarction
- ○ **B.** Air embolus
- ○ **C.** Intrathoracic bleeding
- ○ **D.** Vagal response

196. The nurse calculates the amount of an antibiotic for injection to be given to an infant. The amount of medication to be administered is 1.25mL. The nurse should:

- ○ **A.** Divide the amount into two injections and administer in each vastus lateralis muscle
- ○ **B.** Give the medication in one injection in the dorsogluteal muscle
- ○ **C.** Divide the amount in two injections and give one in the ventrogluteal muscle and one in the vastus lateralis muscle
- ○ **D.** Give the medication in one injection in the ventrogluteal muscle

197. A client with schizophrenia is receiving depot injections of Haldol Deconate (haloperidol decanoate). The client should be told to return for his next injection in:

- ○ **A.** 1 week
- ○ **B.** 2 weeks
- ○ **C.** 4 weeks
- ○ **D.** 6 weeks

198. The physician is preparing to remove a central line. The nurse should tell the client to:

- ○ **A.** Breathe normally
- ○ **B.** Take slow, deep breaths
- ○ **C.** Take a deep breath and hold it
- ○ **D.** Breathe as quickly as possible

199. Cystic fibrosis is an exocrine disorder that affects several systems of the body. The earliest sign associated with a diagnosis of cystic fibrosis is:

- ○ **A.** Steatorrhea
- ○ **B.** Frequent respiratory infections
- ○ **C.** Increased sweating
- ○ **D.** Meconium ileus

200. A 3-year-old is immobilized in a hip spica cast. Which discharge instruction should be given to the parents?

- ○ **A.** Keep the bed flat, with a small pillow beneath the cast.
- ○ **B.** Provide crayons and a coloring book for play activity.
- ○ **C.** Increase her intake of high-calorie foods for healing.
- ○ **D.** Tuck a disposable diaper beneath the cast at the perineal opening.

201. The nurse is caring for a client following the reimplantation of the thumb and index finger. Which finding should be reported to the physician immediately?

- ○ **A.** Temperature of 100°F
- ○ **B.** Coolness and discoloration of the digits
- ○ **C.** Complaints of pain
- ○ **D.** Difficulty moving the digits

202. Which client is at greatest risk for a caesarean section due to cephalopelvic disproportion (CPD)?

- ○ **A.** A 25-year-old gravida 2, para 1
- ○ **B.** A 30-year-old gravida 3, para 2
- ○ **C.** A 17-year-old gravida 1, para 0
- ○ **D.** A 32-year-old gravida 1, para 0

203. The nurse is caring for a client with amyotrophic lateral sclerosis (ALS, Lou Gehrig's disease). The nurse should give priority to:

- ○ **A.** Assessing the client's respiratory status
- ○ **B.** Providing an alternate means of communication
- ○ **C.** Referring the client and family to community support groups
- ○ **D.** Instituting a routine of active range-of-motion exercises

204. The physician has ordered Claforan (cefotaxime) 1g every 6 hours. The pharmacy sends the medication premixed in 100mL of D5W with instructions to infuse the medication over 1 hour. The IV set delivers 20 drops per milliliter. The nurse should set the IV rate at:

- ○ **A.** 50 drops per minute
- ○ **B.** 33 drops per minute
- ○ **C.** 25 drops per minute
- ○ **D.** 12 drops per minute

205. When assessing the urinary output of a client who has had extracorporeal lithotripsy, the nurse can expect to find:

- ○ **A.** Cherry-red urine that gradually becomes clearer
- ○ **B.** Orange-tinged urine containing particles of calculi
- ○ **C.** Dark red urine that becomes cloudy in appearance
- ○ **D.** Dark, smoky-colored urine with high specific gravity

206. A client scheduled for an atherectomy asks the nurse about the procedure. The nurse understands that:

Quick Answer: **133**
Detailed Answer: **154**

- ○ **A.** Plaque will be removed by rotational or directional catheters.
- ○ **B.** Plaque will be destroyed by a laser.
- ○ **C.** A balloon-tipped catheter will compress fatty lesions against the vessel wall.
- ○ **D.** Medication will be used to dissolve the build-up of plaque.

207. An elderly client has a stage II pressure ulcer on her sacrum. During assessment of the client's skin, the nurse would expect to find:

Quick Answer: **133**
Detailed Answer: **154**

- ○ **A.** A deep crater with a nonpainful wound base
- ○ **B.** A craterous area with a nonpainful wound base
- ○ **C.** Cracks and blisters with redness and induration
- ○ **D.** Nonblanchable redness with tenderness and pain

208. The physician has prescribed Cognex (tacrine) for a client with dementia. The nurse should monitor the client for adverse reactions, which include:

Quick Answer: **133**
Detailed Answer: **155**

- ○ **A.** Hypoglycemia
- ○ **B.** Jaundice
- ○ **C.** Urinary retention
- ○ **D.** Tinnitus

209. The suggested diet for a child with cystic fibrosis is one that contains:

Quick Answer: **133**
Detailed Answer: **155**

- ○ **A.** High calories, high protein, moderate fat
- ○ **B.** High calories, moderate protein, low fat
- ○ **C.** Moderate calories, moderate protein, moderate fat
- ○ **D.** Low calories, high protein, low fat

210. The physician has ordered a low-potassium diet for a client with acute glomerulonephritis. Which snack is suitable for the client with potassium restrictions?

Quick Answer: **133**
Detailed Answer: **155**

- ○ **A.** Raisins
- ○ **B.** Oranges
- ○ **C.** Apricots
- ○ **D.** Bananas

211. A client with increased intracranial pressure is placed on mechanical ventilation with hyperventilation. The nurse knows that the purpose of the hyperventilation is to:

- ○ **A.** Prevent the development of acute respiratory failure
- ○ **B.** Decrease cerebral blood flow
- ○ **C.** Increase systemic tissue perfusion
- ○ **D.** Prevent cerebral anoxia

212. The physician has ordered a blood test for *H. pylori.* The nurse should prepare the client by:

- ○ **A.** Withholding oral intake after midnight
- ○ **B.** Telling the client that no special preparation is needed
- ○ **C.** Explaining that a small dose of radioactive isotope will be used
- ○ **D.** Giving an oral suspension of glucose 1 hour before the test

213. The nurse is preparing to give an oral potassium supplement. The nurse should give the medication:

- ○ **A.** Without diluting it
- ○ **B.** With 4oz. of juice
- ○ **C.** With water only
- ○ **D.** On an empty stomach

214. A client with acute alcohol intoxication is being treated for hypomagnesemia. During assessment of the client, the nurse would expect to find:

- ○ **A.** Bradycardia
- ○ **B.** Negative Chvostek's sign
- ○ **C.** Hypertension
- ○ **D.** Positive Trousseau's sign

215. The physician has ordered cultures for cytomegalovirus (CMV). Which statement is true of the collection of cultures for cytomegalovirus?

- ○ **A.** Stool cultures are preferred for definitive diagnosis.
- ○ **B.** Pregnant caregivers may obtain cultures.
- ○ **C.** Collection of one specimen is sufficient.
- ○ **D.** Accurate diagnosis depends on fresh specimens.

216. A home health nurse has four clients assigned for morning visits. The nurse should give priority to visiting the client with:

Quick Answer: **133**
Detailed Answer: **155**

- ○ **A.** Diabetes mellitus with a nongranulated ulcer of the right foot
- ○ **B.** Congestive heart failure who reports coughing up frothy sputum
- ○ **C.** Hemiplegia with tenderness in the right flank and cloudy urine
- ○ **D.** Rheumatoid arthritis with soft tissue swelling behind the right knee

217. Four clients are admitted to a medical unit. If only one private room is available, it should be assigned to:

Quick Answer: **133**
Detailed Answer: **155**

- ○ **A.** The client with ulcerative colitis
- ○ **B.** The client with neutropenia
- ○ **C.** The client with cholecystitis
- ○ **D.** The client with polycythemia vera

218. The RN is making assignments for the morning staff. Which client should be cared for by the RN?

Quick Answer: **133**
Detailed Answer: **155**

- ○ **A.** A client with hemianopsia
- ○ **B.** A client with asterixis
- ○ **C.** A client with akathesia
- ○ **D.** A client with hemoptysis

219. The nurse is reviewing the lab reports on several clients. Which one should be reported to the physician immediately?

Quick Answer: **133**
Detailed Answer: **156**

- ○ **A.** A serum creatinine of 5.2mg/dL in a client with chronic renal failure
- ○ **B.** A positive C reactive protein in a client with rheumatic fever
- ○ **C.** A hematocrit of 52% in a client with gastroenteritis
- ○ **D.** A white cell count of 2,200cu/mm in a client taking Dilantin phenytoin

Quick Answer: **133**
Detailed Answer: **156**

220. The following clients are to be assigned for daily care. The newly licensed nurse should not be assigned to provide primary care for the client with:

- ○ **A.** Full-thickness burns of the abdomen and upper thighs
- ○ **B.** A fractured hip scheduled for hip replacement
- ○ **C.** Ileal reservoir following a cystectomy
- ○ **D.** Noncardiogenic pulmonary edema (ARDS)

221. The RN is making assignments for clients hospitalized on a neurological unit. Which client should be assigned to the LPN?

Quick Answer: **133**
Detailed Answer: **156**

- ○ **A.** A client with a C3 injury immobilized by Crutchfield tongs
- ○ **B.** A client with exacerbation of multiple sclerosis
- ○ **C.** A client with a lumbar laminectomy
- ○ **D.** A client with hemiplegia and a urinary tract infection

222. The nurse has just received the change of shift report. The nurse should give priority to assessing the client with:

Quick Answer: **133**
Detailed Answer: **156**

- ○ **A.** A thoracotomy with 110mL of drainage in the past hour
- ○ **B.** A cholecystectomy with an oral temperature of 100°F
- ○ **C.** A transurethral prostatectomy who complains of urgency to void
- ○ **D.** A stapedectomy who reports diminished hearing in the past hour

223. A client with primary sclerosing cholangitis has received a liver transplant. The nurse should give priority to assessing the client for complications. Which findings are associated with an acute rejection of the new liver?

Quick Answer: **133**
Detailed Answer: **156**

- ○ **A.** Increased jaundice and prolonged prothrombin time
- ○ **B.** Fever and foul-smelling bile drainage
- ○ **C.** Abdominal distention and clay-colored stools
- ○ **D.** Increased uric acid and increased creatinine

224. The nurse is planning care for a client with adrenal insufficiency. Which nursing diagnosis should receive priority?

Quick Answer: **133**
Detailed Answer: **156**

- ○ **A.** Fluid volume deficit
- ○ **B.** Sleep pattern disturbance
- ○ **C.** Altered nutrition
- ○ **D.** Alterations in body image

225. A pediatric client with burns to the hands and arms has dressing changes with Sulfamylon (mafenide acetate) cream. The nurse is aware that the medication:

Quick Answer: **133**
Detailed Answer: **156**

- ○ **A.** Will cause dark staining of the surrounding skin
- ○ **B.** Produces a cooling sensation when applied
- ○ **C.** Can alter the function of the thyroid
- ○ **D.** Produces a burning sensation when applied

226. The physician has ordered Dilantin (phenytoin) for a client with generalized seizures. When planning the client's care the nurse should:

Quick Answer: **133**
Detailed Answer: **156**

- ○ **A.** Maintain strict intake and output
- ○ **B.** Check the pulse before giving the medication
- ○ **C.** Administer the medication 30 minutes before meals
- ○ **D.** Provide oral hygiene and gum care every shift

227. The nurse is caring for a client receiving Capoten (captopril). The nurse should be alert for adverse reactions to the drug, which include:

Quick Answer: **133**
Detailed Answer: **156**

- ○ **A.** Increased red cell count
- ○ **B.** Decreased sodium level
- ○ **C.** Decreased white cell count
- ○ **D.** Increased calcium level

228. A client receiving chemotherapy for breast cancer has an order for Zofran (ondansetron) 8mg PO to be given 30 minutes before induction of the chemotherapy. The purpose of the medication is to:

Quick Answer: **133**
Detailed Answer: **156**

- ○ **A.** Prevent anemia
- ○ **B.** Promote relaxation
- ○ **C.** Prevent nausea
- ○ **D.** Increase neutrophil counts

229. The physician has ordered cortisporin ear drops for a 2-year-old. To administer the ear drops, the nurse should:

Quick Answer: **133**
Detailed Answer: **157**

- ○ **A.** Pull the ear down and back
- ○ **B.** Pull the ear straight out
- ○ **C.** Pull the ear up and back
- ○ **D.** Leave the ear undisturbed

230. A client with Lyme's disease is being treated with Achromycin (tetracycline HCl). The nurse should tell the client that the medication will be rendered ineffective if taken with:

Quick Answer: **133**
Detailed Answer: **157**

- ○ **A.** Antacids
- ○ **B.** Salicylates
- ○ **C.** Antihistamines
- ○ **D.** Sedative-hypnotics

231. A client with schizophrenia has been taking Thorazine (chlorpromazine) 200mg four times a day. Which finding should be reported to the doctor immediately?

Quick Answer: 133
Detailed Answer: 157

   ○ **A.** The client complains of thirst.
   ○ **B.** The client has gained 4 pounds in the past 2 months.
   ○ **C.** The client complains of a sore throat.
   ○ **D.** The client naps throughout the day.

232. The doctor has prescribed Claratin (loratidine) for a client with seasonal allergies. The feature that separates Claratin from other antihistamines such as diphenhydramine is that the medication:

Quick Answer: 133
Detailed Answer: 157

   ○ **A.** Is nonsedating
   ○ **B.** Stimulates appetite
   ○ **C.** Is used for motion sickness
   ○ **D.** Is less expensive

233. A 6-month-old is being treated for thrush with Nystatin (mycostatin) oral suspension. The nurse should administer the medication by:

Quick Answer: 133
Detailed Answer: 157

   ○ **A.** Placing it in a small amount of applesauce
   ○ **B.** Using a cotton-tipped swab
   ○ **C.** Adding it to the infant's formula
   ○ **D.** Placing it in 2–3oz. of water

234. A client with iron-deficiency anemia is taking an oral iron supplement. The nurse should tell the client to take the medication with:

Quick Answer: 133
Detailed Answer: 157

   ○ **A.** Orange juice
   ○ **B.** Water only
   ○ **C.** Milk
   ○ **D.** Apple juice

235. A child is admitted to the emergency room following ingestion of a bottle of Children's Tylenol. The nurse is aware that Tylenol poisoning is treated with:

Quick Answer: 133
Detailed Answer: 157

   ○ **A.** Acetylcysteine
   ○ **B.** Deferoximine
   ○ **C.** Edetate calcium disodium
   ○ **D.** Activated charcoal

236. The nurse knows that a client with right-sided hemiplegia understands teaching regarding ambulation with a cane if she states:

- ○ **A.** "I will hold the cane in my right hand."
- ○ **B.** "I will advance my cane and my right leg at the same time."
- ○ **C.** "I will be able to walk only by using a walker."
- ○ **D.** "I will hold the cane in my left hand."

237. A nursing assistant assigned to care for a client receiving linear accelerator radium therapy for laryngeal cancer states, "I don't want to be assigned to that radioactive patient." The best response by the nurse is to:

- ○ **A.** Tell the nursing assistant that the client is not radioactive
- ○ **B.** Tell the nursing assistant to wear a radiation badge to detect the amount of radiation that she is receiving
- ○ **C.** Instruct her regarding the use of a lead-lined apron
- ○ **D.** Ask a co-worker to care for the client

238. The nurse caring for a client scheduled for an angiogram should prepare the client for the procedure by telling him to expect:

- ○ **A.** Dizziness as the dye is injected
- ○ **B.** Nausea and vomiting after the procedure is completed
- ○ **C.** A decreased heart rate for several hours after the procedure is completed
- ○ **D.** A warm sensation as the dye is injected

239. A client with Parkinson's disease complains of "choking" when he swallows. Which intervention will improve the client's ability to swallow?

- ○ **A.** Withholding liquids until after meals
- ○ **B.** Providing semiliquid foods when possible
- ○ **C.** Providing a fully liquid diet
- ○ **D.** Offering small, more frequent meals

240. Which of the following statements best explains the rationale for placing the client in Trendelenburg position during the insertion of a central line catheter?

- ○ **A.** It will facilitate catheter insertion.
- ○ **B.** It will make the client more comfortable during the insertion.
- ○ **C.** It will prevent the occurrence of ventricular tachycardia.
- ○ **D.** It will prevent the development of pulmonary emboli.

241. The doctor has ordered the removal of a Davol drain. Which of the following instructions should the nurse give to the client before removing the drain?

Quick Answer: **133**
Detailed Answer: **158**

- ○ **A.** The client should be told to breathe normally.
- ○ **B.** The client should be told to take two or three deep breaths as the drain is being removed.
- ○ **C.** The client should be told to hold his breath as the drain is being removed.
- ○ **D.** The client should breathe slowly as the drain is being removed.

242. Which of the following findings is associated with right-sided heart failure?

Quick Answer: **133**
Detailed Answer: **158**

- ○ **A.** Shortness of breath
- ○ **B.** Nocturnal polyuria
- ○ **C.** Daytime oliguria
- ○ **D.** Crackles in the lungs

243. A client returns from surgery with a total knee replacement. Which of the following findings requires immediate nursing intervention?

Quick Answer: **133**
Detailed Answer: **158**

- ○ **A.** Bloody drainage of 30mL from the Davol drain is present.
- ○ **B.** The CPM is set on 90° flexion.
- ○ **C.** The client is unable to ambulate to the bathroom.
- ○ **D.** The client is complaining of muscle spasms.

244. Which of the following postpartal clients is at greatest risk for hemorrhage?

Quick Answer: **133**
Detailed Answer: **158**

- ○ **A.** A gravida 1 para 1 with an uncomplicated delivery of a 7-pound infant
- ○ **B.** A gravida 1 para 0 with a history of polycystic ovarian disease
- ○ **C.** A gravida 3 para 3 with a history of low–birth weight infants
- ○ **D.** A gravida 4 para 3 with a Caesarean section

245. An infant with a ventricular septal defect is discharged with a prescription for lanoxin elixir 0.01mg PO q 12hrs. The bottle is labeled 0.10mg per 1/2 tsp. The nurse should instruct the mother to:

Quick Answer: **133**
Detailed Answer: **158**

- ○ **A.** Administer the medication using a nipple
- ○ **B.** Administer the medication using the calibrated dropper in the bottle
- ○ **C.** Administer the medication using a plastic baby spoon
- ○ **D.** Administer the medication in a baby bottle with 1oz. of water

246. An elderly client with glaucoma is scheduled for a cholecystectomy. Which medication order should the nurse question?

- ○ **A.** Meperidine
- ○ **B.** Cimetadine
- ○ **C.** Atropine
- ○ **D.** Promethazine

247. Which instruction would *not* be included in the discharge teaching of the client receiving chlorpromazine (Thorazine)?

- ○ **A.** "You will need to wear protective clothing or a sunscreen when you are outside."
- ○ **B.** "You will need to avoid eating aged cheese."
- ○ **C.** "You should carry hard candy with you to decrease dryness of the mouth."
- ○ **D.** "You should report a sore throat immediately."

248. An elderly client who experiences nighttime confusion wanders from his room into the room of another client. The nurse can best help with decreasing the client's confusion by:

- ○ **A.** Assigning a nursing assistant to sit with him until he falls asleep
- ○ **B.** Allowing the client to room with another elderly client
- ○ **C.** Administering a bedtime sedative
- ○ **D.** Leaving a nightlight on during the evening and night shifts

249. A 4-year-old is scheduled for a routine tonsillectomy. Which of the following lab findings should be reported to the doctor?

- ○ **A.** A hemoglobin of 12Gm
- ○ **B.** A platelet count of 200,000
- ○ **C.** A white blood cell count of 16,000
- ○ **D.** A urine specific gravity of 1.010

250. A client with psychotic depression is receiving haloperidol (Haldol). Which of the following adverse effects is associated with haloperidol?

- ○ **A.** Akathisia
- ○ **B.** Cataracts
- ○ **C.** Diaphoresis
- ○ **D.** Polyuria

Quick Check Answer Key

1. A	31. D	61. B
2. A	32. A	62. B
3. D	33. A	63. D
4. C	34. B	64. D
5. B	35. B	65. D
6. A	36. D	66. C
7. D	37. B	67. A
8. A	38. C	68. C
9. A	39. C	69. D
10. D	40. A	70. B
11. A	41. D	71. A
12. C	42. C	72. C
13. B	43. B	73. B
14. A	44. D	74. C
15. B	45. B	75. C
16. A	46. B	76. A
17. D	47. C	77. C
18. B	48. C	78. A
19. A	49. D	79. B
20. B	50. D	80. B
21. D	51. C	81. D
22. C	52. A	82. C
23. C	53. D	83. D
24. D	54. A	84. B
25. A	55. B	85. B
26. C	56. C	86. A
27. A	57. B	87. A
28. B	58. A	88. D
29. C	59. C	89. C
30. A	60. C	90. B

91. C	**123.** B	**155.** C
92. A	**124.** A	**156.** A
93. A	**125.** D	**157.** B
94. D	**126.** B	**158.** A
95. C	**127.** A	**159.** B
96. B	**128.** C	**160.** C
97. B	**129.** D	**161.** A
98. D	**130.** B	**162.** B
99. A	**131.** C	**163.** C
100. C	**132.** B	**164.** D
101. B	**133.** C	**165.** D
102. D	**134.** A	**166.** C
103. A	**135.** C	**167.** A
104. A	**136.** D	**168.** A
105. B	**137.** D	**169.** D
106. C	**138.** B	**170.** B
107. D	**139.** D	**171.** A
108. C	**140.** A	**172.** B
109. A	**141.** D	**173.** B
110. B	**142.** B	**174.** D
111. D	**143.** D	**175.** D
112. A	**144.** C	**176.** B
113. B	**145.** A	**177.** C
114. C	**146.** B	**178.** A
115. B	**147.** B	**179.** B
116. A	**148.** A	**180.** D
117. A	**149.** A	**181.** A
118. B	**150.** B	**182.** D
119. D	**151.** A	**183.** B
120. C	**152.** B	**184.** A
121. D	**153.** D	**185.** D
122. D	**154.** D	**186.** C

187. A	**209.** A	**231.** C
188. B	**210.** C	**232.** A
189. A	**211.** B	**233.** B
190. D	**212.** B	**234.** A
191. C	**213.** B	**235.** A
192. C	**214.** D	**236.** D
193. D	**215.** D	**237.** A
194. A	**216.** B	**238.** D
195. B	**217.** B	**239.** B
196. A	**218.** B	**240.** A
197. C	**219.** D	**241.** B
198. C	**220.** D	**242.** B
199. D	**221.** C	**243.** B
200. D	**222.** A	**244.** D
201. B	**223.** A	**245.** B
202. C	**224.** A	**246.** C
203. A	**225.** D	**247.** B
204. B	**226.** D	**248.** D
205. A	**227.** C	**249.** C
206. A	**228.** C	**250.** A
207. C	**229.** A	
208. B	**230.** A	

Answers and Rationales

1. **Answer A is correct.** The major complication of SLE is lupus nephritis, which results in end-stage renal disease. SLE affects the musculoskeletal, integumentary, renal, nervous, and cardiovascular systems, but the major complication is renal involvement; therefore, answers B and D are incorrect. Answer C is incorrect because the SLE produces a "butterfly" rash, not desquamation.

2. **Answer A is correct.** Finasteride is an androgen inhibitor; therefore, women who are pregnant or who might become pregnant should be told to avoid touching the tablets. Answer B is incorrect because there are no benefits to giving the medication with food. Answer C is incorrect because the medication can take 6 months to a year to be effective. Answer D is not an accurate statement; therefore, it is incorrect.

3. **Answer D is correct.** The nurse can expect to find the presence of Trendelenburg sign. (While bearing weight on the affected hip, the pelvis tilts downward on the unaffected side instead of tilting upward, as expected with normal stability). Scarf sign is a characteristic of the preterm newborn; therefore, answer A is incorrect. Harlequin sign can be found in normal newborns and indicates transient changes in circulation; therefore, answer B is incorrect. Answer C is incorrect because Cullen's sign is an indication of intra-abdominal bleeding.

4. **Answer C is correct.** A diet that is high in fat and refined carbohydrates increases the risk of colorectal cancer. High fat content results in an increase in fecal bile acids, which facilitate carcinogenic changes. Refined carbohydrates increase the transit time of food through the gastrointestinal tract and increase the exposure time of the intestinal mucosa to cancer-causing substances. Answers A, B, and D do not relate to the question; therefore, they are incorrect.

5. **Answer B is correct.** The nurse should avoid giving the infant a pacifier or bottle because sucking is not permitted. Holding the infant cradled in the arms, providing a mobile, and offering sterile water using a Breck feeder are permitted; therefore, answers A, C, and D are incorrect.

6. **Answer A is correct.** The client with asterixis or "flapping tremors" will have irregular flexion and extension of the wrists when the arms are extended and the wrist is hyperextended with the fingers separated. Asterixis is associated with hepatic encephalopathy. Answers B, C, and D do not relate to asterixis; therefore, they are incorrect.

7. **Answer D is correct.** The client with esophageal varices might develop spontaneous bleeding from the mechanical irritation caused by taking capsules; therefore, the nurse should request the medication in an alternative form such as a suspension. Answer A is incorrect because it does not best meet the client's needs. Answer B is incorrect because it is not the best means of preventing bleeding. Answer C is incorrect because the medications should not be given with milk or antacids.

8. **Answer A is correct.** Surgical repair of an inguinal hernia is recommended to prevent strangulation of the bowel, which could result in intestinal obstruction and necrosis. Answer B does not relate to an inguinal hernia; therefore, it is incorrect. Bile salts,

which are important to the digestion of fats, are produced by the liver, not the intestines; therefore, answer C is incorrect. Repair of the inguinal hernia will prevent swelling and obstruction associated with strangulation, but it will not increase intestinal motility; therefore, answer D is incorrect.

9. **Answer A is correct.** Tomatoes are a poor source of iron, although they are an excellent source of vitamin C, which increases iron absorption. Answers B, C, and D are good sources of iron; therefore, they are incorrect.

10. **Answer D is correct.** Serum amylase levels greater than 200 units/dL help confirm the diagnosis of acute pancreatitis. Elevations of blood glucose occur with conditions other than acute pancreatitis; therefore, answer A is incorrect. Elevations in WBC are associated with infection and are not specific to acute pancreatitis; therefore, answer B is incorrect. Answer C is within the normal range; therefore, it is incorrect.

11. **Answer A is correct.** Periodically lying in a prone position without a pillow will help prevent the flexion of the spine that occurs with Parkinson's disease. Answers B and C flex the spine; therefore, they are incorrect. Answer D is not realistic because position changes during sleep; therefore, it is incorrect.

12. **Answer C is correct.** The medication should be administered slowly (no more than 50mg per minute); otherwise, cardiac arrhythmias can occur. Answer A is incorrect because the medication must be given slowly. Dextrose solutions cause the medication to crystallize in the line and the medication should be given through a large vein to prevent "purple glove" syndrome; therefore, answers B and D are incorrect.

13. **Answer B is correct.** The client recovering from acute pancreatitis needs a diet that is high in calories and low in fat. Answers A, C, and D are incorrect because they can increase the client's discomfort.

14. **Answer A is correct.** The client with polycythemia vera has an abnormal increase in the number of circulating red blood cells that results in increased viscosity of the blood. Increases in blood pressure further tax the overworked heart. Answers B, C, and D do not directly relate to the condition; therefore, they are incorrect.

15. **Answer B is correct.** Dressing in extra layers of clothing will help decrease the feeling of being cold that is experienced by the client with hypothyroidism. Decreased sensation and decreased alertness are common in the client with hypothyroidism. The use of electric blankets and heating pads can result in burns, making answers A and C incorrect. Answer D is incorrect because the client with hypothyroidism has dry skin, and a hot bath morning and evening would make her condition worse.

16. **Answer A is correct.** An ICP of 17mmHg should be reported to the doctor because it is elevated. (The ICP normally ranges from 4mmHg to 10mmHg, with upper limits of 15mmHg.) Answer B is incorrect because the pressure is not normal. Answer C is incorrect because the pressure is not low. Answer D is incorrect because the ICP reading provides a more reliable measurement than the Glascow coma scale.

17. **Answer D is correct.** A history of frequent alcohol and tobacco use is the most significant factor in the development of cancer of the larynx. Answers A, B, and C are also factors in the development of laryngeal cancer but they are not the most significant; therefore, they are incorrect.

18. **Answer B is correct.** Numbness and tingling in the extremities is common in the client with pernicious anemia, but not those with other types of anemia. Answers A, C, and D are incorrect because they are symptoms of all types of anemia.

19. **Answer A is correct.** Lying prone and allowing the feet to hang over the end of the mattress will help prevent flexion contractures. The client should be told to do this several times a day. Answers B, C, and D do not help prevent flexion contractures; therefore, they are incorrect.

20. **Answer B is correct.** The client with echolalia will repeat words or phrases used by others. Answer A is incorrect because it refers to clang association. Answer C is incorrect because it refers to circumstantiality. Answer D is incorrect because it refers to neologisms.

21. **Answer D is correct.** The presence of fetal hemoglobin until about 6 months of age protects affected infants from episodes of sickling. Answer A is incorrect because it is an untrue statement. Answer B is incorrect because infants do have insensible fluid loss. Answer C is incorrect because respiratory infections such as bronchiolitis and otitis media can cause fever and dehydration, which cause sickle cell crisis.

22. **Answer C is correct.** The warmth from holding a cup of coffee or hot chocolate helps to relieve the pain and stiffness in the hands of the client with rheumatoid arthritis. Answers A, B, and D do not relieve the symptoms of rheumatoid arthritis; therefore, they are incorrect.

23. **Answer C is correct.** If the client's own blood type and Rh are not available, the safest transfusion is O negative blood. Answers A, B, and D are incorrect because they can cause reactions that can prove fatal to the client.

24. **Answer D is correct.** Narcan is a narcotic antagonist that blocks the effects of the client's pain medication; therefore, the client will experience sudden, intense pain. Answers A, B, and C do not relate to the client's condition and the administration of Narcan; therefore, they are incorrect.

25. **Answer A is correct.** The infant's birth weight should double by 6 months of age. Answers B, C, and D are incorrect because they are greater than the expected weight gain by 6 months of age.

26. **Answer C is correct.** The symptoms of nontropical sprue as well as those of celiac are caused by the ingestion of gluten, found in wheat, oats, barley, and rye. Creamed soup and crackers as well as some cold cuts contain gluten. Answers A, B, and D do not contain gluten; therefore, they are incorrect.

27. **Answer A is correct.** Lanoxin slows and strengthens the contraction of the heart. An increase in urinary output shows that the medication is having a desired effect by eliminating excess fluid from the body. Answer B is incorrect because the weight would decrease. Answer C is not related to the medication; therefore, it is incorrect. Answer D is incorrect because pedal edema would decrease, not increase.

28. **Answer B is correct.** The toddler has gross motor skills suited to playing with a ball, which can be kicked forward or thrown overhand. Answers A and C are incorrect because they require fine motor skills. Answer D is incorrect because the toddler lacks gross motor skills for play on the swing set.

29. **Answer C is correct.** Jitteriness and irritability are signs of alcohol withdrawal in the newborn. Answer A is incorrect because it would be associated with use more recent than 1 day ago. Answers B and D are characteristics of a newborn with fetal alcohol syndrome, but they are not a priority at this time; therefore, they are incorrect.

30. **Answer A is correct.** Antacids containing aluminum tend to cause constipation. Answers B, C, and D are not common side effects of the medication.

31. **Answer D is correct.** The client with an abdominal aortic aneurysm frequently complains of pulsations or feeling the heart beat in the abdomen. Answers A and C are incorrect because they are not associated with abdominal aortic aneurysm. Answer B is incorrect because back pain is not affected by changes in position.

32. **Answer A is correct.** The client with nephotic syndrome will be treated with immunosuppressive drugs. Limiting visitors will decrease the chance of infection. Answer B is incorrect because the client needs additional protein. Answer C is incorrect because dialysis is not indicated for the client with nephrotic syndrome. Answer D is incorrect because additional fluids are not needed until the client begins diuresis.

33. **Answer A is correct.** The client with acute adrenal crisis has symptoms of hypovolemia and shock; therefore, the blood pressure would be low. Answer B is incorrect because the pulse would be rapid and irregular. Answer C is incorrect because the skin would be cool and pale. Answer D is incorrect because the urinary output would be decreased.

34. **Answer B is correct.** Tenseness of the anterior fontanel indicates an increase in intracranial pressure. Answer A is incorrect because periorbital edema is not associated with meningitis. Answer C is incorrect because a positive Babinski reflex is normal in the infant. Answer D is incorrect because it relates to the preterm infant, not the infant with meningitis.

35. **Answer B is correct.** The client's priority nursing diagnosis is based on his risk for self-injury. Answers A, C, and D focus on the client's psychosocial needs, which do not take priority over physiological needs; therefore, they are incorrect.

36. **Answer D is correct.** The recommended dose ranges from 175mg to 350mg per day based on the infant's weight. The order as written calls for 400mg per day for an infant weighing 7kg; therefore, the nurse should check the order with the doctor before giving the medication. Answer A is incorrect because the dosage exceeds the recommended amount. Answers B and C are incorrect choices because they involve changing the doctor's order.

37. **Answer B is correct.** Bright red bleeding with many clots indicates arterial bleeding that requires surgical intervention. Answer A is within normal limits, answer C indicates venous bleeding, which can be managed by nursing intervention, and answer D does not indicate excessive need for pain management that requires the doctor's attention; therefore, they are incorrect.

38. **Answer C is correct.** The child will need additional fluids in summer to prevent dehydration that could lead to a sickle cell crises. Answer A is not a true statement; therefore, it is incorrect. Answer B is incorrect because the activity will create a greater oxygen demand and precipitate sickle cell crises. Answer D is not a true statement; therefore, it is incorrect.

39. **Answer C is correct.** The client should be assessed following completion of antibiotic therapy to determine whether the infection has cleared. Answer A would be done if there are repeated instances of otitis media, answer B is incorrect because it will not determine whether the child has completed the medication, and answer D is incorrect because the purpose of the recheck is to determine whether the infection is gone.

40. **Answer A is correct.** The child with Sydenham's chorea will exhibit irregular movements of the extremities, facial grimacing, and labile moods. Answer B is incorrect because it describes subcutaneous nodules. Answer C is incorrect because it describes erythema marginatum. Answer D is incorrect because it describes polymigratory arthritis.

41. **Answer D is correct.** The primary reason for placing a child with croup under a mist tent is to liquefy secretions and relieve laryngeal spasms. Answers A, B, and C are inaccurate statements; therefore, they are incorrect.

42. **Answer C is correct.** The recommended setting for performing tracheostomy suctioning on the adult client is 80–120mmHg. Answers A and B are incorrect because the amount of suction is too low. Answer D is incorrect because the amount of suction is excessive.

43. **Answer B is correct.** Symptoms of myxedema include weight gain, lethargy, slow speech, and decreased respirations. Answers A and D do not describe symptoms associated with myxedema; therefore, they are incorrect. Answer C describes symptoms associated with Graves's disease.

44. **Answer D is correct.** The contagious stage of varicella begins 24 hours before the onset of the rash and lasts until all the lesions are crusted. Answers A, B, and C are inaccurate regarding the time of contagion.

45. **Answer B is correct.** The child with cystic fibrosis has sweat concentrations of chloride greater than 60mEq/L. Answers A and C are incorrect because they refer to potassium concentrations that are not used in making a diagnosis of cystic fibrosis. Answer D is incorrect because the sweat concentration of chloride is too low to be diagnostic.

46. **Answer B is correct.** The nurse should question the order because administering a narcotic so close to the time of delivery can result in respiratory depression in the newborn. Answers A, C, and D are incorrect because giving the medication prior to or during delivery can cause respiratory depression in the newborn.

47. **Answer C is correct.** During concrete operations, the child's thought processes become more logical and coherent. Answers A, B, and D are incorrect because they describe other types of development: sensorimotor, intuitive, and formal.

48. **Answer C is correct.** Delusions of grandeur are associated with feelings of low self-esteem. Answer A is incorrect because reaction formation, a defense mechanism, is characterized by outward emotions that are the opposite of internal feelings. Answers B and D can cause an increase in the client's delusions but do not explain their purpose; therefore, they are incorrect.

49. **Answer D is correct.** According to Kohlberg, in the preconventional stage of development, the behavior of the preschool child is determined by the consequences of the behavior. Answers A, B, and C describe other stages of moral development; therefore, they are incorrect.

50. **Answer D is correct.** Respiratory stridor is a symptom of partial airway obstruction. Answers A, B, and C are expected with a tonsillectomy; therefore, they are incorrect.

51. **Answer C is correct.** Pain associated with duodenal ulcers is lessened if the client eats a meal or snack. Answer A is incorrect because it makes the pain worse. Answer B lessens the discomfort of dumping syndrome; therefore, it is incorrect. Answer D lessens the discomfort of gastroesophageal reflux; therefore, it is incorrect.

52. **Answer A is correct.** Diminished femoral pulses are a sign of coarctation of the aorta. Answers B, C, and D are found in normal newborns and are not associated with cardiac anomaly.

53. **Answer D is correct.** A severe complication associated with Kawasaki's disease is the development of a giant aneurysm. Answers A, B, and C are incorrect because they have no relationship to Kawasaki's disease.

54. **Answer A is correct.** A nosebleed in the client with mild preeclampsia may indicate that the client's blood pressure is elevated. Answers B, C, and D are incorrect because the client will not need strict bed rest, pedal edema is common in the client with preeclampsia, and the client does not need to avoid sodium, although the client should limit or avoid high-sodium foods.

55. **Answer B is correct.** The client taking an MAO inhibitor should avoid over-the-counter medications for colds and hayfever because many contain pseudoephedrine. Combining an MAO inhibitor with pseudoephedrine can result in extreme elevations in blood pressure. Answer A is incorrect because it refers to the client taking an antipsychotic medication such as Thorazine. Answer C is not specific to the client taking an MAO inhibitor and answer D does not apply to the question.

56. **Answer C is correct.** Foods containing rice or millet are permitted in the diet of the client with celiac disease. Answers A, B, and D are not permitted because they contain gluten, which exacerbates the symptoms of celiac disease; therefore, they are incorrect.

57. **Answer B is correct.** Increased thirst and increased urination are signs of lithium toxicity. Answers A and D are not associated with the use of lithium; therefore, they are incorrect. Answer C is an expected side effect of the medication; therefore, it is incorrect.

58. **Answer A is correct.** During dehydration, the kidneys compensate for electrolyte imbalance by retaining potassium. The nurse should check for urinary output before adding potassium to the IV fluid. Answer B is incorrect because it measures respiratory compensation caused by dehydration. Answers C and D do not apply to the use of intravenous fluid with potassium; therefore, they are incorrect.

59. **Answer C is correct.** The immunization protects the child against diphtheria, pertussis, tetanus, and *H. influenza b.* Answer A is incorrect because a second injection is given before 4 years of age. Answer B is not a true statement and answer D is not a one-time injection, nor does it protect against measles, mumps, rubella, or varicella.

60. **Answer C is correct.** A weight gain of 6 pounds in a week in the client taking glucocorticoids indicates that the dosage should be modified. Answers A and B are not specific to the question; therefore, they are incorrect. Answer D is an expected side effect of the medication; therefore, it is incorrect.

61. **Answer B is correct.** Assessing fetal heart tones reveals whether fetal distress occurred with rupture of the membranes. Answers A, C, and D are later interventions; therefore, they are incorrect.

62. **Answer B is correct.** Synthroid (levothyroxine) increases metabolic rate and cardiac output. Adverse reactions include tachycardia and dysrhythmias; therefore, the client should be taught to check her heart rate before taking the medication. Answer A is incorrect because the client does not have to take the medication after breakfast. Answer C does not relate to the medication; therefore, it is incorrect. The medication should not be stopped because of gastric upset; therefore, Answer D is incorrect.

63. **Answer D is correct.** The nurse should wear a special badge when taking care of the client with a radioactive implant, to measure the amount of time spent in the room. The nurse should limit the time of radiation exposure; therefore, answer A is incorrect. Standing at the foot of the bed of a client with a radioactive cervical implant increases the nurse's exposure to radiation; therefore, answer B is incorrect. The nurse does not have to avoid handling items used by the client; therefore, answer C is incorrect.

64. **Answer D is correct.** The milkshake will provide needed calories and nutrients for the client with mania. Answers A, B, and C are incorrect choices because they do not provide as many calories or nutrients as the milkshake.

65. **Answer D is correct.** The maximal effects from tricyclic antidepressants might not be achieved for up to 6 months after the medication is started. Answers A and B are incorrect because the time for maximal effects is too brief. Answer C is incorrect because it refers to the initial symptomatic relief rather than maximal effects.

66. **Answer C is correct.** Beta blockers such as timolol (Timoptic) can cause bronchospasms in the client with chronic obstructive lung disease. Timoptic is not contraindicated for use in the client with diabetes, gastric ulcers, or pancreatitis; therefore, answers A, B, and D are incorrect.

67. **Answer A is correct.** The child with intussusception has stools that contain blood and mucus, which are described as "currant jelly" stools. Answer B is a symptom of pyloric stenosis; therefore, it is incorrect. Answer C is a symptom of Hirschsprungs; therefore, it is incorrect. Answer D is a symptom of Wilms tumor; therefore, it is incorrect.

68. **Answer C is correct.** The infant with biliary atresia has abdominal distention, poor weight gain, and clay-colored stools. Answers A, B, and D do describe the symptoms associated with biliary atresia; therefore, they are incorrect.

69. **Answer D is correct.** The nurse should not use water, soap, or lotion on the area marked for radiation therapy. Answer A is incorrect because it would remove the marking. Answers B and C are not necessary for the client receiving radiation; therefore, they are incorrect.

70. **Answer B is correct.** Blood alcohol concentrations of 400–600mg/dL are associated with respiratory depression, coma, and death. Answer A occurs with blood alcohol concentrations of 50mg/dL, which affects coordination and speech but does not cause respiratory depression; therefore, it is incorrect. Answers C and D are associated with alcohol withdrawal, not overdose; therefore, they are incorrect.

71. **Answer A is correct.** Following a hypophysectomy, the nurse should check the client's blood sugar because insulin levels may rise rapidly resulting in hypoglycemia. Answer B is incorrect because suctioning should be avoided. Answer C is incorrect because the client's head should be elevated to reduce pressure on the operative site. Answer D is incorrect because coughing increases pressure on the operative site that can lead to a leak of cerebral spinal fluid.

72. **Answer C is correct.** Acarbose is to be taken with the first bite of a meal. Answers A, B, and D are incorrect because they specify the wrong schedule for taking the medication.

73. **Answer B is correct.** The client going for therapy in the hyperbaric oxygen chamber requires no special skin care; therefore, washing the skin with water and patting it dry are suitable. Lotions, petroleum products, perfumes, and occlusive dressings interfere with oxygenation of the skin; therefore, answers A, C, and D are incorrect.

74. **Answer C is correct.** Diabetes insipidus is characterized by excessive production of dilute urine. A decline in urinary output shows that the medication is having its intended effect. Answers A and D do not relate to the question; therefore, they are incorrect. Answer B refers to diabetes mellitus; therefore, it is incorrect.

75. **Answer C is correct.** Positioning the client on her left side will take pressure off the vena cava and allow better oxygenation of the fetus. Answers A and B do not relieve pressure on the vena cava; therefore, they are incorrect. Answer D is the preferred position for the client with a prolapsed cord; therefore, it is incorrect for this situation.

76. **Answer A is correct.** Prothrombin time measures the therapeutic level of Coumadin. Answer B is incorrect because it measures the quantity of each specific clotting factor. Answer C is incorrect because it measures the therapeutic level of heparin. Answer D is incorrect because it evaluates the vascular and platelet factors associated with hemostasis.

77. **Answer C is correct.** Accutane is made from concentrated vitamin A, a fat-soluble vitamin. Fat-soluble vitamins have the potential of being hepatotoxic, so a liver panel is needed. Answers A, B, and D do not relate to therapy with Accutane; therefore, they are incorrect.

78. **Answer A is correct.** The client's WBC is only slightly elevated and is most likely due to the birth process. Answer B is incorrect because the WBC would be more elevated if an acute bacterial infection was present. Answer C is incorrect because viral infections usually do not cause elevations in WBC. Answer D is incorrect because dehydration is not reflected by changes in the WBC.

79. **Answer B is correct.** PKU screening is usually done on the third day of life. Answer A is incorrect because the baby will not have had sufficient time to ingest protein sources of phenylalanine. Answer C is incorrect because blood is obtained from a heel stick, not from cord blood. Answer D is incorrect because the first immunizations are done at 6 weeks of age, and by that time, brain damage will already have occurred if the baby has PKU.

80. **Answer B is correct.** The client's blood gases indicate respiratory alkalosis. Answers A, C, and D are not reflected by the client's blood gases or present condition; therefore, they are incorrect.

81. **Answer D is correct.** Cor pulmonale, or right-sided heart failure, is characterized by edema of the legs and feet, enlarged liver, and distended neck veins. Answer A is incorrect because the symptoms are those of left-sided heart failure and pulmonary edema. Answer B is not specific to the question; therefore, it is incorrect. Answer C is incorrect because it does not relate to cor pulmonale.

82. **Answer C is correct.** The primary reason for the NG to is to allow for nourishment without contamination of the suture line. Answer A is not a true statement; therefore, it is incorrect. Answer B is incorrect because there is no mention of suction. Answer D is incorrect because the oral mucosa was not involved in the laryngectomy.

83. **Answer D is correct.** The client's complaints are due to swelling associated with surgery and catheter placement. Answer A is incorrect because it will not relieve the client's symptoms of pain and dribbling. Answer B is incorrect because perineal exercises will not help relieve the post-operative pain. Answer C is incorrect because the client's complaints do not indicate the need for catheter reinsertion.

84. **Answer B is correct.** The chest-drainage system can be disconnected from suction, but the chest tube should remain unclamped to prevent a tension pneumothorax. Answer A is incorrect because it could result in a tension pneumothorax. Answer C is not a true statement; therefore, it is not correct. Answer D is incorrect because the chest-drainage system should be kept lower than the client's chest and shoulders.

85. **Answer B is correct.** Cardiac dysrhythmias are the most common complication for the client with a myocardial infarction. Answers A and C do not relate to myocardial infarction; therefore, they are incorrect. Answer D is incorrect because it is not the most common complication following a myocardial infarction.

86. **Answer A is correct.** Elevations in temperature increase the cardiac output. Answer B is incorrect because temperature elevations are not associated with cardiac tamponade. Answer C is incorrect because temperature elevation does not decrease cardiac output. Answer D is incorrect because elevations in temperature in the client with a coronary artery bypass graft indicate inflammation, not necessarily graft rejection.

87. **Answer A is correct.** The client with expressive aphasia has trouble forming words that are understandable. Answer B is incorrect because it describes receptive aphasia. Answer C refers to apraxia and answer D refers to agnosia, so they are incorrect.

88. **Answer D is correct.** The client taking MAOI, including Parnate, should avoid eating aged cheeses, such as cheddar cheese, because a hypertensive crisis can result. Answer A is incorrect because processed cheese is less likely to produce a hypertensive crisis. Answers B and C do not cause a hypertensive crisis in the client taking an MAOI; therefore, they are incorrect.

89. **Answer C is correct.** The client with rheumatoid arthritis needs to continue moving affected joints within the limits of pain. Answer A and D are incorrect because they will increase stiffness and joint disuse. Answer B is incorrect because, if done correctly, passive range-of-motion exercises will improve the use of affected joints.

90. **Answer B is correct.** Exposed abdominal visera should be covered with a sterile saline-soaked gauze, and the doctor should be notified immediately. Answer A is incorrect because the dressing should be sterile, not clean. Answer C is incorrect because attempting to replace abdominal contents can cause greater injury and should be done only surgically. Answer D is incorrect because the area is kept moist only with sterile normal saline.

91. **Answer C is correct.** Using the ABCD approach to the client with multiple trauma the nurse in the ER would: establish an airway, determine whether the client is breathing, check circulation (control hemorrhage), and check for deficits (head injuries). Answers A, B, and D are incorrect because they are not in the appropriate sequence for maintaining life.

92. **Answer A is correct.** Stimulant medications such as Ritalin tend to cause anorexia and weight loss in some children with ADHD. Providing high-calorie snacks will help the child maintain an appropriate weight. Answer B is incorrect because the medication does not mask infection. Answer C is incorrect because the medication is a central nervous system stimulant, not a depressant. Answer D has no relationship to the medication; therefore, it is incorrect.

93. **Answer A is correct.** The most likely victim of elder abuse is the elderly female with a chronic, debilitating illness. Answers B, C, and D are less likely to be victims of elder abuse; therefore, they are incorrect.

94. **Answer D is correct.** Sunscreens of at least an SPF of 15 should be applied 20–30 minutes before going into the sun. Answers A, B, and C are incorrect because they do not allow sufficient time for sun protection.

95. **Answer C is correct.** Retinal hemorrhages are characteristically found in the child who has been violently shaken. Answers A, B, and D may result from trauma other than that related to abuse; therefore, they are incorrect.

96. **Answer B is correct.** The combination of the two medications produces a synergistic effect (an effect greater than that of either drug used alone). Agonist effects are similar to those produced by chemicals normally present in the body; therefore, answer A is incorrect. Antagonist effects are those in which the actions of the drugs oppose one another; therefore, answer C is incorrect. Answer D is incorrect because the drugs would have a combined depressing, not excitatory effect.

97. **Answer B is correct.** The client with a history of diabetes is most likely to deliver a preterm large for gestational age newborn. These newborns often lack sufficient surfactant levels to prevent respiratory distress syndrome. Answers A, C, and D are less likely to have newborns with respiratory distress syndrome so they are incorrect choices.

98. **Answer D is correct.** Nursing care of the client with cervical tongs includes performance of sterile pin care and assessment of the site. Answers A, B, and C alter the traction and could result in serious injury or death of the client; therefore, they are incorrect.

99. **Answer A is correct.** Chest drainage greater than 100mL per hour is excessive, and the doctor should be notified regarding possible hemorrhage. Confusion and restlessness could be in response to pain, changes in oxygenation, or the emergence from anesthesia; therefore, answer B is incorrect. Answer C is incorrect because it is an expected finding in the client recently returning from a CABG. Answer D is within normal limits; therefore, it is incorrect.

100. **Answer C is correct.** The medication should be withheld and the doctor should be notified. Answers A, B, and D are incorrect because they do not provide for the client's safety.

101. **Answer B is correct.** Solid foods should be added to the diet one at a time, with intervals of 4–7 days between new foods. The extrusion reflex fades at 3–4 months of age; therefore, answer A is incorrect. Answer C is incorrect because solids should not be added to the bottle and the use of infant feeders is discouraged. Answer D is incorrect because the first food added to the infant's diet is rice cereal.

102. **Answer D is correct.** At 32 weeks gestation the fetus can be expected to be active. Answers A, B, and C are not typical findings during the Leopold maneuver of a client who is 32 weeks gestation; therefore, they are incorrect.

103. **Answer A is correct.** The client needs to avoid using sweeteners containing aspartame. Answers B, C, and D indicate that the client understands the nurse's teaching; therefore, they are incorrect.

104. **Answer A is correct.** The treatment of galactosemia consists of eliminating all milk and lactose-containing foods, including breast milk. Answers B and D contain inaccurate information; therefore, they are incorrect. Galactosemia is inherited as an autosomal recessive disorder. There is a one-in-four chance that future children will be affected; therefore, answer C is incorrect.

105. **Answer B is correct.** The child with Tay Sachs disease has cherry-red spots on the macula of the eye. Answer A is incorrect because it is associated with anemia. Answer C is incorrect because it is associated with osteogenesis imperfecta. Answer D is incorrect because it is associated with Down syndrome.

106. **Answer C is correct.** The client's symptoms suggest an adverse reaction to the medication known as neuroleptic malignant syndrome. Answers A, B, and D are not appropriate interventions for the client; therefore, they are incorrect.

107. **Answer D is correct.** The client with HIV should adhere to a low-bacteria diet by avoiding raw fruits and vegetables. Answers A, B, and C are incorrect because they are permitted in the client's diet.

108. **Answer C is correct.** The child with leukemia has low platelet counts, which contribute to spontaneous bleeding. Answers A, B, and D, common in the child with leukemia, are not life-threatening.

109. **Answer A is correct.** The nurse should prevent the infant with atopic dermatitis (eczema) from scratching, which can lead to skin infections. Answer B is incorrect because fever is not associated with atopic dermatitis. Answers C and D are incorrect because they increase dryness of the skin, which worsens the symptoms of atopic dermatitis.

110. **Answer B is correct.** Pavulon is a neuromuscular blocking agent that paralyzes skeletal muscles, making it impossible for the client to fight the ventilator. Sublimaze is an analgesic used to control operative pain; therefore, answer A is incorrect. Versed is a benzodiazepine used to produce conscious sedation; therefore, answer C is incorrect. Answer D is wrong because Atarax is used to treat post-operative nausea.

111. **Answer D is correct.** Symptoms associated with diverticulitis are usually reported after eating foods like popcorn, celery, raw vegetables, whole grains, and nuts. Answers A, B, and C are incorrect because they are allowed in the diet of the client with diverticulitis.

112. **Answer A is correct.** The client with Paget's disease has problems with mobility. Keeping the environment free of clutter will help prevent falls. Answers B, C, and D will improve the client's overall health but are not specific to Paget's disease; therefore, they are incorrect.

113. **Answer B is correct.** The Whipple procedure is performed for cancer located in the head of the pancreas. Answers A, C, and D are not correct because of the location of the cancer.

114. **Answer C is correct.** Side effects of Pulmozyme include sore throat, hoarseness, and laryngitis. Answers A, B, and D are not associated with Pulmozyme; therefore, they are incorrect.

115. **Answer B is correct.** Retained placental fragments are the major cause of late postpartal hemorrhage. Uterine atony is the major cause of early postpartal hemorrhage; therefore, answer A is incorrect. Answers C and D result in slow, steady bleeding; therefore, they are incorrect.

116. **Answer A is correct.** The nurse has a legal responsibility to report suspected abuse and neglect. The nurse does not have the authority to remove the children from the home; therefore, answers B and C are incorrect. Answer D is incorrect because it is unrealistic.

117. **Answer A is correct.** Providing a caring attitude and supportive environment will make the client feel safe. Answer B is incorrect because the client needs to feel free to express anger. Answer C is incorrect because it will increase the client's anxiety. Answer D is incorrect because it is not the most important aspect of care for the client with PTSD.

118. **Answer B is correct.** The nurse should be concerned with alleviating the client's pain. Answers A, C, and D are not primary objectives in the care of the client receiving an opiate analgesic; therefore, they are incorrect.

119. **Answer D is correct.** The therapeutic range for aminophylline is 10–20 micrograms/mL. Levels greater than 20 micrograms/mL can produce signs of toxicity. Answer A is incorrect because it is too low to be therapeutic. Answers B and C are within the therapeutic range; therefore, they are incorrect.

120. **Answer C is correct.** Changes in breath sounds are the best indication of the need for suctioning in the client with ineffective airway clearance. Answers A, B, and D are incorrect because they can be altered by other conditions.

121. **Answer D is correct.** An adverse reaction to Myambutol is changes in visual acuity or color vision. Answer A is incorrect because it does not relate to the medication. Answer B is incorrect because it is an adverse reaction to Streptomycin. Answer C is incorrect because it is a side effect of Rifampin.

122. **Answer D is correct.** Insufficient erythropoietin production is the primary cause of anemia in the client with chronic renal failure. Answers A, B, and C do not relate to the anemia seen in clients with chronic renal failure; therefore, they are incorrect.

123. **Answer B is correct.** The nurse's highest priority should be asking the client about allergies to shellfish and iodine. The contrast media used during an intravenous pyelogram contains iodine, which can result in an anaphylactic reaction. Answers A, C, and D do not relate specifically to the test; therefore, they are incorrect.

124. **Answer A is correct.** Ataxia affects the client's mobility, making falls more likely. Answers B, C, and D are incorrect because they do not relate to the problem of ataxia.

125. **Answer D is correct.** Aspirin decreases platelet aggregation or clumping, thereby preventing clots. Answer A is incorrect because the low-dose aspirin will not prevent headaches. Answers B and C are untrue statements; therefore, they are incorrect.

126. **Answer B is correct.** Insulin molecules adhere to glass and plastic; therefore, the IV set and entire tubing should be flushed and 50mL discarded before administering the infusion to the client. Answers A and D are incorrect because insulin is mixed using 0.9% or 0.45% normal saline. Answer C is incorrect because the infusion is given using a pump or controller.

127. **Answer A is correct.** A serologic marker of HB8 AG that is present 6 months after acute infection with hepatitis B indicates that the client is a carrier or has chronic hepatitis. Answer B is incorrect because the HB8 AG would normally decline and disappear. Answer C is incorrect because the client can still be infected with hepatitis C. Answer D is incorrect because the client is a carrier.

128. **Answer C is correct.** The usual course of treatment using combined therapy with isoniazid and rifampin is 6 months. Answers A and D are incorrect because the treatment time is too brief. Answer B is incorrect because the medication is not needed for life.

129. **Answer D is correct.** At 4 months of age, the infant can roll over, which makes it vulnerable to falls from dressing tables or beds without rails. Answer A is incorrect because it does not prove a threat to safety. Answers B and C are incorrect choices because the 4-month-old is not capable of crawling or standing.

130. **Answer B is correct.** Rhinitis, maculopapular rash, and hepatosplenomegaly are associated with congenital syphilis. Answer A is incorrect because it describes symptoms of scarlet fever. Answer C is incorrect because it describes symptoms of Fifth's disease. Answer D is incorrect because it describes the symptoms of Down syndrome.

131. **Answer C is correct.** It is recommended that infants up to 20 pounds be restrained in a car seat in a semireclining position facing the rear of the car. Answers A and B are incorrect because the child is young enough to require the rear-facing position. Answer D is incorrect because the child can be placed in an upright position in an approved safety seat facing forward.

132. **Answer B is correct.** The client with irritable bowel syndrome has bouts of constipation and diarrhea. Answer A is incorrect because it describes changes associated with diverticulosis. Answer C is incorrect because it describes changes associated with Crohn's disease. Answer D is incorrect because it describes findings associated with ulcerative colitis.

133. **Answer C is correct.** Adverse side effects of Dilantin include agranulocytosis and aplastic anemia; therefore, the client will need regularly scheduled blood work. Answer A is incorrect because the medication does not cause dental staining. Answer B is incorrect because the medication does not interfere with the metabolism of carbohydrates. Answer D is incorrect because the medication does not cause drowsiness.

134. **Answer A is correct.** The infant with hypospadias should not be circumcised because the foreskin is used in reconstruction. Answers B and C are incorrect because surgical correction is done when the infant is 16 to 18 months of age. Answer D is incorrect because the infant with hypospadias should not be circumcised.

135. **Answer C is correct.** Coconut oil is high in saturated fat and is not appropriate for the client on a low-cholesterol diet. Answers A, B, and D are incorrect because they are suggested for the client with elevated cholesterol levels.

136. **Answer D is correct.** Increased blood pressure following a renal transplant is an early sign of transplant failure. Answers A, B, and C are expected with successful renal transplant; therefore, they are incorrect.

137. **Answer D is correct.** The time it takes for alcohol to be fully metabolized is calculated by dividing the blood alcohol level on admission by 20mg/dL (amount metabolized in an hour). Answers A, B, and C are incorrect because there has not been sufficient time for the alcohol to be fully metabolized.

138. **Answer B is correct.** In stage III of Alzheimer's disease, the client develops agnosia, or failure to recognize familiar objects. Answer A is incorrect because it appears in stage I. Answer C is incorrect because it appears in stage II. Answer D is incorrect because it appears in stage IV.

139. **Answer D is correct.** The client taking steroid medication should receive an annual influenza vaccine. Answer A is incorrect because the medication should be taken with food. Answer B is incorrect because increased appetite and weight gain are expected side effects of the medication. Answer C is incorrect because wearing sunglasses will not prevent the development of cataracts in the client taking steroids.

140. **Answer A is correct.** The client with an above-the-knee amputation should be placed in a prone position 15–30 minutes twice a day to prevent contractures. Answers B and D are incorrect choices because elevation of the extremity one day post amputation promotes the development of contractures. Use of a trochanter roll will prevent rotation of the extremity but will not prevent contracture; therefore, answer C is incorrect.

141. **Answer D is correct.** All 20 primary, or deciduous, teeth should be present by age 30 months. Answers A, B, and C are incorrect because the ages are wrong.

142. **Answer B is correct.** Displacement of the esophageal balloon is the most likely cause of respiratory distress in the client with an esophageal tamponade. The nurse should deflate both the gastric and esophageal balloons before removing the tube. Answers A and C are incorrect because applying nasal oxygen and elevating the head will not relieve airway obstruction. Answer D is incorrect because it would cause further obstruction of the airway.

143. **Answer D is correct.** The mitral valve is heard loudest at the fourth intercostal space midclavicular line, which is the apex of the heart. Answer A is incorrect because it is the location for the aortic valve. Answer B is incorrect because it is the location for the pulmonic valve. Answer C is wrong because it is the location for the tricuspid valve.

144. **Answer C is correct.** The radioactive implant should be picked up with tongs and returned to the lead-lined container. Answer A is incorrect because radioactive materials are placed in lead-lined containers, not plastic ones, and they are returned to the radiation department, not the lab. Answer B is incorrect because the client should not touch the implant or try to reinsert it. Answer D is incorrect because the implant should not be placed in the commode for disposal.

145. **Answer A is correct.** Following a laparoscopic cholecystectomy, the client should avoid a tub bath for 48 hours. Answer B is incorrect because the stools should not be clay colored. Answer C is incorrect because pain is usually located in the shoulders. Answer D is incorrect because pain in the back and shoulders is expected following laparoscopic surgery.

146. **Answer B is correct.** The client recovering from mononeucleosis should avoid contact sports and other activities that could result in injury or rupture of the spleen. Answer A is incorrect because the client does not need additional fluids. Hypoglycemia is not associated with mononeucleosis; therefore, answer C is incorrect. Answer D is incorrect because antibiotics are not usually indicated in the treatment of mononeucleosis.

147. **Answer B is correct.** Pancreatic enzyme replacement is given with meals and snacks. Answers A, C, and D do not specify a relationship to meals; therefore, they are incorrect.

148. **Answer A is correct.** Meat, eggs, and dairy products are good sources of vitamin B12. Answer B is incorrect because peanut butter, raisins, and molasses are good sources of iron. Answer C is incorrect because broccoli, cauliflower, and cabbage are good sources of vitamin K. Answer D is incorrect because shrimp, legumes, and bran cereals are good sources of magnesium.

149. **Answer A is correct.** The client's aerobic workout should be 20–30 minutes long three times a week. Answers B, C, and D exceed the recommended time for the client beginning an aerobic program; therefore, they are incorrect.

150. **Answer B is correct.** Demadex is a loop diuretic that depletes potassium. Answers A, C, and D are incorrect because they are potassium-sparing diuretics.

151. **Answer A is correct.** Following a total mastectomy, the client's right arm should be elevated on pillows to facilitate lymph drainage. Answers B, C, and D are incorrect because they would not help facilitate lymph drainage and would create increased edema in the affected extremity.

152. **Answer B is correct.** Nitroglycerin is used to dilate coronary blood vessels, which provides improved circulation to the myocardium. Answers A, C, and D describe the effects of digoxin, not nitroglycerin; therefore, they are incorrect.

153. **Answer D is correct.** The client with flail chest will exhibit paradoxical respirations. (With inspiration, the affected side will move inward; with expiration, the affected side will move outward. Flail chest is frequently associated with high-speed motor vehicle accidents.) Answer A is incorrect because air or blood would be present in the thoracic cavity. Answer B is incorrect because the trachea would be shifted to the affected side. Answer C is incorrect because interstitial edema would be present.

154. **Answer D is correct.** Absence seizures, formerly known as petit mal seizures, are characterized by brief lapses in consciousness accompanied by rapid eye blinking, lip smacking, and minor myoclonus of the upper extremities. Answer A refers to myoclonic seizure; therefore, it is incorrect. Answer B refers to tonic clonic, formerly known as grand mal seizures; therefore, it is incorrect. Answer C refers to atonic seizures; therefore, it is incorrect.

155. **Answer C is correct.** Keeping the room quiet and the lights dimmed will decrease sensory stimulation and help keep the client oriented during withdrawal from alcohol. Answer A is incorrect because darkness would increase confusion and disorientation in the client during withdrawal. Answers B and D are incorrect because they can contribute to the development of seizures.

156. **Answer A is correct.** A side effect of antipsychotic medication is the development of Parkinsonian symptoms. Answers B and C are incorrect choices because they are used to reverse Parkinsonian symptoms in the client taking antipsychotic medication. Answer D is incorrect because the medication is an anticonvulsant used to stabilize mood. Parkinsonian symptoms are not associated with anticonvulsant medication.

157. **Answer B is correct.** Exercises, such as swimming, that provide light passive resistance are best for the child with juvenile rheumatoid arthritis. Answers A and C require movement of the hands and fingers that could be too painful for the child with juvenile rheumatoid arthritis; therefore, they are incorrect. Answer D is incorrect because it requires the use of larger joints affected by the disease.

158. **Answer A is correct.** Reports of cough and fever in the client with AIDS suggest infection with pneumocystis carinii, which requires immediate intervention. Answers B, C, and D have conditions with more predictable outcomes; therefore, they are incorrect.

159. **Answer B is correct.** The client's diabetes is well under control. Answer A is incorrect because it will lead to elevated glucose levels. Answer C is incorrect because the diet and insulin dose are appropriate for the client. Answer D is incorrect because the desired range for glycosylated hemoglobin in the adult client is 2.5%–5.9%.

160. **Answer C is correct.** The purpose of the dexamethasone-suppression test is to identify clients who will benefit from therapy with antidepressants and electroconvulsive therapy rather than psychological or social interventions. Answers A, B, and D contain inaccurate statements; therefore, they are incorrect.

161. **Answer A is correct.** Stadol reduces the perception of pain, which allows the post-operative client to rest. Answers B and C are not affected by the medication; therefore, they are incorrect. Relief of pain generally results in less nausea, but it is not the intended effect of the medication; therefore, answer D is incorrect.

162. **Answer B is correct.** Children with cystic fibrosis are susceptible to chronic sinusitis and nasal polyps, which might require surgical removal. Answer A is incorrect because it is a congenital condition in which there is a bony obstruction between the nares and the pharynx. Answers C and D are not specific to the child with cystic fibrosis; therefore, they are incorrect.

163. **Answer C is correct.** During the emergent phase, the nursing priority for a client with burns confined to the lower body would focus on the risk for fluid volume deficit. Answers A and B are incorrect because there is no indication that the airway is involved. Answer D is incorrect because pain does not take priority over the management of hypovolemia.

164. **Answer D is correct.** Lipid-lowering agents are contraindicated in the client with active liver disease. Answers A, B, and C are incorrect because they are not contraindicated in the client with active liver disease.

165. **Answer D is correct.** An appropriate activity for the client who has recently had an MI is sitting on the side of the bed for 5 minutes three times a day with assistance. Answers A and C are incorrect because they increase the workload on the heart too soon after the MI. Answer B is incorrect because it does not allow the client enough activity.

166. **Answer C is correct.** The client with hypertension should be placed on a low sodium, low cholesterol, high fiber diet. Oatmeal is low in sodium and high in fiber. Answer A is incorrect because cornflakes and whole milk are higher in sodium and are poor sources of fiber. Answers B and D are incorrect choices because they contain animal proteins that are high in both cholesterol and sodium.

167. **Answer A is correct.** Following hypospadias repair, the child will need to avoid straddle toys, such as a rocking horse, until allowed by the surgeon. Answers B, C, and D do not relate to the post-operative care of the child with hypospadias; therefore, they are incorrect.

168. **Answer A is correct.** Eating carbohydrates such as dry crackers or toast before arising helps to alleviate morning sickness. Answer B is incorrect because the additional fat might increase the client's nausea. Answer C is incorrect because the client does not need to skip meals. Answer D is the treatment of hypoglycemia, not morning sickness; therefore, it is incorrect.

169. **Answer D is correct.** An esophageal tamponade is used to control bleeding in the client with esophageal varices. Answers A, B, and C are incorrect because they can be assigned to either the novice RN or the LPN with assisted care by the nursing assistant.

170. **Answer B is correct.** The modified Blalock Taussig procedure is a palliative procedure in which the subclavian artery is joined to the pulmonary artery, thus allowing more blood to reach the lungs. Answers A, C, and D contain inaccurate statements; therefore, they are incorrect.

171. **Answer A is correct.** The stethoscope should be left in the client's room for future use. The stethoscope should not be returned to the exam room or the nurse's station; therefore, answers B and D are incorrect. The stethoscope should not be used to assess other clients; therefore, answer C is incorrect.

172. **Answer B is correct.** The medication will be needed throughout the child's lifetime. Answers A, C, and D contain inaccurate statements; therefore, they are incorrect.

173. **Answer B is correct.** Glucotrol XL is given once a day with breakfast. Answer A is incorrect because the client would develop hypoglycemia while sleeping. Answers C and D are incorrect choices because the client would develop hypoglycemia later in the day or evening.

174. **Answer D is correct.** The client with myasthenia develops progressive weakness that worsens during the day. Answer A is incorrect because it refers to symptoms of multiple sclerosis. Answer B is incorrect because it refers to symptoms of Guillain Barre syndrome. Answer C is incorrect because it refers to Parkinson's disease.

175. **Answer D is correct.** Immaturity of the kidneys places the preterm infant at greater risk for toxicity to aminoglycosides. Answers A, B, and C are true regarding the preterm infant, but they do not increase the risk for toxicity to the drug; therefore, they are incorrect.

176. **Answer B is correct.** To prevent fractures, the parents should lift the infant by the buttocks rather than the ankles when diapering. Answer A is incorrect because infants with osteogenesis imperfecta have normal calcium and phosphorus levels. Answer C is incorrect because the condition is not temporary. Answer D is incorrect because the teeth and the sclera are also affected.

177. **Answer C is correct.** Following a hip replacement, the client should avoid hip flexion. Sitting on a soft, low sofa permits hip flexion and increases the difficulty of standing. Having a pet is important to the client's emotional well-being; therefore, answer A is incorrect. Answers B and D indicate that the nurse's teaching has been effective; therefore, they are incorrect.

178. **Answer A is correct.** Withholding oral intake will help stop the inflammatory process by reducing the secretion of pancreatic enzymes. Answer B is incorrect because the client requires exogenous insulin. Answer C is incorrect because it does not prevent the secretion of gastric acid. Answer D is incorrect because it does not eliminate the need for pain medication.

179. **Answer B is correct.** A rigid or boardlike abdomen is suggestive of peritonitis, which is a complication of diverticulitis. Answers A, C, and D are common findings in diverticulitis; therefore, they are incorrect.

180. **Answer D is correct.** Vancomycin should be administered slowly to prevent "redman" syndrome. Answer A is incorrect because the medication is not given IV push. Answers B and C are incorrect choices because they allow the medication to be given too rapidly.

181. **Answer A is correct.** Protigmine is used to treat clients with myasthenia gravis. Answer B is incorrect because it is used to reverse the effects of neostigmine. Answer C is incorrect because the drug is unrelated to the treatment of myasthenia gravis. Answer D is incorrect because it is the test for myasthenia gravis.

182. **Answer D is correct.** The suggested diet for the client with AIDS is one that is high calorie, high protein, and low fat. Clients with AIDS have a reduced tolerance to fat because of the disease, as well as side effects from some antiviral medications; therefore, answers A and C are incorrect. Answer B is incorrect because the client needs a high-protein diet.

183. **Answer B is correct.** The nurse can help ready the child with cerebral palsy for speech therapy by providing activities that help the child develop tongue control. Most children with cerebral palsy have visual and auditory difficulties that require glasses or hearing devices rather than rehabilitative training; therefore, answers A and C are incorrect. Answer D is incorrect because video games are not appropriate to the age or developmental level for the child with cerebral palsy.

184. **Answer A is correct.** The client with duodenal ulcers commonly complains of epigastric pain that is relieved by eating a meal or snack. Answer B is incorrect because the client with a duodenal ulcer frequently reports weight gain. Answers C and D are incorrect because they describe symptoms associated with gastric ulcers.

185. **Answer D is correct.** Complications following a stapedectomy include damage to the seventh cranial nerve that results in changes in taste or facial sensation. Answers A and B are incorrect because they are expected immediately following a stapedectomy. Answer C is incorrect because it involves the twelfth cranial nerve (hypoglossal nerve).

186. **Answer C is correct.** Most infants begin nocturnal sleep lasting 9–11 hours by 3–4 months of age. Answers A and B are incorrect because the infant is still waking for nighttime feedings. Answer D is incorrect because it does not answer the question.

187. **Answer A is correct.** The goal of oxygen therapy for the client with emphysema is maintaining a PaO2 of 50 to 60mmHg. Answers B, C, and D are incorrect because the PaO2 levels are too high.

188. **Answer B is correct.** The medication is having its intended effect when the client's urine specific gravity is within the normal range. Answers A and D refer to the client with diabetes mellitus not diabetes insipidus; therefore, they are incorrect. Answer C is incorrect because it is not related to diabetes insipidus.

189. **Answer A is correct.** The child with myelomeningocele is at greatest risk for the development of latex allergy because of repeated exposure to latex products during surgery and from numerous urinary catheterizations. The clients in answers B, C, and D are much less likely to be exposed to latex; therefore, they are incorrect.

190. **Answer D is correct.** The therapeutic range for aminophylline is 10–20 micrograms/mL. Answers A, B, and C are incorrect because they are too low to be therapeutic.

191. **Answer C is correct.** The priority nursing diagnosis for a client with acromegaly focuses on the risk for ineffective airway clearance. Answers A, B, and D apply to the client with acromegaly but do not take priority; therefore, they are incorrect.

192. **Answer C is correct.** The nurse can help increase ventilation and perfusion to all areas of the lungs by turning the client every hour. Rocking beds can also be used to keep the client in constant motion. Answer A is incorrect because the client with ARDS will have respirations controlled by the ventilator. Answer B is incorrect because the nurse must have a physician's order to increase the PEEP. Answer D is incorrect because it will not increase ventilation and perfusion.

193. **Answer D is correct.** The nurse or parent should use a cupped hand when performing chest percussion. Answer A is incorrect because the hand should be cupped. Answer B is incorrect because the child's position should be changed every 5–10 minutes, and the whole session should be limited to 20 minutes. Answer C is incorrect because chest percussion should be done before meals.

194. **Answer A is correct.** The client with Addison's disease requires lifetime management with steroids. The nurse should stress the importance of taking the medication exactly as directed by the physician, as well as reporting adverse reactions to the medication. The client should be cautioned not to skip doses or to abruptly discontinue the medication. Answers B, C, and D should be included in the client's teaching but do not pose life-threatening consequences; therefore, they are incorrect.

195. **Answer B is correct.** Air embolus can occur with insertion, maintenance, and removal of central line catheters. The client's history of recent removal of a central line and the development of dyspnea, substernal chest pain, confusion, and fear suggest an air embolus. Answer A is incorrect because it is not associated with central line use. Answer C is incorrect because the symptoms do not suggest bleeding. Answer D is incorrect because it is not a complication of central line use.

196. **Answer A is correct.** No more than 1mL should be given in the vastus lateralis of the infant. Answers B, C, and D are incorrect because the dorsogluteal and ventrogluteal muscles are not used for injections in the infant.

197. **Answer C is correct.** Depot injections of Haldol are administered every 4 weeks. Answers A and B are incorrect because the medication is still in the client's system. Answer D is incorrect because the medication has been eliminated from the client's system, which allows the symptoms of schizophrenia to return.

198. **Answer C is correct.** The client should take a deep breath and hold it (Valsalva maneuver) when the central line is being removed. This increases the intrathoracic pressure and decreases the likelihood of having an air embolus. Answers A and B do not increase intrathoracic pressure; therefore, they are incorrect for the situation. Answer D increases the likelihood of air embolus; therefore, it is incorrect.

199. **Answer D is correct.** The earliest sign of cystic fibrosis is meconium ileus, which may be present in the newborn with the disease. Answers A, B, and C are later manifestations; therefore, they are incorrect.

200. **Answer D is correct.** Tucking a disposable diaper at the perineal opening will help prevent soiling of the cast by urine and stool. Answer A is incorrect because the head of the bed should be elevated. Answer B is incorrect because the child can place the crayons beneath the cast, causing pressure areas to develop. Answer C is incorrect because the child does not need high-calorie foods that would cause weight gain while she is immobilized by the cast.

201. **Answer B is correct.** Coolness and discoloration of the reimplanted digits indicates compromised circulation, which should be reported immediately to the physician. The temperature should be monitored, but the client would receive antibiotics to prevent infection; therefore, answer A is incorrect. Answers C and D are expected following amputation and reimplantation; therefore, they are incorrect.

202. **Answer C is correct.** The obstetrical client under age 18 is at greatest risk for CPD because pelvic growth is not fully completed. Answers A, B, and D are incorrect because these clients are not as likely to have CPD.

203. **Answer A is correct.** Priority of care should focus on maintaining the client's airway. Answers B and C are important to the client's care, but they do not take priority over maintaining the client's airway; therefore, they are incorrect. Answer D is incorrect because the client will require a passive range of motion exercise.

204. **Answer B is correct.** Answers A, C, and D are incorrect because they are inaccurate amounts.

205. **Answer A is correct.** Following extracorporeal lithotripsy, the urine will appear cherry red in color but will gradually change to clear urine. Answer B is incorrect because the urine will be red, not orange. Answer C is incorrect because the urine will be not be dark red or cloudy in appearance. Answer D is incorrect because it describes the urinary output of the client with acute glomerulonephritis.

206. **Answer A is correct.** Special rotational or directional catheters will be used to remove the plaque. Answer B is incorrect because it describes ablation. Answer C is incorrect because it describes percutaneous transluminal coronary angioplasty. Answer D is incorrect because it refers to lipid-lowering agents.

207. **Answer C is correct.** A stage II pressure ulcer has cracks and blisters with areas of redness and induration. Answer A is incorrect because it describes the appearance of a stage IV pressure ulcer. Answer B is incorrect because it describes the appearance of a stage III pressure ulcer. Answer D is incorrect because it describes the appearance of a stage I pressure ulcer.

208. **Answer B is correct.** An adverse reaction to Cognex is drug-induced hepatitis. The nurse should monitor the client for signs of jaundice. Answers A, C, and D are incorrect because they are not associated with the use of Cognex.

209. **Answer A is correct.** The child with cystic fibrosis needs a diet that is high in calories, with high protein and moderate amounts of fat. Answers B, C, and D are incorrect because they do not meet the nutritional requirements imposed by the disease.

210. **Answer C is correct.** Apricots are low in potassium; therefore, this is a suitable snack for the client on a potassium-restricted diet. Raisins, oranges, and bananas are all high in potassium; therefore, answers A, B, and D are incorrect.

211. **Answer B is correct.** Hyperventilation reduces swelling and increased intracranial pressure by decreasing cerebral blood flow. Answers A, C, and D do not pertain to the situation; therefore, they are incorrect.

212. **Answer B is correct.** No special preparation is needed for the blood test for *H. pylori*. Answer A is incorrect because the client is not NPO before the test. Answer C is incorrect because it refers to preparation for the breath test. Answer D is incorrect because glucose is not administered before the test.

213. **Answer B is correct.** Oral potassium supplements should be given in at least 4oz of juice or other liquid such as fruit punch to disguise the unpleasant taste. Answers A, C, and D are incorrect because they cause gastric upset.

214. **Answer D is correct.** The client with hypomagnesemia will have a positive Trousseau's sign. Answer A is incorrect because the client would have tachycardia. Answer B is incorrect because the client would have a positive Chvostek's sign. Answer C is incorrect because the client would have hypotension.

215. **Answer D is correct.** Fresh specimens are essential for an accurate diagnosis of CMV. Answer A is incorrect because cultures of urine, sputum, and oral swab are preferred. Answer B is incorrect because pregnant caregivers should not be assigned to care for clients with suspected or known infection with CMV. Answer C is incorrect because a convalescent culture is obtained 2–4 weeks after diagnosis.

216. **Answer B is correct.** The client with congestive heart failure who reports coughing up frothy sputum should be carefully evaluated for increasing pulmonary edema, which requires immediate treatment. Answers A, C, and D involve chronic conditions with complications that require skilled nursing care and assessment, but they do not present immediate life-threatening situations; therefore, they are incorrect.

217. **Answer B is correct.** The client with neutropenia needs to be placed in a private room in protective isolation. The other clients can be placed in the room with other clients; therefore, answers A, C, and D are incorrect.

218. **Answer B is correct.** Asterixis is a symptom of impending liver failure, so the client should be cared for by the RN. The remaining clients can be cared for by the LPN; therefore, answers A, C, and D are incorrect.

219. **Answer D is correct.** Adverse reactions to phenytoin include agranulocytosis. The client's WBC is abnormally low and should be reported to the physician immediately. Answer A is incorrect because elevations in serum creatinine are expected in the client with chronic renal failure. Answer B is wrong because a positive C reactive protein is usually present in those with rheumatic fever. Answer C is wrong because a hematocrit of 52% in a client with gastroenteritis can be expected due to dehydration.

220. **Answer D is correct.** The newly licensed nurse should not be assigned to provide primary care for the client with noncardiogenic pulmonary edema (ARDS) because the client's condition warrants care by an experienced RN. Answers A, B, and C are incorrect because the newly licensed nurse could assume primary care for clients with those conditions.

221. **Answer C is correct.** The client with a lumbar laminectomy can be safely cared for by the LPN. Answer A is incorrect because the client with a high cervical injury immobilized by skeletal traction is best cared for by the RN. Answers B and D are incorrect choices because these clients have conditions that require intravenous medication, which requires the skill of the RN.

222. **Answer A is correct.** The client with a thoracotomy who has 110mL of drainage in the past hour has excessive bleeding that should be evaluated and reported to the physician immediately. A temperature of 100°F following a surgery is not unusual; therefore, answer B is incorrect. Feelings of urinary urgency are normal after a transurethral prostatectomy; therefore, answer C is incorrect. Diminished loss of hearing in the hours following a stapedectomy is expected due to the swelling and accumulation of blood in the inner ear; therefore, answer D is incorrect.

223. **Answer A is correct.** Increased jaundice and prolonged prothrombin time are indications that the liver is not working. Answer B is incorrect because the symptoms suggest infection. Answer C is incorrect because the symptoms suggest obstruction. Answer D is incorrect because the symptoms are associated with renal failure.

224. **Answer A is correct.** The client with adrenal insufficiency suffers from fluid volume deficit and acidosis. Answers B, C, and D are incorrect because they do not pose a life-threatening acid-based imbalance.

225. **Answer D is correct.** Sulfamylon produces a burning sensation when applied; therefore, the client should receive pain medication 30 minutes before application. Answer A is incorrect because it refers to therapy with silver nitrate. Answer B is incorrect because it refers therapy with Silvadene. Answer C is incorrect because it refers therapy with to Betadine.

226. **Answer D is correct.** Gingival hyperplasia is a side effect of Dilantin, so the nurse should provide oral hygiene and gum care every shift. Answers A, B, and C do not apply to the medication; therefore, they are incorrect.

227. **Answer C is correct.** Adverse reactions to Captoten include a decreased white cell count. Answers A, B, and D are incorrect because they are associated with the medication.

228. **Answer C is correct.** Zofran is given before chemotherapy to prevent nausea. Answers A, B, and D are not associated with the medication; therefore, they are incorrect.

229. **Answer A is correct.** When administering ear drops to a child under 3 years of age, the nurse should pull the ear down and back to straighten the ear canal. Answers B and D are incorrect positions for administering ear drops. Answer C is used for administering ear drops to the adult client.

230. **Answer A is correct.** Antibiotics such as Achromycin should not be taken with antacids. Answers B, C, and D may be taken with antibiotics; therefore, they are incorrect.

231. **Answer C is correct.** The nurse should carefully monitor the client taking Thorazine for signs of infection that can quickly become overwhelming. Answers A, B, and D are incorrect because they are expected side effects of the medication.

232. **Answer A is correct.** Claratin does not produce sedation like other antihistamines. Answers B, C, and D are inaccurate statements; therefore, they are incorrect.

233. **Answer B is correct.** A cotton-tipped swab is used to apply the suspension to the affected areas. Answers A, C, and D are incorrect because they do not ensure that the medication reaches the affected areas.

234. **Answer A is correct.** Iron is better absorbed when taken with ascorbic acid. Orange juice is an excellent source of ascorbic acid. Answer B is incorrect because the medication should be taken with orange juice or tomato juice. Answer C is incorrect because iron should not be taken with milk because it interferes with absorption. Answer D is incorrect because apple juice does not contain high amounts of ascorbic acid.

235. **Answer A is correct.** Acetylcysteine is the antidote for acetaminophen poisoning. Answer B is incorrect because it is the antidote for iron poisoning. Answer C is incorrect because it is the treatment for lead poisoning. Answer D is incorrect because it is used for noncorrosive poisonings.

236. **Answer D is correct.** The client should hold the cane in the unaffected side. Answer A is incorrect because this answer instructs the client to hold the cane in the affected side. It will not be necessary for the client to use a walker, and advancing the cane with the affected leg is not correct; thus, answers B and C are incorrect.

237. **Answer A is correct.** Linear accelerator therapy is done in the radium department and does not make the client radioactive. Answer B is incorrect because there is no radiation emitted from the client. Answer C is incorrect because it is not necessary for the nursing assistant to wear an apron when caring for this client. Answer D is incorrect because there is no need to reassign the nursing assistant.

238. **Answer D is correct.** The client undergoing an angiogram will experience a warm sensation as the dye is injected. Answers A, B, and C are not associated with an angiogram.

239. **Answer B is correct.** Semi-liquids are more easily swallowed by the client with dysphagia than either liquids or solids. Answers A, C, and D do not improve the client's ability to swallow, so they are incorrect choices.

240. **Answer A is correct.** Placing the client in the Trendelenburg position will engorge the vessels, make insertion of the catheter easier, and lessen the likelihood of air entering the central line. Answer B is incorrect because the client will not be more comfortable in the Trendelenburg position. Answers C and D are not correct statements.

241. **Answer B is correct.** Taking deep breaths will decrease the discomfort experienced during removal of the drain. Answers A, C, and D are incorrect statements because they do not decrease the discomfort during removal of the drain.

242. **Answer B is correct.** Increased voiding at night is a symptom of right-sided heart failure. Answers A, C, and D are incorrect because they are symptoms of left-sided heart failure.

243. **Answer B is correct.** The CPM machine should not be set at 90° flexion until the fifth post-operative day. Answers A, C, and D are expected findings and do not require immediate nursing intervention; therefore, they are incorrect.

244. **Answer D is correct.** The multiparous client with a large newborn has the greatest risk for postpartal hemorrhage. Answers A, B, and C are incorrect choices because they do not have a greater risk for postpartal hemorrhage.

245. **Answer B is correct.** The medication should be administered using the calibrated dropper that comes with the medication. Answers A and C are incorrect because part or all of the medication could be lost during administration. Answer D is incorrect because part or all of the medication will be lost if the child does not finish the bottle.

246. **Answer C is correct.** Atropine is contraindicated in the client with glaucoma because the medication increases intraocular pressure. Answers A, B, and D are not contraindicated in the client with glaucoma; therefore, they are incorrect answers.

247. **Answer B is correct.** Aged cheese, wine, and smoked or pickled meats should be avoided by the client taking an MAOI, not a phenothiazine. Answers A, C, and D are included in the discharge teaching of a client receiving chlorpromazine (Thorazine).

248. **Answer D is correct.** Leaving a nightlight on during the evening and night shifts helps the client remain oriented to the environment and fosters independence. Answers A and B will not decrease the client's confusion. Answer C will increase the likelihood of confusion in an elderly client.

249. **Answer C is correct.** Elevations in white cell count indicate the presence of infection, which requires treatment before surgery. Answers A, B, and D are within normal limits and require no intervention.

250. **Answer A is correct.** Akathisia is an adverse extrapyramidal side effect of many older antipsychotic medications such as haloperidol and chlorpromazine. Answers B, C, and D are not associated with the use of haloperidol.

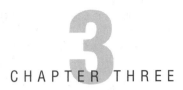

CHAPTER THREE

Practice Exam 3 and Rationales

1. A 43-year-old African American male is admitted with sickle cell anemia. The nurse plans to assess circulation in the lower extremities every 2 hours. Which of the following outcome criteria would the nurse use?

   ○ **A.** Body temperature of 99°F or less

   ○ **B.** Toes moved in active range of motion

   ○ **C.** Sensation reported when soles of feet are touched

   ○ **D.** Capillary refill of < 3 seconds

2. A 30-year-old male from Haiti is brought to the emergency department in sickle cell crisis. What is the best position for this client?

   ○ **A.** Side-lying with knees flexed

   ○ **B.** Knee-chest

   ○ **C.** High Fowler's with knees flexed

   ○ **D.** Semi-Fowler's with legs extended on the bed

3. A 25-year-old male is admitted in sickle cell crisis. Which of the following interventions would be of highest priority for this client?

   ○ **A.** Taking hourly blood pressures with mechanical cuff

   ○ **B.** Encouraging fluid intake of at least 200mL per hour

   ○ **C.** Position in high Fowler's with knee gatch raised

   ○ **D.** Administering Tylenol as ordered

4. Which of the following foods would the nurse encourage the client in sickle cell crisis to eat?

   ○ **A.** Peaches

   ○ **B.** Cottage cheese

   ○ **C.** Popsicle

   ○ **D.** Lima beans

5. A newly admitted client has sickle cell crisis. He is complaining of pain in his feet and hands. The nurse's assessment findings include a pulse oximetry of 92. Assuming that all the following interventions are ordered, which should be done first?

   ○ **A.** Adjust the room temperature

   ○ **B.** Give a bolus of IV fluids

   ○ **C.** Start O_2

   ○ **D.** Administer meperidine (Demerol) 75mg IV push

6. The nurse is instructing a client with iron-deficiency anemia. Which of the following meal plans would the nurse expect the client to select?

   ○ **A.** Roast beef, gelatin salad, green beans, and peach pie

   ○ **B.** Chicken salad sandwich, coleslaw, French fries, ice cream

   ○ **C.** Egg salad on wheat bread, carrot sticks, lettuce salad, raisin pie

   ○ **D.** Pork chop, creamed potatoes, corn, and coconut cake

7. Clients with sickle cell anemia are taught to avoid activities that cause hypoxia and hypoxemia. Which of the following activities would the nurse recommend?

   ○ **A.** A family vacation in the Rocky Mountains

   ○ **B.** Chaperoning the local boys club on a snow-skiing trip

   ○ **C.** Traveling by airplane for business trips

   ○ **D.** A bus trip to the Museum of Natural History

8. The nurse is conducting an admission assessment of a client with vitamin B12 deficiency. Which finding reinforces the diagnosis of B12 deficiency?

   ○ **A.** Enlarged spleen

   ○ **B.** Elevated blood pressure

   ○ **C.** Bradycardia

   ○ **D.** Beefy tongue

9. The body part that would most likely display jaundice in the dark-skinned individual is the:

   ○ **A.** Conjunctiva of the eye

   ○ **B.** Soles of the feet

   ○ **C.** Roof of the mouth

   ○ **D.** Shins

10. The nurse is conducting a physical assessment on a client with anemia. Which of the following clinical manifestations would be most indicative of the anemia?

- ○ **A.** BP 146/88
- ○ **B.** Respirations 28 shallow
- ○ **C.** Weight gain of 10 pounds in 6 months
- ○ **D.** Pink complexion

11. The nurse is teaching the client with polycythemia vera about prevention of complications of the disease. Which of the following statements by the client indicates a need for further teaching?

- ○ **A.** "I will drink 500mL of fluid or less each day."
- ○ **B.** "I will wear support hose."
- ○ **C.** "I will check my blood pressure regularly."
- ○ **D.** "I will report ankle edema."

12. A 33-year-old male is being evaluated for possible acute leukemia. Which of the following findings is most likely related to the diagnosis of leukemia?

- ○ **A.** The client collects stamps as a hobby.
- ○ **B.** The client recently lost his job as a postal worker.
- ○ **C.** The client had radiation for treatment of Hodgkin's disease as a teenager.
- ○ **D.** The client's brother had leukemia as a child.

13. Where is the best site for examining for the presence of petechiae in an African American client?

- ○ **A.** The abdomen
- ○ **B.** The thorax
- ○ **C.** The earlobes
- ○ **D.** The soles of the feet

14. The client is being evaluated for possible acute leukemia. Which inquiry by the nurse is most important?

- ○ **A.** "Have you noticed a change in sleeping habits recently?"
- ○ **B.** "Have you had a respiratory infection in the last 6 months?"
- ○ **C.** "Have you lost weight recently?"
- ○ **D.** "Have you noticed changes in your alertness?"

15. Which of the following would be the priority nursing diagnosis for the adult client with acute leukemia?

Quick Answer: **212**
Detailed Answer: **216**

  ○ **A.** Oral mucous membrane, altered related to chemotherapy

  ○ **B.** Risk for injury related to thrombocytopenia

  ○ **C.** Fatigue related to the disease process

  ○ **D.** Interrupted family processes related to life-threatening illness of a family member

16. A 21-year-old male with Hodgkin's lymphoma is a senior at the local university. He is engaged to be married and is to begin a new job upon graduation. Which of the following diagnoses would be a priority for this client?

Quick Answer: **212**
Detailed Answer: **216**

  ○ **A.** Sexual dysfunction related to radiation therapy

  ○ **B.** Anticipatory grieving related to terminal illness

  ○ **C.** Tissue integrity related to prolonged bed rest

  ○ **D.** Fatigue related to chemotherapy

17. A client has autoimmune thrombocytopenic purpura. To determine the client's response to treatment, the nurse would monitor:

Quick Answer: **212**
Detailed Answer: **216**

  ○ **A.** Platelet count

  ○ **B.** White blood cell count

  ○ **C.** Potassium levels

  ○ **D.** Partial prothrombin time (PTT)

18. The home health nurse is visiting a client with autoimmune thrombocytopenic purpura (ATP). The client's platelet count currently is 80,000. It will be most important to teach the client and family about:

Quick Answer: **212**
Detailed Answer: **216**

  ○ **A.** Bleeding precautions

  ○ **B.** Prevention of falls

  ○ **C.** Oxygen therapy

  ○ **D.** Conservation of energy

19. The client has surgery for removal of a Prolactinoma. Which of the following interventions would be appropriate for this client?

Quick Answer: **212**
Detailed Answer: **216**

  ○ **A.** Place the client in Trendelenburg position for postural drainage

  ○ **B.** Encourage coughing and deep breathing every 2 hours

  ○ **C.** Elevate the head of the bed 30°

  ○ **D.** Encourage the Valsalva maneuver for bowel movements

20. The client with a history of diabetes insipidus is admitted with polyuria, polydipsia, and mental confusion. The priority intervention for this client is:

Quick Answer: **212**
Detailed Answer: **217**

- ○ **A.** Measure the urinary output
- ○ **B.** Check the vital signs
- ○ **C.** Encourage increased fluid intake
- ○ **D.** Weigh the client

21. A client with hemophilia has a nosebleed. Which nursing action is most appropriate to control the bleeding?

Quick Answer: **212**
Detailed Answer: **217**

- ○ **A.** Place the client in a sitting position.
- ○ **B.** Administer acetaminophen (Tylenol).
- ○ **C.** Pinch the soft lower part of the nose.
- ○ **D.** Apply ice packs to the forehead.

22. A client has had a unilateral adrenalectomy to remove a tumor. The most important measurement in the immediate post-operative period for the nurse to take is to.

Quick Answer: **212**
Detailed Answer: **217**

- ○ **A.** Check the blood pressure
- ○ **B.** Monitor the temperature
- ○ **C.** Evaluate the urinary output
- ○ **D.** Check the specific gravity of the urine

23. A client with Addison's disease has been admitted with a history of nausea and vomiting for the past 3 days. The client is receiving IV glucocorticoids (Solu-Medrol). Which of the following interventions would the nurse implement?

Quick Answer: **212**
Detailed Answer: **217**

- ○ **A.** Glucometer readings as ordered
- ○ **B.** Intake/output measurements
- ○ **C.** Evaluate the sodium and potassium levels
- ○ **D.** Daily weights

24. A client had a total thyroidectomy yesterday. The client is complaining of tingling around the mouth and in the fingers and toes. What would the nurses' next action be?

Quick Answer: **212**
Detailed Answer: **217**

- ○ **A.** Obtain a crash cart
- ○ **B.** Check the calcium level
- ○ **C.** Assess the dressing for drainage
- ○ **D.** Assess the blood pressure for hypertension

25. A 32-year-old mother of three is brought to the clinic. Her pulse is 52, there is a weight gain of 30 pounds in 4 months, and the client is wearing two sweaters. The client is diagnosed with hypothyroidism. Which of the following nursing diagnoses is of highest priority?

    Quick Answer: **212**
    Detailed Answer: **217**

    ○ **A.** Impaired physical mobility related to decreased endurance

    ○ **B.** Hypothermia r/t decreased metabolic rate

    ○ **C.** Disturbed thought processes r/t interstitial edema

    ○ **D.** Decreased cardiac output r/t bradycardia

26. The client presents to the clinic with a serum cholesterol of 275mg/dL and is placed on rosuvastatin (Crestor). Which instruction should be given to the client taking rosuvastatin (Crestor)?

    Quick Answer: **212**
    Detailed Answer: **217**

    ○ **A.** Report muscle weakness to the physician.

    ○ **B.** Allow six months for the drug to take effect.

    ○ **C.** Take the medication with fruit juice.

    ○ **D.** Report difficulty sleeping.

27. The client is admitted to the hospital with hypertensive crises. Diazoxide (Hyperstat) is ordered. During administration, the nurse should:

    Quick Answer: **212**
    Detailed Answer: **217**

    ○ **A.** Utilize an infusion pump

    ○ **B.** Check the blood glucose level

    ○ **C.** Place the client in Trendelenburg position

    ○ **D.** Cover the solution with foil

28. The 6-month-old client with a ventral septal defect is receiving Digitalis for regulation of his heart rate. Which finding should be reported to the doctor?

    Quick Answer: **212**
    Detailed Answer: **217**

    ○ **A.** Blood pressure of 126/80

    ○ **B.** Blood glucose of 110mg/dL

    ○ **C.** Heart rate of 60bpm

    ○ **D.** Respiratory rate of 30 per minute

29. The client admitted with angina is given a prescription for nitroglycerine. The client should be instructed to:

    Quick Answer: **212**
    Detailed Answer: **218**

    ○ **A.** Replenish his supply every 3 months

    ○ **B.** Take one every 15 minutes if pain occurs

    ○ **C.** Leave the medication in the brown bottle

    ○ **D.** Crush the medication and take with water

30. The client is instructed regarding foods that are low in fat and choles-
    terol. Which diet selection is lowest in saturated fats?

Quick Answer: **212**
Detailed Answer: **218**

   ○ **A.** Macaroni and cheese

   ○ **B.** Shrimp with rice

   ○ **C.** Turkey breast

   ○ **D.** Spaghetti with meat sauce

31. The client is admitted with left-sided congestive heart failure. In assess-
    ing the client for edema, the nurse should check the:

Quick Answer: **212**
Detailed Answer: **218**

   ○ **A.** Feet

   ○ **B.** Neck

   ○ **C.** Hands

   ○ **D.** Sacrum

32. The nurse is checking the client's central venous pressure. The nurse
    should place the zero of the manometer at the:

Quick Answer: **212**
Detailed Answer: **218**

   ○ **A.** Phlebostatic axis

   ○ **B.** PMI

   ○ **C.** Erb's point

   ○ **D.** Tail of Spence

33. The physician orders lisinopril (Zestril) and furosemide (Lasix) to be
    administered concomitantly to the client with hypertension. The nurse
    should:

Quick Answer: **212**
Detailed Answer: **218**

   ○ **A.** Question the order

   ○ **B.** Administer the medications

   ○ **C.** Administer separately

   ○ **D.** Contact the pharmacy

34. The best method of evaluating the amount of peripheral edema is:

Quick Answer: **212**
Detailed Answer: **218**

   ○ **A.** Weighing the client daily

   ○ **B.** Measuring the extremity

   ○ **C.** Measuring the intake and output

   ○ **D.** Checking for pitting

35. A client with vaginal cancer is being treated with a radioactive vaginal implant. The client's husband asks the nurse if he can spend the night with his wife. The nurse should explain that:

- ○ **A.** Overnight stays by family members is against hospital policy.
- ○ **B.** There is no need for him to stay because staffing is adequate.
- ○ **C.** His wife will rest much better knowing that he is at home.
- ○ **D.** Visitation is limited to 30 minutes when the implant is in place.

36. The nurse is caring for a client hospitalized with a facial stroke. Which diet selection would be suited to the client?

- ○ **A.** Roast beef sandwich, potato chips, pickle spear, iced tea
- ○ **B.** Split pea soup, mashed potatoes, pudding, milk
- ○ **C.** Tomato soup, cheese toast, Jello, coffee
- ○ **D.** Hamburger, baked beans, fruit cup, iced tea

37. The physician has prescribed Novalog insulin for a client with diabetes mellitus. Which statement indicates that the client knows when the peak action of the insulin occurs?

- ○ **A.** "I will make sure I eat breakfast within 10 minutes of taking my insulin."
- ○ **B.** "I will need to carry candy or some form of sugar with me all the time."
- ○ **C.** "I will eat a snack around three o'clock each afternoon."
- ○ **D.** "I can save my dessert from supper for a bedtime snack."

38. The nurse is teaching basic infant care to a group of first-time parents. The nurse should explain that a sponge bath is recommended for the first 2 weeks of life because:

- ○ **A.** New parents need time to learn how to hold the baby.
- ○ **B.** The umbilical cord needs time to separate.
- ○ **C.** Newborn skin is easily traumatized by washing.
- ○ **D.** The chance of chilling the baby outweighs the benefits of bathing.

39. A client with leukemia is receiving Trimetrexate. After reviewing the client's chart, the physician orders Wellcovorin (leucovorin calcium). The rationale for administering leucovorin calcium to a client receiving Trimetrexate is to:

Quick Answer: **212**
Detailed Answer: **219**

- ○ **A.** Treat iron-deficiency anemia caused by chemotherapeutic agents
- ○ **B.** Create a synergistic effect that shortens treatment time
- ○ **C.** Increase the number of circulating neutrophils
- ○ **D.** Reverse drug toxicity and prevent tissue damage

40. A 4-month-old is brought to the well-baby clinic for immunization. In addition to the DPT and polio vaccines, the baby should receive:

Quick Answer: **212**
Detailed Answer: **219**

- ○ **A.** Hib titer
- ○ **B.** Mumps vaccine
- ○ **C.** Hepatitis B vaccine
- ○ **D.** MMR

41. The physician has prescribed Nexium (esomeprazole) for a client with erosive gastritis. The nurse should administer the medication:

Quick Answer: **212**
Detailed Answer: **219**

- ○ **A.** 30 minutes before a meal
- ○ **B.** With each meal
- ○ **C.** In a single dose at bedtime
- ○ **D.** 30 minutes after meals

42. A client on the psychiatric unit is in an uncontrolled rage and is threatening other clients and staff. What is the most appropriate action for the nurse to take?

Quick Answer: **212**
Detailed Answer: **219**

- ○ **A.** Call security for assistance and prepare to sedate the client.
- ○ **B.** Tell the client to calm down and ask him if he would like to play cards.
- ○ **C.** Tell the client that if he continues his behavior he will be punished.
- ○ **D.** Leave the client alone until he calms down.

43. When the nurse checks the fundus of a client on the first postpartum day, she notes that the fundus is firm, is at the level of the umbilicus, and is displaced to the right. The next action the nurse should take is to:

Quick Answer: **212**
Detailed Answer: **219**

- ○ **A.** Check the client for bladder distention
- ○ **B.** Assess the blood pressure for hypotension
- ○ **C.** Determine whether an oxytocic drug was given
- ○ **D.** Check for the expulsion of small clots

44. A client is admitted to the hospital with a temperature of 99.8°F, complaints of blood-tinged hemoptysis, fatigue, and night sweats. The client's symptoms are consistent with a diagnosis of:

Quick Answer: **212**
Detailed Answer: **219**

- ○ **A.** Pneumonia
- ○ **B.** Reaction to antiviral medication
- ○ **C.** Tuberculosis
- ○ **D.** Superinfection due to low CD4 count

45. The client is seen in the clinic for treatment of migraine headaches. The drug Imitrex (sumatriptan succinate) is prescribed for the client. Which of the following in the client's history should be reported to the doctor?

Quick Answer: **212**
Detailed Answer: **219**

- ○ **A.** Diabetes
- ○ **B.** Prinzmetal's angina
- ○ **C.** Cancer
- ○ **D.** Cluster headaches

46. The client with suspected meningitis is admitted to the unit. The doctor is performing an assessment to determine meningeal irritation and spinal nerve root inflammation. A positive Kernig's sign is charted if the nurse notes:

Quick Answer: **212**
Detailed Answer: **220**

- ○ **A.** Pain on flexion of the hip and knee
- ○ **B.** Nuchal rigidity on flexion of the neck
- ○ **C.** Pain when the head is turned to the left side
- ○ **D.** Dizziness when changing positions

47. The client with Alzheimer's disease is being assisted with activities of daily living when the nurse notes that the client uses her toothbrush to brush her hair. The nurse is aware that the client is exhibiting:

Quick Answer: **212**
Detailed Answer: **220**

- ○ **A.** Agnosia
- ○ **B.** Apraxia
- ○ **C.** Anomia
- ○ **D.** Aphasia

48. The client with dementia is experiencing confusion late in the afternoon and before bedtime. The nurse is aware that the client is experiencing what is known as:

Quick Answer: **212**
Detailed Answer: **220**

- ○ **A.** Chronic fatigue syndrome
- ○ **B.** Normal aging
- ○ **C.** Sundowning
- ○ **D.** Delusions

49. The client with confusion says to the nurse, "I haven't had anything to eat all day long. When are they going to bring breakfast?" The nurse saw the client in the day room eating breakfast with other clients 30 minutes before this conversation. Which response would be best for the nurse to make?

Quick Answer: **212**
Detailed Answer: **220**

- ○ **A.** "You know you had breakfast 30 minutes ago."
- ○ **B.** "I am so sorry that they didn't get you breakfast. I'll report it to the charge nurse."
- ○ **C.** "I'll get you some juice and toast. Would you like something else?"
- ○ **D.** "You will have to wait a while; lunch will be here in a little while."

50. The doctor has prescribed Exelon (rivastigmine) for the client with Alzheimer's disease. Which side effect is most often associated with this drug?

Quick Answer: **212**
Detailed Answer: **220**

- ○ **A.** Urinary incontinence
- ○ **B.** Headaches
- ○ **C.** Confusion
- ○ **D.** Nausea

51. A client is admitted to the labor and delivery unit in active labor. During examination, the nurse notes a papular lesion on the perineum. Which initial action is most appropriate?

Quick Answer: **212**
Detailed Answer: **220**

- ○ **A.** Document the finding
- ○ **B.** Report the finding to the doctor
- ○ **C.** Prepare the client for a C-section
- ○ **D.** Continue primary care as prescribed

52. A client with a diagnosis of HPV is at risk for which of the following?

Quick Answer: **212**
Detailed Answer: **220**

- ○ **A.** Hodgkin's lymphoma
- ○ **B.** Cervical cancer
- ○ **C.** Multiple myeloma
- ○ **D.** Ovarian cancer

53. During the initial interview, the client reports that she has a lesion on the perineum. Further investigation reveals a small blister on the vulva that is painful to touch. The nurse is aware that the most likely source of the lesion is:

- ○ **A.** Syphilis
- ○ **B.** Herpes
- ○ **C.** Gonorrhea
- ○ **D.** Condylomata

54. A client visiting a family planning clinic is suspected of having an STI. The best diagnostic test for treponema pallidum is:

- ○ **A.** Venereal Disease Research Lab (VDRL)
- ○ **B.** Rapid plasma reagin (RPR)
- ○ **C.** Florescent treponemal antibody (FTA)
- ○ **D.** Thayer-Martin culture (TMC)

55. A 15-year-old primigravida is admitted with a tentative diagnosis of HELLP syndrome. Which laboratory finding is associated with HELLP syndrome?

- ○ **A.** Elevated blood glucose
- ○ **B.** Elevated platelet count
- ○ **C.** Elevated creatinine clearance
- ○ **D.** Elevated hepatic enzymes

56. The nurse is assessing the deep tendon reflexes of a client with preeclampsia. Which method is used to elicit the biceps reflex?

- ○ **A.** The nurse places her thumb on the muscle inset in the ante-cubital space and taps the thumb briskly with the reflex hammer.
- ○ **B.** The nurse loosely suspends the client's arm in an open hand while tapping the back of the client's elbow.
- ○ **C.** The nurse instructs the client to dangle her legs as the nurse strikes the area below the patella with the blunt side of the reflex hammer.
- ○ **D.** The nurse instructs the client to place her arms loosely at her side as the nurse strikes the muscle insert just above the wrist.

		PLEASE CALL	✓
TELEPHONED	✓	WILL CALL AGAIN	
CAME TO SEE YOU		WANTS TO SEE YOU	
RETURNED YOUR CALL			

MESSAGE

SIGNED

adams
9711

57. A primigravida with diabetes is admitted to the labor and delivery unit at 34 weeks gestation. Which doctor's order should the nurse question?

Quick Answer: 212
Detailed Answer: 221

  ○ **A.** Magnesium sulfate 4gm (25%) IV

  ○ **B.** Brethine 10mcg IV

  ○ **C.** Stadol 1mg IV push every 4 hours as needed prn for pain

  ○ **D.** Ancef 2gm IVPB every 6 hours

58. A diabetic multigravida is scheduled for an amniocentesis at 32 weeks gestation to determine the L/S ratio and phosphatidyl glycerol level. The L/S ratio is 1:1 and the presence of phosphatidylglycerol is noted. The nurse's assessment of this data is:

Quick Answer: 212
Detailed Answer: 221

  ○ **A.** The infant is at low risk for congenital anomalies.

  ○ **B.** The infant is at high risk for intrauterine growth retardation.

  ○ **C.** The infant is at high risk for respiratory distress syndrome.

  ○ **D.** The infant is at high risk for birth trauma.

59. Which observation in the newborn of a diabetic mother would require immediate nursing intervention?

Quick Answer: 212
Detailed Answer: 221

  ○ **A.** Crying

  ○ **B.** Wakefulness

  ○ **C.** Jitteriness

  ○ **D.** Yawning

60. The nurse caring for a client receiving intravenous magnesium sulfate must closely observe for side effects associated with drug therapy. An expected side effect of magnesium sulfate is:

Quick Answer: 212
Detailed Answer: 221

  ○ **A.** Decreased urinary output

  ○ **B.** Hypersomnolence

  ○ **C.** Absence of knee jerk reflex

  ○ **D.** Decreased respiratory rate

61. The client has elected to have epidural anesthesia to relieve labor pain. If the client experiences hypotension, the nurse would:

Quick Answer: 212
Detailed Answer: 221

  ○ **A.** Place her in Trendelenburg position

  ○ **B.** Decrease the rate of IV infusion

  ○ **C.** Administer oxygen per nasal cannula

  ○ **D.** Increase the rate of the IV infusion

62. A client has cancer of the pancreas. The nurse should be most concerned about which nursing diagnosis?

- ○ **A.** Alteration in nutrition
- ○ **B.** Alteration in bowel elimination
- ○ **C.** Alteration in skin integrity
- ○ **D.** Ineffective individual coping

Quick Answer: **212**
Detailed Answer: **221**

63. The nurse is caring for a client with uremic frost. The nurse is aware that uremic frost is often seen in clients with:

- ○ **A.** Severe anemia
- ○ **B.** Arteriosclcrosis
- ○ **C.** Liver failure
- ○ **D.** Parathyroid disorder

Quick Answer: **212**
Detailed Answer: **221**

64. The client arrives in the emergency department after a motor vehicle accident. Nursing assessment findings include BP 80/34, pulse rate 120, and respirations 20. Which is the client's most appropriate priority nursing diagnosis?

- ○ **A.** Alteration in cerebral tissue perfusion
- ○ **B.** Fluid volume deficit
- ○ **C.** Ineffective airway clearance
- ○ **D.** Alteration in sensory perception

Quick Answer: **212**
Detailed Answer: **222**

65. The home health nurse is visiting an 18-year-old with osteogenesis imperfecta. Which information obtained on the visit would cause the most concern? The client:

- ○ **A.** Likes to play football
- ○ **B.** Drinks carbonated drinks
- ○ **C.** Has two sisters
- ○ **D.** Is taking acetaminophen for pain

Quick Answer: **212**
Detailed Answer: **222**

66. The nurse working the organ transplant unit is caring for a client with a white blood cell count of 450. During evening visitation, a visitor brings a basket of fruit. What action should the nurse take?

- ○ **A.** Allow the client to keep the fruit
- ○ **B.** Place the fruit next to the bed for easy access by the client
- ○ **C.** Offer to wash the fruit for the client
- ○ **D.** Ask the family members to take the fruit home

Quick Answer: **212**
Detailed Answer: **222**

67. The nurse is caring for the client following a laryngectomy when suddenly the client becomes nonresponsive and pale, with a BP of 90/40. The initial nurse's action should be to:

  ◯ **A.** Place the client in Trendelenburg position

  ◯ **B.** Increase the infusion of normal saline

  ◯ **C.** Administer atropine intravenously

  ◯ **D.** Move the emergency cart to the bedside

68. The client admitted 2 days earlier with a lung resection accidentally pulls out the chest tube. Which action by the nurse indicates understanding of the management of chest tubes?

  ◯ **A.** Order a chest x-ray

  ◯ **B.** Reinsert the tube

  ◯ **C.** Cover the insertion site with a Vaseline gauze

  ◯ **D.** Call the doctor

69. A client being treated with sodium warfarin (Coumadin) has a Protime of 120 seconds. Which intervention would be most important to include in the nursing care plan?

  ◯ **A.** Assess for signs of abnormal bleeding

  ◯ **B.** Anticipate an increase in the Coumadin dosage

  ◯ **C.** Instruct the client regarding the drug therapy

  ◯ **D.** Increase the frequency of neurological assessments

70. Which selection would provide the most calcium for the client who is 4 months pregnant?

  ◯ **A.** A granola bar

  ◯ **B.** A bran muffin

  ◯ **C.** A cup of yogurt

  ◯ **D.** A glass of fruit juice

71. The client with preeclampsia is admitted to the unit with an order for magnesium sulfate. Which action by the nurse indicates the understanding of magnesium toxicity?

  ◯ **A.** The nurse performs a vaginal exam every thirty minutes.

  ◯ **B.** The nurse places a padded tongue blade at the bedside.

  ◯ **C.** The nurse inserts a Foley catheter.

  ◯ **D.** The nurse darkens the room.

72. The best size cathlon for administration of a blood transfusion to a six year old is:

    Quick Answer: **212**
    Detailed Answer: **222**

    - ○ **A.** 18 gauge
    - ○ **B.** 19 gauge
    - ○ **C.** 22 gauge
    - ○ **D.** 20 gauge

73. A client is admitted to the unit 2 hours after an explosion causes burns to the face. The nurse would be most concerned with the client developing which of the following?

    Quick Answer: **212**
    Detailed Answer: **222**

    - ○ **A.** Hypovolemia
    - ○ **B.** Laryngeal edema
    - ○ **C.** Hypernatremia
    - ○ **D.** Hyperkalemia

74. The client has recently been diagnosed with diabetes. Which of the following indicates understanding of the management of diabetes?

    Quick Answer: **212**
    Detailed Answer: **222**

    - ○ **A.** The client selects a balanced diet from the menu.
    - ○ **B.** The client can tell the nurse the normal blood glucose level.
    - ○ **C.** The client asks for brochures on the subject of diabetes.
    - ○ **D.** The client demonstrates correct insulin injection technique.

75. The client is admitted following cast application for a fractured ulna. Which finding should be reported to the doctor?

    Quick Answer: **212**
    Detailed Answer: **222**

    - ○ **A.** Pain at the site
    - ○ **B.** Warm fingers
    - ○ **C.** Pulses rapid
    - ○ **D.** Paresthesia of the fingers

76. The client with AIDS should be taught to:

    Quick Answer: **212**
    Detailed Answer: **223**

    - ○ **A.** Avoid warm climates.
    - ○ **B.** Refrain from taking herbals.
    - ○ **C.** Avoid exercising.
    - ○ **D.** Report any changes in skin color.

77. Which action by the healthcare worker indicates a need for further teaching?

- ○ **A.** The nursing assistant ambulates the elderly client using a gait belt.
- ○ **B.** The nurse wears goggles while performing a venopuncture.
- ○ **C.** The nurse washes his hands after changing a dressing.
- ○ **D.** The nurse wears gloves to monitor the IV infusion rate.

78. The client is having electroconvulsive therapy for treatment of severe depression. Prior to the ECT the nurse should:

- ○ **A.** Apply a tourniquet to the client's arm.
- ○ **B.** Administer an anticonvulsant medication.
- ○ **C.** Ask the client if he is allergic to shell fish.
- ○ **D.** Apply a blood pressure cuff to the arm.

79. The 5-year-old is being tested for enterobiasis (pinworms). Which symptom is associated with enterobiasis?

- ○ **A.** Rectal itching
- ○ **B.** Nausea
- ○ **C.** Oral ulcerations
- ○ **D.** Scalp itching

80. The nurse is teaching the mother regarding treatment for pedicalosis capitis. Which instruction should be given regarding the medication?

- ○ **A.** Treatment is not recommended for children less than 10 years of age.
- ○ **B.** Bed linens should be washed in hot water.
- ○ **C.** Medication therapy will continue for 1 year.
- ○ **D.** Intravenous antibiotic therapy will be ordered.

81. The registered nurse is making assignments for the day. Which client should be assigned to the pregnant nurse?

- ○ **A.** The client with HIV
- ○ **B.** The client with a radium implant for cervical cancer
- ○ **C.** The client with RSV (respiratory synctial virus)
- ○ **D.** The client with cytomegalovirus

82. The nurse is planning room assignments for the day. Which client should be assigned to a private room if only one is available?

   - ○ **A.** The client with methcillin resistant-staphylococcus aureas (MRSA)
   - ○ **B.** The client with diabetes
   - ○ **C.** The client with pancreatitis
   - ○ **D.** The client with Addison's disease

Quick Answer: **212**
Detailed Answer: **223**

83. The doctor accidentally cuts the bowel during surgery. As a result of this action, the client develops an infection and suffers brain damage. The doctor can be charged with:

   - ○ **A.** Negligence
   - ○ **B.** Tort
   - ○ **C.** Assault
   - ○ **D.** Malpractice

Quick Answer: **212**
Detailed Answer: **223**

84. Which assignment should not be performed by the nursing assistant?

   - ○ **A.** Feeding the client
   - ○ **B.** Bathing the client
   - ○ **C.** Obtaining a stool
   - ○ **D.** Administering a fleet enema

Quick Answer: **212**
Detailed Answer: **223**

85. The mother calls the clinic to report that her newborn has a rash on his forehead and face. Which action is most appropriate?

   - ○ **A.** Tell the mother to wash the face with soap and apply powder.
   - ○ **B.** Tell her that 30% of newborns have a rash that will go away by one month of life.
   - ○ **C.** Report the rash to the doctor immediately.
   - ○ **D.** Ask the mother if anyone else in the family has had a rash in the last six months.

Quick Answer: **212**
Detailed Answer: **223**

86. Which nurse should not be assigned to care for the client with a radium implant for vaginal cancer?

   - ○ **A.** The LPN who is 6 months postpartum
   - ○ **B.** The RN who is pregnant
   - ○ **C.** The RN who is allergic to iodine
   - ○ **D.** The RN with a 3 year old at home

Quick Answer: **212**
Detailed Answer: **223**

87. Which information should be reported to the state Board of Nursing?

○ **A.** The facility fails to provide literature in both Spanish and English.

○ **B.** The narcotic count has been incorrect on the unit for the past 3 days.

○ **C.** The client fails to receive an itemized account of his bills and services received during his hospital stay.

○ **D.** The nursing assistant assigned to the client with hepatitis fails to feed the client and give the bath.

Quick Answer: **212**
Detailed Answer: **223**

88. The nurse is suspected of charting medication administration that he did not give. After talking to the nurse, the charge nurse should:

○ **A.** Call the Board of Nursing

○ **B.** File a formal reprimand

○ **C.** Terminate the nurse

○ **D.** Charge the nurse with a tort

Quick Answer: **212**
Detailed Answer: **224**

89. The home health nurse is planning for the day's visits. Which client should be seen first?

○ **A.** The 78-year-old who had a gastrectomy 3 weeks ago and has a PEG tube

○ **B.** The 5-month-old discharged 1 week ago with pneumonia who is being treated with amoxicillin liquid suspension

○ **C.** The 50-year-old with MRSA being treated with Vancomycin via a PICC line

○ **D.** The 30-year-old with an exacerbation of multiple sclerosis being treated with cortisone via a centrally placed venous catheter

Quick Answer: **212**
Detailed Answer: **224**

90. The emergency room is flooded with clients injured in a tornado. Which clients can be assigned to share a room in the emergency department during the disaster?

○ **A.** A client having auditory hallucinations and the client with ulcerative colitis

○ **B.** The client who is pregnant and the client with a broken arm

○ **C.** A child who is cyanotic with severe dypsnea and a client with a frontal head injury

○ **D.** The client who arrives with a large puncture wound to the abdomen and the client with chest pain

Quick Answer: **212**
Detailed Answer: **224**

91. Before administering eardrops to a toddler, the nurse should recognize that it is essential to consider which of the following?

    ○ **A.** The age of the child.

    ○ **B.** The child's weight.

    ○ **C.** The developmental level of the child.

    ○ **D.** The IQ of the child.

Quick Answer: **213**
Detailed Answer: **224**

92. The nurse is discussing meal planning with the mother of a 2-year-old. Which of the following statements, if made by the mother, would require a need for further instruction?

    ○ **A.** "It is okay to give my child white grape juice for breakfast."

    ○ **B.** "My child can have a grilled cheese sandwich for lunch."

    ○ **C.** "We are going on a camping trip this weekend, and I have bought hot dogs to grill for his lunch."

    ○ **D.** "For a snack, my child can have ice cream."

Quick Answer: **213**
Detailed Answer: **224**

93. A client with AIDS has a viral load of 200 copies per ml. The nurse should interpret this finding as:

    ○ **A.** The client is at risk for opportunistic diseases.

    ○ **B.** The client is no longer communicable.

    ○ **C.** The client's viral load is extremely low so he is relatively free of circulating virus.

    ○ **D.** The client's T-cell count is extremely low.

Quick Answer: **213**
Detailed Answer: **224**

94. The client has an order for sliding scale insulin at 1900 hours and Lantus insulin at the same hour. The nurse should:

    ○ **A.** Administer the two medications together.

    ○ **B.** Administer the medications in two injections.

    ○ **C.** Draw up the Lantus insulin and then the regular insulin and administer them together.

    ○ **D.** Contact the doctor because these medications should not be given to the same client.

Quick Answer: **213**
Detailed Answer: **224**

95. A priority nursing diagnosis for a child being admitted from surgery following a tonsillectomy is:

    ○ **A.** Altered nutrition

    ○ **B.** Impaired communication

    ○ **C.** Risk for injury/aspiration

    ○ **D.** Altered urinary elimination

Quick Answer: **213**
Detailed Answer: **224**

96. What would the nurse expect the admitting assessment to reveal in a client with glomerulonephritis?

Quick Answer: **213**
Detailed Answer: **224**

- ○ **A.** Hypertension
- ○ **B.** Lassitude
- ○ **C.** Fatigue
- ○ **D.** Vomiting and diarrhea

97. Which action is contraindicated in the client with epiglottis?

Quick Answer: **213**
Detailed Answer: **224**

- ○ **A.** Ambulation
- ○ **B.** Oral airway assessment using a tongue blade
- ○ **C.** Placing a blood pressure cuff on the arm
- ○ **D.** Checking the deep tendon reflexes.

98. A 25-year-old client with a goiter is admitted to the unit. What would the nurse expect the admitting assessment to reveal?

Quick Answer: **213**
Detailed Answer: **224**

- ○ **A.** Slow pulse
- ○ **B.** Anorexia
- ○ **C.** Bulging eyes
- ○ **D.** Weight gain

99. Which of the following foods, if selected by the mother with a child with celiac, would indicate her understanding of the dietary instructions?

Quick Answer: **213**
Detailed Answer: **224**

- ○ **A.** Whole-wheat toast
- ○ **B.** Angel hair pasta
- ○ **C.** Reuben on rye
- ○ **D.** Rice cereal

100. The first action that the nurse should take if she finds the client has an O_2 saturation of 68% is:

Quick Answer: **213**
Detailed Answer: **225**

- ○ **A.** Elevate the head
- ○ **B.** Recheck the O_2 saturation in 30 minutes
- ○ **C.** Apply oxygen by mask
- ○ **D.** Assess the heart rate

101. Which observation would the nurse expect to make after an amniotomy?

Quick Answer: **213**
Detailed Answer: **225**

- ○ **A.** Dark yellow amniotic fluid
- ○ **B.** Clear amniotic fluid
- ○ **C.** Greenish amniotic fluid
- ○ **D.** Red amniotic fluid

102. The client taking Glyburide (Diabeta) should be cautioned to:

Quick Answer: **213**
Detailed Answer: **225**

- ○ **A.** Avoid eating sweets
- ○ **B.** Report changes in urinary pattern
- ○ **C.** Allow 3 hours for onset
- ○ **D.** Check the glucose daily

103. The obstetric client's fetal heart rate is 80–90 during the contractions. The first action the nurse should take is:

Quick Answer: **213**
Detailed Answer: **225**

- ○ **A.** Reposition the monitor
- ○ **B.** Turn the client to her left side
- ○ **C.** Ask the client to ambulate
- ○ **D.** Prepare the client for delivery

104. Arterial ulcers are best described as ulcers that:

Quick Answer: **213**
Detailed Answer: **225**

- ○ **A.** Are smooth in texture
- ○ **B.** Have irregular borders
- ○ **C.** Are cool to touch
- ○ **D.** Are painful to touch

105. A vaginal exam reveals a footling breech presentation. The nurse should take which of the following actions at this time?

Quick Answer: **213**
Detailed Answer: **225**

- ○ **A.** Anticipate the need for a Caesarean section
- ○ **B.** Apply an internal fetal monitor
- ○ **C.** Place the client in Genu Pectoral position
- ○ **D.** Perform an ultrasound

106. A vaginal exam reveals that the cervix is 4cm dilated, with intact membranes and a fetal heart tone rate of 160–170bpm. The nurse decides to apply an external fetal monitor. The rationale for this implementation is:

Quick Answer: **213**
Detailed Answer: **225**

- ○ **A.** The cervix is closed.
- ○ **B.** The membranes are still intact.
- ○ **C.** The fetal heart tones are within normal limits.
- ○ **D.** The contractions are intense enough for insertion of an internal monitor.

107. The following are all nursing diagnoses appropriate for a gravida 1 para 0 in labor. Which one would be most appropriate for the primagravida as she completes the early phase of labor?

- ○ **A.** Impaired gas exchange related to hyperventilation
- ○ **B.** Alteration in placental perfusion related to maternal position
- ○ **C.** Impaired physical mobility related to fetal-monitoring equipment
- ○ **D.** Potential fluid volume deficit related to decreased fluid intake

108. As the client reaches 6cm dilation, the nurse notes late decelerations on the fetal monitor. What is the most likely explanation of this pattern?

- ○ **A.** The baby is sleeping.
- ○ **B.** The umbilical cord is compressed.
- ○ **C.** There is head compression.
- ○ **D.** There is uteroplacental insufficiency.

109. The nurse notes variable decelerations on the fetal monitor strip. The most appropriate initial action would be to:

- ○ **A.** Notify her doctor
- ○ **B.** Start an IV
- ○ **C.** Reposition the client
- ○ **D.** Readjust the monitor

110. Which of the following is a characteristic of an ominous periodic change in the fetal heart rate?

- ○ **A.** A fetal heart rate of 120–130bpm
- ○ **B.** A baseline variability of 6–10bpm
- ○ **C.** Accelerations in FHR with fetal movement
- ○ **D.** A recurrent rate of 90–100bpm at the end of the contractions.

111. The rationale for inserting a French catheter every hour for the client with epidural anesthesia is:

- ○ **A.** The bladder fills more rapidly because of the medication used for the epidural.
- ○ **B.** Her level of consciousness is such that she is in a trancelike state.
- ○ **C.** The sensation of the bladder filling is diminished or lost.
- ○ **D.** She is embarrassed to ask for the bedpan that frequently.

112. A client in the family planning clinic asks the nurse about the most likely time for her to conceive. The nurse explains that conception is most likely to occur when:

    ○ **A.** Estrogen levels are low.

    ○ **B.** Lutenizing hormone is high.

    ○ **C.** The endometrial lining is thin.

    ○ **D.** The progesterone level is low.

Quick Answer: **213**
Detailed Answer: **226**

113. A client tells the nurse that she plans to use the rhythm method of birth control. The nurse is aware that the success of the rhythm method depends on the:

    ○ **A.** Age of the client

    ○ **B.** frequency of intercourse

    ○ **C.** Regularity of the menses

    ○ **D.** Range of the client's temperature

Quick Answer: **213**
Detailed Answer: **226**

114. A client with diabetes asks the nurse for advice regarding methods of birth control. Which method of birth control is most suitable for the client with diabetes?

    ○ **A.** Intrauterine device

    ○ **B.** Oral contraceptives

    ○ **C.** Diaphragm

    ○ **D.** Contraceptive sponge

Quick Answer: **213**
Detailed Answer: **226**

115. The doctor suspects that the client has an ectopic pregnancy. Which symptom is consistent with a diagnosis of a ruptured ectopic pregnancy?

    ○ **A.** Painless vaginal bleeding

    ○ **B.** Abdominal cramping

    ○ **C.** Throbbing pain in the upper quadrant

    ○ **D.** Sudden, stabbing pain in the lower quadrant

Quick Answer: **213**
Detailed Answer: **226**

116. The nurse is teaching a pregnant client about nutritional needs during pregnancy. Which menu selection will best meet the nutritional needs of the pregnant client?

    ○ **A.** Hamburger pattie, green beans, French fries, and iced tea

    ○ **B.** Roast beef sandwich, potato chips, baked beans, and cola

    ○ **C.** Baked chicken, fruit cup, potato salad, coleslaw, yogurt, and iced tea

    ○ **D.** Fish sandwich, gelatin with fruit, and coffee

Quick Answer: **213**
Detailed Answer: **226**

117. The client with hyperemesis gravidarum is at risk for developing:

    ○ **A.** Respiratory alkalosis without dehydration

    ○ **B.** Metabolic acidosis with dehydration

    ○ **C.** Respiratory acidosis without dehydration

    ○ **D.** Metabolic alkalosis with dehydration

Quick Answer: **213**
Detailed Answer: **226**

118. A client tells the doctor that she is about 20 weeks pregnant. The most definitive sign of pregnancy is:

    ○ **A.** Elevated human choronic gonadatropin

    ○ **B.** The presence of fetal heart tones

    ○ **C.** Uterine enlargement

    ○ **D.** Breast enlargement and tenderness

Quick Answer: **213**
Detailed Answer: **226**

119. The nurse is caring for a neonate whose mother is diabetic. The nurse will expect the neonate to be:

    ○ **A.** Hypoglycemic, small for gestational age

    ○ **B.** Hyporglyccmic, large for gestational age

    ○ **C.** Hypoglycemic, large for gestational age

    ○ **D.** Hyperglycemic, small for gestational age

Quick Answer: **213**
Detailed Answer: **227**

120. Which of the following instructions should be included in the nurse's teaching regarding oral contraceptives?

    ○ **A.** Weight gain should be reported to the physician.

    ○ **B.** An alternate method of birth control is needed when taking antibiotics.

    ○ **C.** If the client misses one or more pills, two pills should be taken per day for 1 week.

    ○ **D.** Changes in the menstrual flow should be reported to the physician.

Quick Answer: **213**
Detailed Answer: **227**

121. The nurse is discussing breastfeeding with a postpartum client. Breastfeeding is contraindicated in the postpartum client with:

    ○ **A.** Diabetes

    ○ **B.** HIV

    ○ **C.** Hypertension

    ○ **D.** Thyroid disease

Quick Answer: **213**
Detailed Answer: **227**

122. A client is admitted to the labor and delivery unit complaining of vaginal bleeding with very little discomfort. The nurse's first action should be to:

- ○ **A.** Assess the fetal heart tones
- ○ **B.** Check for cervical dilation
- ○ **C.** Check for firmness of the uterus
- ○ **D.** Obtain a detailed history

Quick Answer: **213**
Detailed Answer: **227**

123. A client telephones the emergency room stating that she thinks that she is in labor. The nurse should tell the client that labor has probably begun when:

- ○ **A.** Her contractions are 2 minutes apart.
- ○ **B.** She has back pain and a bloody discharge.
- ○ **C.** She experiences abdominal pain and frequent urination.
- ○ **D.** Her contractions are 5 minutes apart.

Quick Answer: **213**
Detailed Answer: **227**

124. The nurse is teaching a group of prenatal clients about the effects of cigarette smoke on fetal development. Which characteristic is associated with babies born to mothers who smoked during pregnancy?

- ○ **A.** Low birth weight
- ○ **B.** Large for gestational age
- ○ **C.** Preterm birth, but appropriate size for gestation
- ○ **D.** Growth retardation in weight and length

Quick Answer: **213**
Detailed Answer: **227**

125. The physician has ordered an injection of RhoGam for the postpartum client whose blood type is A negative but whose baby is O positive. To provide postpartum prophylaxis, RhoGam should be administered:

- ○ **A.** Within 72 hours of delivery
- ○ **B.** Within 1 week of delivery
- ○ **C.** Within 2 weeks of delivery
- ○ **D.** Within 1 month of delivery

Quick Answer: **213**
Detailed Answer: **227**

126. After the physician performs an amniotomy, the nurse's first action should be to assess the:

- ○ **A.** Degree of cervical dilation
- ○ **B.** Fetal heart tones
- ○ **C.** Client's vital signs
- ○ **D.** Client's level of discomfort

Quick Answer: **213**
Detailed Answer: **227**

127. A client is admitted to the labor and delivery unit. The nurse performs a vaginal exam and determines that the client's cervix is 5cm dilated with 75% effacement. Based on the nurse's assessment the client is in which phase of labor?

- ○ **A.** Active
- ○ **B.** Latent
- ○ **C.** Transition
- ○ **D.** Early

128. A newborn with narcotic abstinence syndrome is admitted to the nursery. Nursing care of the newborn should include:

- ○ **A.** Teaching the mother to provide tactile stimulation
- ○ **B.** Wrapping the newborn snugly in a blanket
- ○ **C.** Placing the newborn in the infant seat
- ○ **D.** Initiating an early infant-stimulation program

129. A client elects to have epidural anesthesia to relieve the discomfort of labor. Following the initiation of epidural anesthesia, the nurse should give priority to:

- ○ **A.** Checking for cervical dilation
- ○ **B.** Placing the client in a supine position
- ○ **C.** Checking the client's blood pressure
- ○ **D.** Obtaining a fetal heart rate

130. The nurse is aware that the best way to prevent post-operative wound infection in the surgical client is to:

- ○ **A.** Administer a prescribed antibiotic
- ○ **B.** Wash her hands for 2 minutes before care
- ○ **C.** Wear a mask when providing care
- ○ **D.** Ask the client to cover her mouth when she coughs

131. The elderly client is admitted to the emergency room. Which symptom is the client with a fractured hip most likely to exhibit?

- ○ **A.** Pain
- ○ **B.** Disalignment
- ○ **C.** Cool extremity
- ○ **D.** Absence of pedal pulses

132. The nurse knows that a 60-year-old female client's susceptibility to osteoporosis is most likely related to:

- ○ **A.** Lack of exercise
- ○ **B.** Hormonal disturbances
- ○ **C.** Lack of calcium
- ○ **D.** Genetic predisposition

133. A 2-year-old is admitted for repair of a fractured femur and is placed in Bryant's traction. Which finding by the nurse indicates that the traction is working properly?

- ○ **A.** The infant no longer complains of pain.
- ○ **B.** The buttocks are 15° off the bed.
- ○ **C.** The legs are suspended in the traction.
- ○ **D.** The pins are secured within the pulley.

134. Which statement is true regarding balanced skeletal traction? Balanced skeletal traction:

- ○ **A.** Utilizes a Steinman pin
- ○ **B.** Requires that both legs be secured
- ○ **C.** Utilizes Kirschner wires
- ○ **D.** Is used primarily to heal the fractured hips

135. The client is admitted for an open reduction internal fixation of a fractured hip. Immediately following surgery, the nurse should give priority to assessing the:

- ○ **A.** Serum collection (Davol) drain
- ○ **B.** Client's pain
- ○ **C.** Nutritional status
- ○ **D.** Immobilizer

136. Which statement made by the family member caring for the client with a percutaneous gastrostomy tube indicates understanding of the nurse's teaching?

- ○ **A.** "I must flush the tube with water after feedings and clamp the tube."
- ○ **B.** "I must check placement four times per day."
- ○ **C.** "I will report to the doctor any signs of indigestion."
- ○ **D.** "If my father is unable to swallow, I will discontinue the feeding and call the clinic."

137. The nurse is assessing the client with a total knee replacement 2 hours post-operative. Which information requires notification of the doctor?

- ○ **A.** Scant bleeding on the dressing.
- ○ **B.** Low-grade temperature.
- ○ **C.** Hemoglobin of 7gm
- ○ **D.** The urinary output has been 120ml during the last hour.

138. The nurse is caring for the client with a 5-year-old diagnosis of plumbism. Which information in the health history is most likely related to the development of plumbism?

- ○ **A.** The client has traveled out of the country in the last 6 months.
- ○ **B.** The client's parents are skilled stained-glass artists.
- ○ **C.** The client lives in a house built in 1990.
- ○ **D.** The client has several brothers and sisters.

139. A client with a total hip replacement requires special equipment. Which equipment would assist the client with a total hip replacement with activities of daily living?

- ○ **A.** High-seat commode
- ○ **B.** Recliner
- ○ **C.** TENS unit
- ○ **D.** Abduction pillow

140. An elderly client with an abdominal surgery is admitted to the unit following surgery. In anticipation of complications of anesthesia and narcotic administration, the nurse should:

- ○ **A.** Administer oxygen via nasal cannula
- ○ **B.** Have narcan (naloxane) available
- ○ **C.** Prepare to administer blood products
- ○ **D.** Prepare to do cardioresuscitation

141. Which roommate would be most suitable for the 6-year-old male with a fractured femur in Russell's traction?

- ○ **A.** 16-year-old female with scoliosis
- ○ **B.** 12-year-old male with a fractured femur
- ○ **C.** 10-year-old male with sarcoma
- ○ **D.** 6-year-old male with osteomylitis

142. A client with osteoarthritis has a prescription for Celebrex (celecoxib). Which instruction should be included in the discharge teaching?

Quick Answer: 213
Detailed Answer: 229

   ○ **A.** Take the medication with milk.

   ○ **B.** Report chest pain.

   ○ **C.** Remain upright after taking for 30 minutes.

   ○ **D.** Allow 6 weeks for optimal effects.

143. A client with a fractured tibia has a plaster-of-Paris cast applied to immobilize the fracture. Which action by the nurse indicates understanding of a plaster-of-Paris cast?
The nurse:

Quick Answer: 213
Detailed Answer: 229

   ○ **A.** Handles the cast with the fingertips

   ○ **B.** Petals the cast

   ○ **C.** Dries the cast with a hair dryer

   ○ **D.** Allows 24 hours before bearing weight

144. The teenager with a fiberglass cast asks the nurse if it will be okay to allow his friends to autograph his cast. Which response would be best?

Quick Answer: 213
Detailed Answer: 230

   ○ **A.** "It will be alright for your friends to autograph the cast."

   ○ **B.** "Because the cast is made of plaster, autographing can weaken the cast."

   ○ **C.** "If they don't use chalk to autograph, it is okay."

   ○ **D.** "Autographing or writing on the cast in any form will harm the cast."

145. The nurse is assigned to care for the client with a Steinmen pin. During pin care, she notes that the LPN uses sterile gloves and Q-tips to clean the pin. Which action should the nurse take at this time?

Quick Answer: 213
Detailed Answer: 230

   ○ **A.** Assisting the LPN with opening sterile packages and peroxide

   ○ **B.** Telling the LPN that clean gloves are allowed

   ○ **C.** Telling the LPN that the registered nurse should perform pin care

   ○ **D.** Asking the LPN to clean the weights and pulleys with peroxide

146. A child with scoliosis has a spica cast applied. Which action specific to the spica cast should be taken?

    ○ **A.** Check the bowel sounds

    ○ **B.** Assess the blood pressure

    ○ **C.** Offer pain medication

    ○ **D.** Check for swelling

Quick Answer: **213**
Detailed Answer: **230**

147. The client with a cervical fracture is placed in traction. Which type of traction will be utilized at the time of discharge?

    ○ **A.** Russell's traction

    ○ **B.** Buck's traction

    ○ **C.** Halo traction

    ○ **D.** Crutchfield tong traction

Quick Answer: **213**
Detailed Answer: **230**

148. A client with a total knee replacement has a CPM (continuous passive motion device) applied during the post-operative period. Which statement made by the nurse indicates understanding of the CPM machine?

    ○ **A.** "Use of the CPM will permit the client to ambulate during the therapy."

    ○ **B.** "The CPM machine controls should be positioned distal to the site."

    ○ **C.** "If the client complains of pain during the therapy, I will turn off the machine and call the doctor."

    ○ **D.** "Use of the CPM machine will alleviate the need for physical therapy after the client is discharged."

Quick Answer: **213**
Detailed Answer: **230**

149. A client with a fractured hip is being taught correct use of the walker. The nurse is aware that the correct use of the walker is achieved if the:

    ○ **A.** Palms rest lightly on the handles

    ○ **B.** Elbows are flexed 0°

    ○ **C.** Client walks to the front of the walker

    ○ **D.** Client carries the walker

Quick Answer: **213**
Detailed Answer: **230**

150. When assessing a laboring client, the nurse finds a prolapsed cord. The nurse should:

Quick Answer: **213**
Detailed Answer: **230**

- ○ **A.** Attempt to replace the cord
- ○ **B.** Place the client on her left side
- ○ **C.** Elevate the client's hips
- ○ **D.** Cover the cord with a dry, sterile gauze

151. The nurse is caring for a 30-year-old male admitted with a stab wound. While in the emergency room, a chest tube is inserted. Which of the following explains the primary rationale for insertion of chest tubes?

Quick Answer: **213**
Detailed Answer: **230**

- ○ **A.** The tube will allow for equalization of the lung expansion.
- ○ **B.** Chest tubes serve as a method of draining blood and serous fluid and assist in reinflating the lungs.
- ○ **C.** Chest tubes relieve pain associated with a collapsed lung.
- ○ **D.** Chest tubes assist with cardiac function by stabilizing lung expansion.

152. A client who delivered this morning tells the nurse that she plans to breastfeed her baby. The nurse is aware that successful breastfeeding is most dependent on the:

Quick Answer: **213**
Detailed Answer: **230**

- ○ **A.** Mother's educational level
- ○ **B.** Infant's birth weight
- ○ **C.** Size of the mother's breast
- ○ **D.** Mother's desire to breastfeed

153. The nurse is monitoring the progress of a client in labor. Which finding should be reported to the physician immediately?

Quick Answer: **213**
Detailed Answer: **231**

- ○ **A.** The presence of scant bloody discharge
- ○ **B.** frequent urination
- ○ **C.** The presence of green-tinged amniotic fluid
- ○ **D.** Moderate uterine contractions

154. The nurse is measuring the duration of the client's contractions. Which statement is true regarding the measurement of the duration of contractions?

- ○ **A.** Duration is measured by timing from the beginning of one contraction to the beginning of the next contraction.
- ○ **B.** Duration is measured by timing from the end of one contraction to the beginning of the next contraction.
- ○ **C.** Duration is measured by timing from the beginning of one contraction to the end of the same contraction.
- ○ **D.** Duration is measured by timing from the peak of one contraction to the end of the same contraction.

155. The physician has ordered an intravenous infusion of Pitocin for the induction of labor. When caring for the obstetric client receiving intravenous Pitocin, the nurse should monitor for:

- ○ **A.** Maternal hypoglycemia
- ○ **B.** Fetal bradycardia
- ○ **C.** Maternal hyperreflexia
- ○ **D.** Fetal movement

156. A client with diabetes visits the prenatal clinic at 28 weeks gestation. Which statement is true regarding insulin needs during pregnancy?

- ○ **A.** Insulin requirements moderate as the pregnancy progresses.
- ○ **B.** A decreased need for insulin occurs during the second trimester.
- ○ **C.** Elevations in human choronic gonadotrophin decrease the need for insulin.
- ○ **D.** Fetal development depends on adequate insulin regulation.

157. A client in the prenatal clinic is assessed to have a blood pressure of 180/96. The nurse should give priority to:

- ○ **A.** Providing a calm environment
- ○ **B.** Obtaining a diet history
- ○ **C.** Administering an analgesic
- ○ **D.** Assessing fetal heart tones

158. A primigravida, age 42, is 6 weeks pregnant. Based on the client's age, her infant is at risk for:

- ○ **A.** Down syndrome
- ○ **B.** Respiratory distress syndrome
- ○ **C.** Turner's syndrome
- ○ **D.** Pathological jaundice

159. A client with a missed abortion at 29 weeks gestation is admitted to the hospital. The client will most likely be treated with:

- ○ **A.** Magnesium sulfate
- ○ **B.** Calcium gluconate
- ○ **C.** Dinoprostone (Prostin E.)
- ○ **D.** Bromocrystine (Parlodel)

160. A client with preeclampsia has been receiving an infusion containing magnesium sulfate for a blood pressure that is 160/80; deep tendon reflexes are 1 plus, and the urinary output for the past hour is 100mL. The nurse should:

- ○ **A.** Continue the infusion of magnesium sulfate while monitoring the client's blood pressure
- ○ **B.** Stop the infusion of magnesium sulfate and contact the physician
- ○ **C.** Slow the infusion rate and turn the client on her left side
- ○ **D.** Administer calcium gluconate IV push and continue to monitor the blood pressure

161. Which statement made by the nurse describes the inheritance pattern of autosomal recessive disorders?

- ○ **A.** An affected newborn has unaffected parents.
- ○ **B.** An affected newborn has one affected parent.
- ○ **C.** Affected parents have a one in four chance of passing on the defective gene.
- ○ **D.** Affected parents have unaffected children who are carriers.

162. A pregnant client, age 32, asks the nurse why her doctor has recommended a serum alpha fetoprotein. The nurse should explain that the doctor has recommended the test:

- ○ **A.** Because it is a state law
- ○ **B.** To detect cardiovascular defects
- ○ **C.** Because of her age
- ○ **D.** To detect neurological defects

163. A client with hypothyroidism asks the nurse if she will still need to take thyroid medication during the pregnancy. The nurse's response is based on the knowledge that:

- ○ **A.** There is no need to take thyroid medication because the fetus's thyroid produces a thyroid-stimulating hormone.
- ○ **B.** Regulation of thyroid medication is more difficult because the thyroid gland increases in size during pregnancy.
- ○ **C.** It is more difficult to maintain thyroid regulation during pregnancy due to a slowing of metabolism.
- ○ **D.** Fetal growth is arrested if thyroid medication is continued during pregnancy.

164. The nurse is responsible for performing a neonatal assessment on a full-term infant. At 1 minute, the nurse could expect to find:

- ○ **A.** An apical pulse of 100
- ○ **B.** An absence of tonus
- ○ **C.** Cyanosis of the feet and hands
- ○ **D.** Jaundice of the skin and sclera

165. A client with sickle cell anemia is admitted to the labor and delivery unit during the first phase of labor. The nurse should anticipate the client's need for:

- ○ **A.** Supplemental oxygen
- ○ **B.** Fluid restriction
- ○ **C.** Blood transfusion
- ○ **D.** Delivery by Caesarean section

166. A client with diabetes has an order for ultrasonography. Preparation for an ultrasound includes:

- ○ **A.** Increasing fluid intake
- ○ **B.** Limiting ambulation
- ○ **C.** Administering an enema
- ○ **D.** Withholding food for 8 hours

167. An infant who weighs 8 pounds at birth would be expected to weigh how many pounds at 1 year?

- ○ **A.** 14 pounds
- ○ **B.** 16 pounds
- ○ **C.** 18 pounds
- ○ **D.** 24 pounds

168. A pregnant client with a history of alcohol addiction is scheduled for a nonstress test. The nonstress test:

Quick Answer: **213**
Detailed Answer: **232**

- ○ **A.** Determines the lung maturity of the fetus
- ○ **B.** Measures the activity of the fetus
- ○ **C.** Shows the effect of contractions on the fetal heart rate
- ○ **D.** Measures the neurological well-being of the fetus

169. A full-term male has hypospadias. Which statement describes hypospadias?

Quick Answer: **213**
Detailed Answer: **232**

- ○ **A.** The urethral opening is absent.
- ○ **B.** The urethra opens on the top side of the penis.
- ○ **C.** The urethral opening is enlarged.
- ○ **D.** The urethra opens on the under side of the penis.

170. A gravida III para II is admitted to the labor unit. Vaginal exam reveals that the client's cervix is 8cm dilated, with complete effacement. The priority nursing diagnosis at this time is:

Quick Answer: **213**
Detailed Answer: **232**

- ○ **A.** Alteration in coping related to pain
- ○ **B.** Potential for injury related to precipitate delivery
- ○ **C.** Alteration in elimination related to anesthesia
- ○ **D.** Potential for fluid volume deficit related to NPO status

171. The client with varicella will most likely have an order for which category of medication?

Quick Answer: **213**
Detailed Answer: **232**

- ○ **A.** Antibiotics
- ○ **B.** Antipyretics
- ○ **C.** Antivirals
- ○ **D.** Anticoagulants

172. A client is admitted complaining of chest pain. Which of the following drug orders should the nurse question?

Quick Answer: **213**
Detailed Answer: **232**

- ○ **A.** Nitroglycerin
- ○ **B.** Ampicillin
- ○ **C.** Propranolol
- ○ **D.** Verapamil

173. Which of the following instructions should be included in the teaching for the client with rheumatoid arthritis?

Quick Answer: **213**
Detailed Answer: **233**

- ○ **A.** Avoid exercise because it fatigues the joints.
- ○ **B.** Take prescribed anti-inflammatory medications with meals.
- ○ **C.** Alternate hot and cold packs to affected joints.
- ○ **D.** Avoid weight-bearing activity.

174. A client with acute pancreatitis is experiencing severe abdominal pain. Which of the following orders should be questioned by the nurse?

- ○ **A.** Meperidine 100mg IM m 4 hours PRN pain
- ○ **B.** Mylanta 30 ccs m 4 hours via NG
- ○ **C.** Cimetadine 300mg PO m.i.d.
- ○ **D.** Morphine 8mg IM m 4 hours PRN pain

175. The client is admitted to the chemical dependence unit with an order for continuous observation. The nurse is aware that the doctor has ordered continuous observation because:

- ○ **A.** Hallucinogenic drugs create both stimulant and depressant effects.
- ○ **B.** Hallucinogenic drugs induce a state of altered perception.
- ○ **C.** Hallucinogenic drugs produce severe respiratory depression.
- ○ **D.** Hallucinogenic drugs induce rapid physical dependence.

176. A client with a history of abusing barbiturates abruptly stops taking the medication. The nurse should give priority to assessing the client for:

- ○ **A.** Depression and suicidal ideation
- ○ **B.** Tachycardia and diarrhea
- ○ **C.** Muscle cramping and abdominal pain
- ○ **D.** Tachycardia and euphoric mood

177. During the assessment of a laboring client, the nurse notes that the FHT are loudest in the upper-right quadrant. The infant is most likely in which position?

- ○ **A.** Right breech presentation
- ○ **B.** Right occipital anterior presentation
- ○ **C.** Left sacral anterior presentation
- ○ **D.** Left occipital transverse presentation

178. The primary physiological alteration in the development of asthma is:

- ○ **A.** Bronchiolar inflammation and dyspnea
- ○ **B.** Hypersecretion of abnormally viscous mucus
- ○ **C.** Infectious processes causing mucosal edema
- ○ **D.** Spasm of bronchiolar smooth muscle

179. A client with mania is unable to finish her dinner. To help her maintain sufficient nourishment, the nurse should:

- ○ **A.** Serve high-calorie foods she can carry with her
- ○ **B.** Encourage her appetite by sending out for her favorite foods
- ○ **C.** Serve her small, attractively arranged portions
- ○ **D.** Allow her in the unit kitchen for extra food whenever she pleases

180. To maintain Bryant's traction, the nurse must make certain that the child's:

- ○ **A.** Hips are resting on the bed, with the legs suspended at a right angle to the bed
- ○ **B.** Hips are slightly elevated above the bed and the legs are suspended at a right angle to the bed
- ○ **C.** Hips are elevated above the level of the body on a pillow and the legs are suspended parallel to the bed
- ○ **D.** Hips and legs are flat on the bed, with the traction positioned at the foot of the bed

181. Which action by the nurse indicates understanding of herpes zoster?

- ○ **A.** The nurse covers the lesions with a sterile dressing.
- ○ **B.** The nurse wears gloves when providing care.
- ○ **C.** The nurse administers a prescribed antibiotic.
- ○ **D.** The nurse administers oxygen.

182. The client has an order for a trough to be drawn on the client receiving Vancomycin. The nurse is aware that the nurse should contact the lab for them to collect the blood:

- ○ **A.** 15 minutes after the infusion
- ○ **B.** 30 minutes before the fourth infusion
- ○ **C.** 1 hour after the infusion
- ○ **D.** 2 hours after the infusion

183. The client using a diaphragm should be instructed to:

- ○ **A.** Refrain from keeping the diaphragm in longer than 4 hours
- ○ **B.** Keep the diaphragm in a cool location
- ○ **C.** Have the diaphragm resized if she gains 5 pounds
- ○ **D.** Have the diaphragm resized if she has any surgery

184. The nurse is providing postpartum teaching for a mother planning to breastfeed her infant. Which of the client's statements indicates the need for additional teaching?

○ **A.** "I'm wearing a support bra."

○ **B.** "I'm expressing milk from my breast."

○ **C.** "I'm drinking four glasses of fluid during a 24-hour period."

○ **D.** "While I'm in the shower, I'll allow the water to run over my breasts."

185. Damage to the VII cranial nerve results in:

○ **A.** Facial pain

○ **B.** Absence of ability to smell

○ **C.** Absence of eye movement

○ **D.** Tinnitus

186. A client is receiving Pyridium (phenazopyridine hydrochloride) for a urinary tract infection. The client should be taught that the medication may:

○ **A.** Cause diarrhea

○ **B.** Change the color of her urine

○ **C.** Cause mental confusion

○ **D.** Cause changes in taste

187. Which of the following tests should be performed before beginning a prescription of Accutane?

○ **A.** Check the calcium level

○ **B.** Perform a pregnancy test

○ **C.** Monitor apical pulse

○ **D.** Obtain a creatinine level

188. A client with AIDS is taking Zovirax (acyclovir). Which nursing intervention is most critical during the administration of acyclovir?

○ **A.** Limit the client's activity

○ **B.** Encourage a high-carbohydrate diet

○ **C.** Utilize an incentive spirometer to improve respiratory function

○ **D.** Encourage fluids

189. A client is admitted for an CAT scan. The nurse should question the client regarding:

Quick Answer: **214**
Detailed Answer: **234**

- ○ **A.** Pregnancy
- ○ **B.** A titanium hip replacement
- ○ **C.** Allergies to antibiotics
- ○ **D.** Inability to move his feet

190. The nurse is caring for the client receiving Amphotericin B. Which of the following indicates that the client has experienced toxicity to this drug?

Quick Answer: **214**
Detailed Answer: **234**

- ○ **A.** Changes in vision
- ○ **B.** Nausea
- ○ **C.** Urinary frequency
- ○ **D.** Changes in skin color

191. The nurse should visit which of the following clients first?

Quick Answer: **214**
Detailed Answer: **235**

- ○ **A.** The client with diabetes with a blood glucose of 95mg/dL
- ○ **B.** The client with hypertension being maintained on Lisinopril
- ○ **C.** The client with chest pain and a history of angina
- ○ **D.** The client with Raynaud's disease

192. A client with cystic fibrosis is taking pancreatic enzymes. The nurse should administer this medication:

Quick Answer: **214**
Detailed Answer: **235**

- ○ **A.** Once per day in the morning
- ○ **B.** Three times per day with meals
- ○ **C.** Once per day at bedtime
- ○ **D.** Four times per day

193. Cataracts result in opacity of the crystalline lens. Which of the following best explains the functions of the lens?

Quick Answer: **214**
Detailed Answer: **235**

- ○ **A.** The lens controls stimulation of the retina.
- ○ **B.** The lens orchestrates eye movement.
- ○ **C.** The lens focuses light rays on the retina.
- ○ **D.** The lens magnifies small objects.

194. A client who has glaucoma is to have miotic eyedrops instilled in both eyes. The nurse knows that the purpose of the medication is to:

Quick Answer: **214**
Detailed Answer: **235**

- ○ **A.** Anesthetize the cornea
- ○ **B.** Dilate the pupils
- ○ **C.** Constrict the pupils
- ○ **D.** Paralyze the muscles of accommodation

195. A client with a severe corneal ulcer has an order for Gentamycin gtt. q 4 hours and Neomycin 1 gtt q 4 hours. Which of the following schedules should be used when administering the drops?

- ○ **A.** Allow 5 minutes between the two medications.
- ○ **B.** The medications may be used together.
- ○ **C.** The medications should be separated by a cycloplegic drug.
- ○ **D.** The medications should not be used in the same client.

196. The client with color blindness will most likely have problems distinguishing which of the following colors?

- ○ **A.** Orange
- ○ **B.** Violet
- ○ **C.** Red
- ○ **D.** White

197. The client with a pacemaker should be taught to:

- ○ **A.** Report ankle edema
- ○ **B.** Check his blood pressure daily
- ○ **C.** Refrain from using a microwave oven
- ○ **D.** Monitor his pulse rate

198. The client with enuresis is being taught regarding bladder retraining. The nurse should advise the client to refrain from drinking after:

- ○ **A.** 1900
- ○ **B.** 1200
- ○ **C.** 1000
- ○ **D.** 0700

199. Which of the following diet instructions should be given to the client with recurring urinary tract infections?

- ○ **A.** Increase intake of meats.
- ○ **B.** Avoid citrus fruits.
- ○ **C.** Perform pericare with hydrogen peroxide.
- ○ **D.** Drink a glass of cranberry juice every day.

200. The physician has prescribed NPH insulin for a client with diabetes mellitus. Which statement indicates that the client knows when the peak action of the insulin occurs?

- ○ **A.** "I will make sure I eat breakfast within 2 hours of taking my insulin."
- ○ **B.** "I will need to carry candy or some form of sugar with me all the time."
- ○ **C.** "I will eat a snack around three o'clock each afternoon."
- ○ **D.** "I can save my dessert from supper for a bedtime snack."

201. A client with pneumacystis carini pneumonia is receiving Methotrexate. The rationale for administering leucovorin calcium to a client receiving Methotrexate is to:

- ○ **A.** Treat anemia.
- ○ **B.** Create a synergistic effect.
- ○ **C.** Increase the number of white blood cells.
- ○ **D.** Reverse drug toxicity.

202. A client tells the nurse that she is allergic to eggs, dogs, rabbits, and chicken feathers. Which order should the nurse question?

- ○ **A.** TB skin test
- ○ **B.** Rubella vaccine
- ○ **C.** ELISA test
- ○ **D.** Chest x-ray

203. The physician has prescribed rantidine (Zantac) for a client with erosive gastritis. The nurse should administer the medication:

- ○ **A.** 30 minutes before meals
- ○ **B.** With each meal
- ○ **C.** In a single dose at bedtime
- ○ **D.** 60 minutes after meals

204. A temporary colostomy is performed on the client with colon cancer. The nurse is aware that the proximal end of a double barrel colostomy:

- ○ **A.** Is the opening on the client's left side
- ○ **B.** Is the opening on the distal end on the client's left side
- ○ **C.** Is the opening on the client's right side
- ○ **D.** Is the opening on the distal right side

205. While assessing the postpartal client, the nurse notes that the fundus is displaced to the right. Based on this finding, the nurse should:

- ○ **A.** Ask the client to void
- ○ **B.** Assess the blood pressure for hypotension
- ○ **C.** Administer oxytocin
- ○ **D.** Check for vaginal bleeding

Quick Answer: **214**
Detailed Answer: **236**

206. The physician has ordered an MRI for a client with an orthopedic ailment. An MRI should not be done if the client has:

- ○ **A.** The need for oxygen therapy
- ○ **B.** A history of claustrophobia
- ○ **C.** A permanent pacemaker
- ○ **D.** Sensory deafness

Quick Answer: **214**
Detailed Answer: **236**

207. A 6-month-old client is placed on strict bed rest following a hernia repair. Which toy is best suited to the client?

- ○ **A.** Colorful crib mobile
- ○ **B.** Hand-held electronic games
- ○ **C.** Cars in a plastic container
- ○ **D.** 30-piece jigsaw puzzle

Quick Answer: **214**
Detailed Answer: **236**

208. The nurse is preparing to discharge a client with a long history of polio. The nurse should tell the client that:

- ○ **A.** Taking a hot bath will decrease stiffness and spasticity.
- ○ **B.** A schedule of strenuous exercise will improve muscle strength.
- ○ **C.** Rest periods should be scheduled throughout the day.
- ○ **D.** Visual disturbances can be corrected with prescription glasses.

Quick Answer: **214**
Detailed Answer: **236**

209. A client on the postpartum unit has a proctoepisiotomy. The nurse should anticipate administering which medication?

- ○ **A.** Dulcolax suppository
- ○ **B.** Docusate sodium (Colace)
- ○ **C.** Methyergonovine maleate (Methergine)
- ○ **D.** Bromocriptine sulfate (Parlodel)

Quick Answer: **214**
Detailed Answer: **236**

210. A client with pancreatic cancer has an infusion of TPN (Total Parenteral Nutrition). The doctor has ordered for sliding-scale insulin. The most likely explanation for this order is:

- ○ **A.** Total Parenteral Nutrition leads to negative nitrogen balance and elevated glucose levels.
- ○ **B.** Total Parenteral Nutrition cannot be managed with oral hypo-glycemics.
- ○ **C.** Total Parenteral Nutrition is a high-glucose solution that often elevates the blood glucose levels.
- ○ **D.** Total Parenteral Nutrition leads to further pancreatic disease.

211. An adolescent primigravida who is 10 weeks pregnant attends the antepartal clinic for a first check-up. To develop a teaching plan, the nurse should initially assess:

- ○ **A.** The client's knowledge of the signs of preterm labor
- ○ **B.** The client's feelings about the pregnancy
- ○ **C.** Whether the client was using a method of birth control
- ○ **D.** The client's thought about future children

212. An obstetric client is admitted with dehydration. Which IV fluid would be most appropriate for the client?

- ○ **A.** .45 normal saline
- ○ **B.** Dextrose 1% in water
- ○ **C.** Lactated Ringer's
- ○ **D.** Dextrose 5% in .45 normal saline

213. The physician has ordered a thyroid scan to confirm the diagnosis of a goiter. Before the procedure, the nurse should:

- ○ **A.** Assess the client for allergies
- ○ **B.** Bolus the client with IV fluid
- ○ **C.** Tell the client he will be asleep
- ○ **D.** Insert a urinary catheter

214. The physician has ordered an injection of RhoGam for a client with blood type A negative. The nurse understands that RhoGam is given to:

- ○ **A.** Provide immunity against Rh isoenzymes
- ○ **B.** Prevent the formation of Rh antibodies
- ○ **C.** Eliminate circulating Rh antibodies
- ○ **D.** Convert the Rh factor from negative to positive

215. The nurse is caring for a client admitted to the emergency room after a fall. X-rays reveal that the client has several fractured bones in the foot. Which treatment should the nurse anticipate for the fractured foot?

- ○ **A.** Application of a short inclusive spica cast
- ○ **B.** Stabilization with a plaster-of-Paris cast
- ○ **C.** Surgery with Kirschner wire implantation
- ○ **D.** A gauze dressing only

Quick Answer: **214**
Detailed Answer: **237**

216. A client with bladder cancer is being treated with iridium seed implants. The nurse's discharge teaching should include telling the client to:

- ○ **A.** Strain his urine
- ○ **B.** Increase his fluid intake
- ○ **C.** Report urinary frequency
- ○ **D.** Avoid prolonged sitting

Quick Answer: **214**
Detailed Answer: **237**

217. Following a heart transplant, a client is started on medication to prevent organ rejection. Which category of medication prevents the formation of antibodies against the new organ?

- ○ **A.** Antivirals
- ○ **B.** Antibiotics
- ○ **C.** Immunosuppressants
- ○ **D.** Analgesics

Quick Answer: **214**
Detailed Answer: **237**

218. The nurse is preparing a client for cataract surgery. The nurse is aware that the procedure will use:

- ○ **A.** Mydriatics to facilitate removal
- ○ **B.** Miotic medications such as Timoptic
- ○ **C.** A laser to smooth and reshape the lens
- ○ **D.** Silicone oil injections into the eyeball

Quick Answer: **214**
Detailed Answer: **237**

219. A client with Alzheimer's disease is awaiting placement in a skilled nursing facility. Which long-term plans would be most therapeutic for the client?

- ○ **A.** Placing mirrors in several locations in the home
- ○ **B.** Placing a picture of herself in her bedroom
- ○ **C.** Placing simple signs to indicate the location of the bedroom, bathroom, and so on
- ○ **D.** Alternating healthcare workers to prevent boredom

Quick Answer: **214**
Detailed Answer: **237**

220. A client with an abdominal cholecystectomy returns from surgery with a Jackson-Pratt drain. The chief purpose of the Jackson-Pratt drain is to:

- ○ **A.** Prevent the need for dressing changes
- ○ **B.** Reduce edema at the incision
- ○ **C.** Provide for wound drainage
- ○ **D.** Keep the common bile duct open

221. The nurse is performing an initial assessment of a newborn Caucasian male delivered at 32 weeks gestation. The nurse can expect to find the presence of:

- ○ **A.** Mongolian spots
- ○ **B.** Scrotal rugae
- ○ **C.** Head lag
- ○ **D.** Polyhydramnios

222. The nurse is caring for a client admitted with multiple trauma. Fractures include the pelvis, femur, and ulna. Which finding should be reported to the physician immediately?

- ○ **A.** Hematuria
- ○ **B.** Muscle spasms
- ○ **C.** Dizziness
- ○ **D.** Nausea

223. A client is brought to the emergency room by the police. He is combative and yells, "I have to get out of here. They are trying to kill me." Which assessment is most likely correct in relation to this statement?

- ○ **A.** The client is experiencing an auditory hallucination.
- ○ **B.** The client is having a delusion of grandeur.
- ○ **C.** The client is experiencing paranoid delusions.
- ○ **D.** The client is intoxicated.

224. The nurse is preparing to suction the client with a tracheotomy. The nurse notes a previously used bottle of normal saline on the client's bedside table. There is no label to indicate the date or time of initial use. The nurse should:

- ○ **A.** Lip the bottle and use a pack of sterile 4×4 for the dressing
- ○ **B.** Obtain a new bottle and label it with the date and time of first use
- ○ **C.** Ask the ward secretary when the solution was requested
- ○ **D.** Label the existing bottle with the current date and time

225. An infant's Apgar score is 9 at 5 minutes. The nurse is aware that the most likely cause for the deduction of one point is:

- ○ **A.** The baby is hypothermic.
- ○ **B.** The baby is experiencing bradycardia.
- ○ **C.** The baby's hands and feet are blue.
- ○ **D.** The baby is lethargic.

Quick Answer: **214**
Detailed Answer: **238**

226. The primary reason for rapid continuous rewarming of the area affected by frostbite is to:

- ○ **A.** Lessen the amount of cellular damage
- ○ **B.** Prevent the formation of blisters
- ○ **C.** Promote movement
- ○ **D.** Prevent pain and discomfort

Quick Answer: **214**
Detailed Answer: **238**

227. A client recently started on hemodialysis wants to know how the dialysis will take the place of his kidneys. The nurse's response is based on the knowledge that hemodialysis works by:

- ○ **A.** Passing water through a dialyzing membrane
- ○ **B.** Eliminating plasma proteins from the blood
- ○ **C.** Lowering the pH by removing nonvolatile acids
- ○ **D.** Filtering waste through a dialyzing membrane

Quick Answer: **214**
Detailed Answer: **238**

228. During a home visit, a client with AIDS tells the nurse that he has been exposed to measles. Which action by the nurse is most appropriate?

- ○ **A.** Administer an antibiotic
- ○ **B.** Contact the physician for an order for immune globulin
- ○ **C.** Administer an antiviral
- ○ **D.** Tell the client that he should remain in isolation for 2 weeks

Quick Answer: **214**
Detailed Answer: **238**

229. A client hospitalized with MRSA is placed on contact precautions. Which statement is true regarding precautions for infections spread by contact?

- ○ **A.** The client should be placed in a room with negative pressure.
- ○ **B.** Infection Requires close contact; therefore, the door may remain open.
- ○ **C.** Transmission is highly likely, so the client should wear a mask at all times.
- ○ **D.** Infection Requires skin-to-skin contact and is prevented by hand washing, gloves, and a gown.

Quick Answer: **214**
Detailed Answer: **238**

230. A client who is admitted with an above-the-knee amputation tells the nurse that his foot hurts and itches. Which response by the nurse indicates understanding of phantom limb pain?

Quick Answer: **214**
Detailed Answer: **239**

- ○ **A.** "The pain will go away in a few days."
- ○ **B.** "The pain is due to peripheral nervous system interruptions. I will get you some pain medication."
- ○ **C.** "The pain is psychological because your foot is no longer there."
- ○ **D.** "The pain and itching are due to the infection you had before the surgery."

231. A client with cancer of the pancreas has undergone a Whipple procedure. The nurse is aware that during the Whipple procedure, the doctor will remove the:

Quick Answer: **214**
Detailed Answer: **239**

- ○ **A.** Head of the pancreas
- ○ **B.** Proximal third section of the small intestines
- ○ **C.** Stomach and duodenum
- ○ **D.** Esophagus and jejunum

232. The physician has ordered a minimal-bacteria diet for a client with neutropenia. The client should be taught to avoid eating:

Quick Answer: **214**
Detailed Answer: **239**

- ○ **A.** Fruits
- ○ **B.** Salt
- ○ **C.** Pepper
- ○ **D.** Ketchup

233. A client is discharged home with a prescription for Coumadin (sodium warfarin). The client should be instructed to:

Quick Answer: **214**
Detailed Answer: **239**

- ○ **A.** Have a Protime done monthly
- ○ **B.** Eat more fruits and vegetables
- ○ **C.** Drink more liquids
- ○ **D.** Avoid crowds

234. The nurse is assisting the physician with removal of a central venous catheter. To facilitate removal, the nurse should instruct the client to:

Quick Answer: **214**
Detailed Answer: **239**

- ○ **A.** Perform the Valsalva maneuver as the catheter is advanced
- ○ **B.** Turn his head to the left side and hyperextend the neck
- ○ **C.** Take slow, deep breaths as the catheter is removed
- ○ **D.** Turn his head to the right while maintaining a sniffing position

235. A client has an order for streptokinase. Before administering the medication, the nurse should assess the client for:

   ○ **A.** Allergies to pineapples and bananas

   ○ **B.** A history of streptococcal infections

   ○ **C.** Prior therapy with phenytoin

   ○ **D.** A history of alcohol abuse

Quick Answer: **214**
Detailed Answer: **239**

236. The nurse is providing discharge teaching for the client with leukemia. The client should be told to avoid:

   ○ **A.** Using oil- or cream-based soaps

   ○ **B.** Flossing between the teeth

   ○ **C.** The intake of salt

   ○ **D.** Using an electric razor

Quick Answer: **214**
Detailed Answer: **239**

237. The nurse is changing the ties of the client with a tracheotomy. The safest method of changing the tracheotomy ties is to:

   ○ **A.** Apply the new tie before removing the old one.

   ○ **B.** Have a helper present.

   ○ **C.** Hold the tracheotomy with the nondominant hand while removing the old tie.

   ○ **D.** Ask the doctor to suture the tracheostomy in place.

Quick Answer: **214**
Detailed Answer: **239**

238. The nurse is monitoring a client following a lung resection. The hourly output from the chest tube was 300mL. The nurse should give priority to:

   ○ **A.** Turning the client to the left side

   ○ **B.** Milking the tube to ensure patency

   ○ **C.** Slowing the intravenous infusion

   ○ **D.** Notifying the physician

Quick Answer: **214**
Detailed Answer: **239**

239. The infant is admitted to the unit with Tetralogy of Fallot. The nurse would anticipate an order for which medication?

   ○ **A.** Digoxin

   ○ **B.** Epinephrine

   ○ **C.** Aminophyline

   ○ **D.** Atropine

Quick Answer: **214**
Detailed Answer: **239**

240. The nurse is educating the lady's club in self-breast exam. The nurse is aware that most malignant breast masses occur in the Tail of Spence. On the diagram, place an X on the Tail of Spence.

Quick Answer: **214**
Detailed Answer: **240**

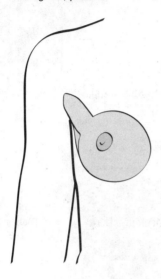

241. The toddler is admitted with a cardiac anomaly. The nurse is aware that the infant with a ventricular septal defect will:

○ **A.** Tire easily

○ **B.** Grow normally

○ **C.** Need more calories

○ **D.** Be more susceptible to viral infections

Quick Answer: **214**
Detailed Answer: **240**

242. The nurse is monitoring a client with a history of stillborn infants. The nurse is aware that a nonstress test can be ordered for this client to:

○ **A.** Determine lung maturity

○ **B.** Measure the fetal activity

○ **C.** Show the effect of contractions on fetal heart rate

○ **D.** Measure the well-being of the fetus

Quick Answer: **214**
Detailed Answer: **240**

243. The nurse is evaluating the client who was admitted 8 hours ago for induction of labor. The following graph is noted on the monitor. Which action should be taken first by the nurse?

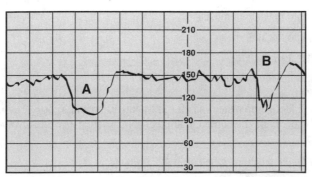

Fetal Heart Rate

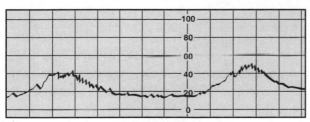

Uterine Contractions

- ○ **A.** Instruct the client to push
- ○ **B.** Perform a vaginal exam
- ○ **C.** Turn off the Pitocin infusion
- ○ **D.** Place the client in a semi-Fowler's position

244. The nurse notes the following on the ECG monitor. The nurse would evaluate the cardiac arrhythmia as:

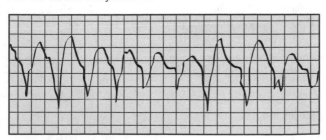

- ○ **A.** Atrial flutter
- ○ **B.** A sinus rhythm
- ○ **C.** Ventricular tachycardia
- ○ **D.** Atrial fibrillation

245. A client with clotting disorder has an order to continue Lovenox (enoxa-parin) injections after discharge. The nurse should teach the client that Lovenox injections should:

Quick Answer: **214**
Detailed Answer: **240**

- ○ **A.** Be injected into the deltoid muscle
- ○ **B.** Be injected into the abdomen
- ○ **C.** Aspirate after the injection
- ○ **D.** Clear the air from the syringe before injections

246. The nurse has a preop order to administer Valium (diazepam) 10mg and Phenergan (promethazine) 25mg. The correct method of administering these medications is to:

Quick Answer: **214**
Detailed Answer: **240**

- ○ **A.** Administer the medications together in one syringe
- ○ **B.** Administer the medication separately
- ○ **C.** Administer the Valium, wait 5 minutes, and then inject the Phenergan
- ○ **D.** Question the order because they cannot be given at the same time

247. A client with frequent urinary tract infections asks the nurse how she can prevent the reoccurrence. The nurse should teach the client to:

Quick Answer: **214**
Detailed Answer: **240**

- ○ **A.** Douche after intercourse
- ○ **B.** Void every 3 hours
- ○ **C.** Obtain a urinalysis monthly
- ○ **D.** Wipe from back to front after voiding

248. Which task should be assigned to the nursing assistant?

Quick Answer: **214**
Detailed Answer: **240**

- ○ **A.** Placing the client in seclusion
- ○ **B.** Emptying the Foley catheter of the preeclamptic client
- ○ **C.** Feeding the client with dementia
- ○ **D.** Ambulating the client with a fractured hip

249. The client has recently returned from having a thyroidectomy. The nurse should keep which of the following at the bedside?

Quick Answer: **214**
Detailed Answer: **240**

- ○ **A.** A tracheotomy set
- ○ **B.** A padded tongue blade
- ○ **C.** An endotracheal tube
- ○ **D.** An airway

Quick Check

Quick Answer: **214**
Detailed Answer: **240**

250. The physician has ordered a histoplasmosis test for the elderly client. The nurse is aware that histoplasmosis is transmitted to humans by:

○ **A.** Cats

○ **B.** Dogs

○ **C.** Turtles

○ **D.** Birds

Quick Check Answer Key

1.	D	31.	B	61.	D
2.	D	32.	A	62.	A
3.	B	33.	B	63.	C
4.	C	34.	B	64.	B
5.	C	35.	D	65.	A
6.	C	36.	B	66.	D
7.	D	37.	A	67.	B
8.	D	38.	B	68.	C
9.	C	39.	D	69.	A
10.	B	40.	A	70.	C
11.	A	41.	A	71.	C
12.	C	42.	A	72.	D
13.	D	43.	A	73.	B
14.	B	44.	C	74.	D
15.	B	45.	B	75.	D
16.	A	46.	A	76.	B
17.	A	47.	B	77.	D
18.	A	48.	C	78.	D
19.	C	49.	C	79.	A
20.	B	50.	D	80.	B
21.	C	51.	B	81.	A
22.	A	52.	B	82.	A
23.	A	53.	B	83.	D
24.	B	54.	C	84.	D
25.	D	55.	D	85.	B
26.	A	56.	A	86.	B
27.	B	57.	B	87.	B
28.	C	58.	C	88.	B
29.	C	59.	C	89.	D
30.	C	60.	B	90.	B

91. A	123. D	**155.** B
92. C	124. A	**156.** D
93. C	125. A	**157.** A
94. B	126. B	**158.** A
95. C	127. A	**159.** C
96. A	128. B	**160.** A
97. B	129. C	**161.** C
98. C	130. B	**162.** D
99. D	131. B	**163.** B
100. C	132. B	**164.** C
101. B	133. B	**165.** A
102. D	134. A	**166.** A
103. B	135. A	**167.** D
104. D	136. A	**168.** B
105. B	137. C	**169.** D
106. B	138. B	**170.** A
107. D	139. A	**171.** C
108. D	140. B	**172.** B
109. C	141. B	**173.** B
110. D	142. B	**174.** D
111. C	143. D	**175.** B
112. B	144. A	**176.** B
113. C	145. A	**177.** A
114. C	146. A	**178.** D
115. D	147. C	**179.** A
116. C	148. B	**180.** B
117. B	149. A	**181.** B
118. B	150. C	**182.** B
119. C	151. B	**183.** B
120. B	152. D	**184.** C
121. B	153. C	**185.** A
122. A	154. C	**186.** B

187. B	**209.** B	**231.** A	**241.** A
188. D	**210.** C	**232.** C	**242.** B
189. A	**211.** B	**233.** A	**243.** C
190. D	**212.** A	**234.** A	**244.** C
191. C	**213.** A	**235.** B	**245.** B
192. B	**214.** B	**236.** B	**246.** B
193. C	**215.** B	**237.** A	**247.** B
194. C	**216.** A	**238.** D	**248.** C
195. A	**217.** C	**239.** A	**249.** A
196. B	**218.** A	**240.** See diagram.	**250.** D
197. D	**219.** C		
198. A	**220.** C		
199. D	**221.** C		
200. C	**222.** A		
201. D	**223.** C		
202. B	**224.** B		
203. B	**225.** C		
204. C	**226.** A		
205. A	**227.** D		
206. C	**228.** B		
207. C	**229.** D		
208. C	**230.** B		

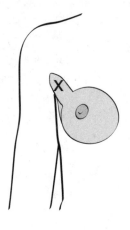

Answers and Rationales

1. **Answer D is correct.** It is important to assess the extremities for blood vessel occlusion in the client with sickle cell anemia because a change in capillary refill would indicate a change in circulation. Body temperature, motion, and sensation would not give information regarding peripheral circulation; therefore, answers A, B, and C are incorrect.

2. **Answer D is correct.** Placing the client in semi-Fowler's position provides the best oxygenation for this client. Flexion of the hips and knees, which includes the knee-chest position, impedes circulation and is not correct positioning for this client. Therefore, answers A, B, and C are incorrect.

3. **Answer B is correct.** It is important to keep the client in sickle cell crisis hydrated to prevent further sickling of the blood. Answer A is incorrect because a mechanical cuff places too much pressure on the arm. Answer C is incorrect because raising the knee gatch impedes circulation. Answer D is incorrect because Tylenol is too mild an analgesic for the client in crisis.

4. **Answer C is correct.** Hydration is important in the client with sickle cell disease to prevent thrombus formation. Popsicles, gelatin, juice, and pudding have high fluid content. The foods in answers A, B, and D do not aid in hydration and are, therefore, incorrect.

5. **Answer C is correct.** The pulse oximetry indicates that oxygen levels are low; thus, oxygenation takes precedence over pain relief. Answer A is incorrect because although a warm environment reduces pain and minimizes sickling, it would not be a priority. Answer B is incorrect because although hydration is important, it would not require a bolus. Answer D is incorrect because Demerol is acidifying to the blood and increases sickling.

6. **Answer C is correct.** Egg yolks, wheat bread, carrots, raisins, and green, leafy vegetables are all high in iron, which is an important mineral for this client. Roast beef, cabbage, and pork chops are also high in iron, but the side dishes accompanying these choices are not; therefore, answers A, B, and D are incorrect.

7. **Answer D is correct.** Taking a trip to the museum is the only answer that does not pose a threat. A family vacation in the Rocky Mountains at high altitudes, cold temperatures, and airplane travel can cause sickling episodes and should be avoided; therefore, answers A, B, and C are incorrect.

8. **Answer D is correct.** The tongue of the client with B12 insufficiency is red and beefy. A, B, and C incorrect because enlarged spleen, elevated BP, and bradycardia are not associated with B12 deficiency.

9. **Answer C is correct.** The oral mucosa and hard palate (roof of the mouth) are the best indicators of jaundice in dark-skinned persons. The conjunctiva can have normal deposits of fat, which give a yellowish hue; thus, answer A is incorrect. The soles of the feet can be yellow if they are calloused, making answer B incorrect; the shins would be an area of darker pigment, so answer D is incorrect.

10. **Answer B is correct.** When there are fewer red blood cells, there is less hemoglobin and less oxygen. Therefore, the client is often short of breath, as indicated in answer B. The client with anemia is often pale in color, has weight loss, and may be hypotensive. Answers A, C, and D are within normal and, therefore, are incorrect.

11. **Answer A is correct.** The client with polycythemia vera is at risk for thrombus formation. Hydrating the client with at least 3L of fluid per day is important in preventing clot formation, so the statement to drink less than 500mL is incorrect. Answers B, C, and D are incorrect because they all contribute to the prevention of complications. Support hose promotes venous return, the electric razor prevents bleeding due to injury, and a diet low in iron is essential to preventing further red cell formation.

12. **Answer C is correct.** Radiation treatment for other types of cancer can contribute to the development of leukemia. Some hobbies and occupations involving chemicals are linked to leukemia, but not the ones in these answers; therefore, answers A and B are incorrect. Answer D is incorrect because the incidence of leukemia is higher in twins not siblings.

13. **Answer D is correct.** Petechiae are not usually visualized on dark skin. The soles of the feet and palms of the hand provide a lighter surface for assessing the client for petichiae. Answers A, B, and C are incorrect because the skin may be too dark to make an assessment.

14. **Answer B is correct.** The client with leukemia is at risk for infection and has often had recurrent respiratory infections during the previous 6 months. Insomnolence, weight loss, and a decrease in alertness also occur in leukemia, but bleeding tendencies and infections are the primary clinical manifestations; therefore, answers A, C, and D are incorrect.

15. **Answer B is correct.** The client with acute leukemia has bleeding tendencies due to decreased platelet counts, and any injury would exacerbate the problem. The client would require close monitoring for hemorrhage, which is of higher priority than the diagnoses in answers A, C, and D, which are incorrect.

16. **Answer A is correct.** Radiation therapy often causes sterility in male clients and would be of primary importance to this client. The psychosocial needs of the client are important to address in light of the age and life choices. Hodgkin's disease, however, has a good prognosis when diagnosed early. Answers B, C, and D are incorrect because they are of lesser priority.

17. **Answer A is correct.** Clients with autoimmune thrombocytopenic purpura (ATP) have low platelet counts, making answer A the correct answer. White cell counts, potassium levels, and PTT are not affected in ATP; thus, answers B, C, and D are incorrect.

18. **Answer A is correct.** The normal platelet count is 120,000–400,000. Bleeding occurs in clients with low platelets. The priority is to prevent and minimize bleeding. Oxygenation in answer C is important, but platelets do not carry oxygen. Answers B and D are of lesser priority and are incorrect in this instance.

19. **Answer C is correct.** A prolactinoma is a type of pituitary tumor. Elevating the head of the bed 30° avoids pressure on the sella turcica and helps to prevent headaches. Answers A, B, and D are incorrect because Trendelenburg, Valsalva maneuver, and coughing all increase the intracranial pressure.

20. **Answer B is correct.** The large amount of fluid loss can cause fluid and electrolyte imbalance that should be corrected. The loss of electrolytes would be reflected in the vital signs. Measuring the urinary output is important, but the stem already says that the client has polyuria, so answer A is incorrect. Encouraging fluid intake will not correct the problem, making answer C incorrect. Answer D is incorrect because weighing the client is not necessary at this time.

21. **Answer C is correct.** C is correct because direct pressure to the nose stops the bleeding. Answers A, B, and D are incorrect because they do not stop bleeding

22. **Answer A is correct.** Blood pressure is the best indicator of cardiovascular collapse in the client who has had an adrenal gland removed. The remaining gland might have been suppressed due to the tumor activity. Temperature would be an indicator of infection, decreased output would be a clinical manifestation but would take longer to occur than blood pressure changes, and specific gravity changes occur with other disorders; therefore, answers B, C, and D are incorrect.

23. **Answer A is correct.** IV glucocorticoids raise the glucose levels and often require coverage with Insulin. Answer B is not necessary at this time, sodium and potassium levels would be monitored when the client is receiving mineral corticoids, and daily weights is unnecessary; therefore, answers B, C, and D are incorrect.

24. **Answer B is correct.** The parathyroid glands are responsible for calcium production and can be damaged during a thyroidectomy. The tingling can be due to low calcium levels. The crash cart would be needed in respiratory distress but would not be the next action to take; thus, answer A is incorrect. Hypertension occurs in thyroid storm and the drainage would occur in hemorrhage, so answers C and D are incorrect.

25. **Answer D is correct.** The decrease in pulse can affect the cardiac output and lead to shock, which would take precedence over the other choices; therefore, answers A, B, and C are incorrect.

26. **Answer A is correct.** The client taking antilipidemics should be encouraged to report muscle weakness because this is a sign of rhabdomyolysis. The medication takes effect within 1 month of beginning therapy, so answer B is incorrect. The medication should be taken with water because fruit juice, particularly grapefruit, can decrease the effectiveness, making answer C incorrect. Liver function studies should be checked before beginning the medication, not after the fact, making answer D incorrect.

27. **Answer B is correct.** Hyperstat is given IV push for hypertensive crises, but it often causes hyperglycemia. The glucose level will drop rapidly when stopped. Answer A is incorrect because the hyperstat is given by IV push. The client should be placed in dorsal recumbent position, not Trendelenburg position, as stated in answer C. Answer D is incorrect because the medication does not have to be covered with foil.

28. **Answer C is correct.** A heart rate of 60 in the baby should be reported immediately. The dose should be held if the heart rate is below 100bpm. The blood glucose, blood pressure, and respirations are within normal limits; thus answers A, B, and D are incorrect.

29. **Answer C is correct.** Nitroglycerine should be kept in a brown bottle (or even a special air- and water-tight, solid or plated silver or gold container) because of its instability and tendency to become less potent when exposed to air, light, or water. The supply should be replenished every 6 months, not 3 months, and one tablet should be taken every 5 minutes until pain subsides, so answers A and B are incorrect. If the pain does not subside, the client should report to the emergency room. The medication should be taken sublingually and should not be crushed, as stated in answer D.

30. **Answer C is correct.** Turkey contains the least amount of fats and cholesterol. Liver, eggs, beef, cream sauces, shrimp, cheese, and chocolate should be avoided by the client; thus, answers A, B, and D are incorrect. The client should bake meat rather than frying to avoid adding fat to the meat during cooking.

31. **Answer B is correct.** The jugular veins in the neck should be assessed for distension. The other parts of the body will be edematous in right-sided congestive heart failure, not left-sided; thus, answers A, C, and D are incorrect.

32. **Answer A is correct.** The phlebostatic axis is located at the fifth intercostals space midaxillary line and is the correct placement of the manometer. The PMI or point of maximal impulse is located at the fifth intercostals space midclavicular line, so answer B is incorrect. Erb's point is the point at which you can hear the valves close simultaneously, making answer C incorrect. The Tail of Spence (the upper outer quadrant of the breast) is the area where most breast cancers are located and has nothing to do with placement of a manometer; thus, answer D is incorrect.

33. **Answer B is correct.** Zestril is an ACE inhibitor and is frequently given with a diuretic such as Lasix for hypertension. Answers A, C, and D are incorrect because the order is accurate. There is no need to question the order, administer the medication separately, or contact the pharmacy.

34. **Answer B is correct.** The best indicator of peripheral edema is measuring the extremity. A paper tape measure should be used rather than one made of plastic or cloth, and the area should be marked with a pen, providing the most objective assessment. Answer A is incorrect because weighing the client will not indicate peripheral edema. Answer C is incorrect because checking the intake and output will not indicate peripheral edema. Answer D is incorrect because checking for pitting edema is less reliable than measuring with a paper tape measure.

35. **Answer D is correct.** Clients with radium implants should have close contact limited to 30 minutes per visit. The general rule is limiting time spent exposed to radium, putting distance between people and the radium source, and using lead to shield against the radium. Teaching the family member these principles is extremely important. Answers A, B, and C are not empathetic and do not address the question; therefore, they are incorrect.

36. **Answer B is correct.** The client with a facial stroke will have difficulty swallowing and chewing, and the foods in answer B provide the least amount of chewing. The foods in answers A, C, and D would require more chewing and, thus, are incorrect.

37. **Answer A is correct.** Novalog insulin onsets very quickly, so food should be available within 10–15 minutes of taking the insulin. Answer B does not address a particular type of insulin, so it is incorrect. NPH insulin peaks in 8–12 hours, so a snack should be eaten at the expected peak time. It may not be 3 p.m. as stated in answer C. Answer D is incorrect because there is no need to save the dessert until bedtime.

38. **Answer B is correct.** The umbilical cord needs time to dry and fall off before putting the infant in the tub. Although answers A, C, and D might be important, they are not the primary answer to the question.

39. **Answer D is correct.** Leucovorin is the antidote for Methotrexate and Trimetrexate which are folic acid antagonists. Leucovorin is a folic acid derivative. Answers A, B, and C are incorrect because Leucovorin does not treat iron deficiency, increase neutrophils, or have a synergistic effect.

40. **Answer A is correct.** The Hemophilus influenza vaccine is given at 4 months with the polio vaccine. Answers B, C, and D are incorrect because these vaccines are given later in life.

41. **Answer A is correct.** Proton pump inhibitors should be taken prior to the meal. Answers B, C, and D are incorrect times for giving proton pump inhibitors like Nexium.

42. **Answer A is correct.** If the client is a threat to the staff and to other clients the nurse should call for help and prepare to administer a medication such as Haldol to sedate him. Answer B is incorrect because simply telling the client to calm down will not work. Answer C is incorrect because telling the client that if he continues he will be punished is a threat and may further anger him. Answer D is incorrect because if the client is left alone he might harm himself.

43. **Answer A is correct.** If the fundus of the client is displaced to the side, this might indicate a full bladder. The next action by the nurse should be to check for bladder distention and catheterize, if necessary. The answers in B, C, and D are actions that relate to postpartal hemorrhage.

44. **Answer C is correct.** A low-grade temperature, blood-tinged sputum, fatigue, and night sweats are symptoms consistent with tuberculosis. If the answer in A had said pneumocystis pneumonia, answer A would have been consistent with the symptoms given in the stem, but just saying pneumonia isn't specific enough to diagnose the problem. Answers B and D are not directly related to the stem.

45. **Answer B is correct.** If the client has a history of Prinzmetal's angina, he should not be prescribed triptan preparations because they cause vasoconstriction and coronary spasms. There is no contraindication for taking triptan drugs in clients with diabetes, cancer, or cluster headaches making answers A, C, and D incorrect.

46. **Answer A is correct.** Kernig's sign is positive if pain occurs on flexion of the hip and knee. The Brudzinski reflex is positive if pain occurs on flexion of the head and neck onto the chest so answer B is incorrect. Answers C and D might be present but are not related to Kernig's sign.

47. **Answer B is correct.** Apraxia is the inability to use objects appropriately. Agnosia is loss of sensory comprehension, anomia is the inability to find words, and aphasia is the inability to speak or understand so answers A, C, and D are incorrect.

48. **Answer C is correct.** Increased confusion at night is known as "sundowning" syndrome. This increased confusion occurs when the sun begins to set and continues during the night. Answer A is incorrect because fatigue is not necessarily present. Increased confusion at night is not part of normal aging; therefore, answer B is incorrect. A delusion is a firm, fixed belief; therefore, answer D is incorrect.

49. **Answer C is correct.** The client who is confused might forget that he ate earlier. Don't argue with the client. Simply get him something to eat that will satisfy him until lunch. Answers A and D are incorrect because the nurse is dismissing the client. Answer B is validating the delusion.

50. **Answer D is correct.** Nausea and gastrointestinal upset are very common in clients taking acetylcholinesterase inhibitors such as Exelon. Other side effects include liver toxicity, dizziness, unsteadiness, and clumsiness. The client might already be experiencing urinary incontinence or headaches, but they are not necessarily associated; and the client with Alzheimer's disease is already confused. Therefore, answers A, B, and C are incorrect.

51. **Answer B is correct.** Any lesion should be reported to the doctor. This can indicate a herpes lesion. Clients with open lesions related to herpes are delivered by Cesarean section because there is a possibility of transmission of the infection to the fetus with direct contact to lesions. It is not enough to document the finding, so answer A is incorrect. The physician must make the decision to perform a C-section, making answer C incorrect. It is not enough to continue primary care, so answer D is incorrect.

52. **Answer B is correct.** The client with HPV is at higher risk for cervical and vaginal cancer related to this STI. She is not at higher risk for the other cancers mentioned in answers A, C, and D, so those are incorrect.

53. **Answer B is correct.** A lesion that is painful is most likely a herpetic lesion. A chancre lesion associated with syphilis is not painful, so answer A is incorrect. Condylomata lesions are painless warts, so answer D is incorrect. In answer C, gonorrhea does not present as a lesion, but is exhibited by a yellow discharge.

54. **Answer C is correct.** Florescent treponemal antibody (FTA) is the test for treponema pallidum. VDRL and RPR are screening tests done for syphilis, so answers A and B are incorrect. The Thayer-Martin culture is done for gonorrhea, so answer D is incorrect.

55. **Answer D is correct.** The criteria for HELLP is hemolysis, elevated liver enzymes, and low platelet count. In answer A, an elevated blood glucose level is not associated with HELLP. Platelets are decreased, not elevated, in HELLP syndrome as stated in answer B. The creatinine levels are elevated in renal disease and are not associated with HELLP syndrome so answer C is incorrect.

56. **Answer A is correct.** Answer B elicits the triceps reflex, so it is incorrect. Answer C elicits the patella reflex, making it incorrect. Answer D elicits the radial nerve, so it is incorrect.

57. **Answer B is correct.** Brethine is used cautiously because it raises the blood glucose levels. Answers A, C, and D are all medications that are commonly used in the diabetic client, so they are incorrect.

58. **Answer C is correct.** When the L/S ratio reaches 2:1, the lungs are considered to be mature. The infant will most likely be small for gestational age and will not be at risk for birth trauma, so answer D is incorrect. The L/S ratio does not indicate congenital anomalies, as stated in answer A, and the infant is not at risk for intrauterine growth retardation, making answer B incorrect.

59. **Answer C is correct.** Jitteriness is a sign of seizure in the neonate. Crying, wakefulness, and yawning are expected in the newborn, so answers A, B, and D are incorrect.

60. **Answer B is correct.** The client is expected to become sleepy, have hot flashes, and be lethargic. A decreasing urinary output, absence of the knee-jerk reflex, and decreased respirations indicate toxicity, so answers A, C, and D are incorrect.

61. **Answer D is correct.** If the client experiences hypotension after an injection of epidural anesthetic, the nurse should turn her to the left side, apply oxygen by mask, and speed the IV infusion. If the blood pressure does not return to normal, the physician should be contacted. Epinephrine should be kept for emergency administration. Answer A is incorrect because placing the client in Trendelenburg position (head down) will allow the anesthesia to move up above the respiratory center, thereby decreasing the diaphragm's ability to move up and down and ventilate the client. In answer B, the IV rate should be increased, not decreased. In answer C, the oxygen should be applied by mask, not cannula.

62. **Answer A is correct.** Cancer of the pancreas frequently leads to severe nausea and vomiting and altered glucose levels. The other problems are of lesser concern; thus, answers B, C, and D are incorrect.

63. **Answer C is correct.** Uremic frost is most likely related to liver disease. It is not related to anemia, arteriosclerosis, or parathyroid disorders, therefore A, B, and D are incorrect.

64. **Answer B is correct.** The vital signs indicate hypovolemic shock. They do not indicate cerebral tissue perfusion, airway clearance, or sensory perception alterations, so answers A, C, and D are incorrect.

65. **Answer A is correct.** The client with osteogenesis imperfecta is at risk for pathological fractures and is likely to experience these fractures if he participates in contact sports. Answers B, C, and D are not factors for concern.

66. **Answer D is correct.** The client with neutropenia should not have fresh fruit because it should be peeled and/or cooked before eating. Any source of bacteria should be eliminated, if possible. Answers A, B, and C will not help prevent bacterial invasions.

67. **Answer B is correct.** The client's BP is low so increasing the IV is priority. Answers A, C, and D are not the first priority therefore they are incorrect.

68. **Answer C is correct.** If the client pulls the chest tube out of the chest, the nurse's first action should be to cover the insertion site with an occlusive dressing. Afterward, the nurse should call the doctor, who will order a chest x-ray and possibly reinsert the tube. Answers A, B, and D are not the first action to be taken.

69. **Answer A is correct.** The normal Protime is approximately 12–20 seconds. A Protime of 120 seconds indicates an extremely prolonged Protime and can result in a spontaneous bleeding episode. Answers B, C, and D may be needed at a later time but are not the most important actions to take first.

70. **Answer C is correct.** The food with the most calcium is the yogurt. Answers A, B, and D are good choices, but not as good as the yogurt, which has approximately 400mg of calcium.

71. **Answer C is correct.** The client receiving magnesium sulfate should have a Foley catheter in place, and hourly intake and output should be checked. Answers A, B, and D are incorrect because they do not indicate understanding of $MgSO_4$ toxicity.

72. **Answer D is correct.** D is correct because the best size cathlon to use in a child receiving blood is a 20 gauge. A, B, and C are incorrect because the size is either too large or too small.

73. **Answer B is correct.** The nurse should be most concerned with laryngeal edema because of the area of burn. The next priority should be answer A, as well as hyponatremia and hypokalemia in C and D, but these answers are not of primary concern so are incorrect.

74. **Answer D is correct.** The client with diabetes indicates understanding of his illness by correctly demonstrating the technique for administration. A, B, and C are incorrect because they do not indicate understanding.

75. **Answer D is correct.** At this time, pain beneath the cast is normal. The client's fingers should be warm to the touch, and pulses should be present. Paresthesia is not normal and might indicate compartment syndrome. Therefore, Answers A, B, and C are incorrect.

76. **Answer B is correct.** Herbals can prolong bleeding times or interfere with antiviral medications, therefore the client should avoid the use of herbals. A and D are not contraindicated for the client with AIDS. C is incorrect because there is no need to report all changes in skin color.

77. **Answer D is correct.** It is not necessary to wear gloves to check the IV drip rate. The healthcare workers in answers A, B, and C indicate knowledge by their actions.

78. **Answer D is correct.** The client that is having ECT is given a sedative. When the blood pressure cuff is inflated the fingers twitch when he has a grand mal seizure. A, B, and C are incorrect because there is no need for the nurse to take these interventions prior to ECT.

79. **Answer A is correct.** Pinworms cause rectal itching. B, C, and D are incorrect because they are not signs of pinworms.

80. **Answer B is correct.** Bed linen should be washed in hot water. A is incorrect because special shampoos can be used by children under age 10. Answers C and D are incorrect statements therefore they are wrong.

81. **Answer A is correct.** The pregnant nurse can care for the client with HIV if she uses standard precautions. The clients in answers B, C, and D pose a risk to the pregnant nurse.

82. **Answer A is correct.** The client with MRSA is placed on contact precautions. The clients in answers B, C, and D pose no risk to themselves or others.

83. **Answer D is correct.** The doctor could be charged with malpractice, which is failing to perform, or performing an act that causes harm to the client. Answers A, B, and C are incorrect because they apply to other wrongful acts. Negligence is failing to perform care for the client; a tort is a wrongful act committed on the client or their belongings; and assault is a violent physical or verbal attack.

84. **Answer D is correct.** The nursing assistant should not be assigned to administer a Fleets enema. They can administer a soap suds or tap water enema. The other tasks can be performed by the nursing assistant, therefore A, B, and C are incorrect.

85. **Answer B is correct.** The mother is most likely describing a newborn rash. About 30% of all newborns have a rash on the face and forehead that dissipates in approximately one month. A, C, and D are incorrect actions.

86. **Answer B is correct.** The nurse who is pregnant should not be assigned to the client with a radium implant. The other nurses are not at risk when caring for this client, so A, C, and D are incorrect.

87. **Answer B is correct.** The Joint Commission on Accreditation of Hospitals will probably be interested in the problems in answers A and C. The failure of the nursing assistant to care for the client with hepatitis might result in termination, but is not of interest to the Joint Commission.

88. **Answer B is correct.** The next action after discussing the problem with the nurse is to document the incident by filing a formal reprimand. If the behavior continues or if harm has resulted to the client, the nurse may be terminated and reported to the Board of Nursing, but these are not the first actions requested in the stem. A tort is a wrongful act to the client or his belongings and is not indicated in this instance. Therefore, Answers A, C, and D are incorrect.

89. **Answer D is correct.** The client at highest risk for complications is the client with multiple sclerosis who is being treated with cortisone via the central line. The clients in answers A, B, and C are more stable and can be seen later.

90. **Answer B is correct.** The pregnant client and the client with a broken arm are the best choices for placing in the same room. The clients in answers A, C, and D need to be placed in separate rooms due to the serious natures of their injuries.

91. **Answer A is correct.** Before instilling the eardrops, the nurse should consider the age of the child because the ear should be pulled down and out to best deliver the drops in the ear canal. B, C, and D are not considerations when instilling eardrops in a small child.

92. **Answer C is correct.** Remember the ABCs (airway, breathing, circulation) when answering this question. Answer C is correct because a hotdog is the size and shape of the child's trachea and poses a risk of aspiration. Answers A, B, and D are incorrect because white grape juice, a grilled cheese sandwich, and ice cream do not pose a risk of aspiration for a child.

93. **Answer C is correct.** A viral load of 200 is extremely low. This indicates that the client has a low risk for opportunistic illnesses. A, B, and D do not indicate understanding.

94. **Answer B is correct.** Lantus insulin cannot be mixed with other insulins, but can be taken by the client taking regular insulin. A, C, and D are not correct methods of administering Lantus insulin with regular insulin.

95. **Answer C is correct.** Always remember your ABCs (airway, breathing, circulation) when selecting an answer. A, B, and D are incorrect because they are not the priority.

96. **Answer A is correct.** The client with glomerulonephritis will probably have hypertension. B and C are vague answers and are therefore incorrect. D does not directly relate to glomerulonephritis.

97. **Answer B is correct.** A child with epiglottis has the possibility of complete obstruction of the airway. For this reason the nurse should not evaluate the airway using a tongue blade. A, C, and D are allowed actions and are therefore incorrect.

98. **Answer C is correct.** Exophthalmos (protrusion of eyeballs) often occurs with hyperthyroidism. The client with hyperthyroidism will often exhibit tachycardia, increased appetite, and weight loss; therefore, answers A, B, and D are incorrect.

99. **Answer D is correct.** The child with celiac disease should be on a gluten-free diet. Answers A, B, and C all contain gluten, while answer D gives the only choice of foods that does not contain gluten.

100. **Answer C is correct.** Remember the ABCs (airway, breathing, circulation) when answering this question. Before notifying the physician or assessing the pulse, oxygen should be applied to increase the oxygen saturation, so answers A and D are incorrect. The normal oxygen saturation is 92%–100%, making answer B incorrect.

101. **Answer B is correct.** An amniotomy is an artificial rupture of membranes and normal amniotic fluid is straw-colored and odorless. A, C, and D are abnormal findings.

102. **Answer D is correct.** Diabeta is an antidiabetic medication that can result in hypoglycemia. A, B, and D are incorrect because they are not related to Diabeta.

103. **Answer B is correct.** The normal fetal heart rate is 120–160bpm; 100–110bpm is bradycardia. The first action would be to turn the client to the left side and apply oxygen. Answer A is not indicated at this time. Answer C is not the best action for clients experiencing bradycardia. There is no data to indicate the need to move the client to the delivery room at this time.

104. **Answer D is correct.** Arterial ulcers are painful. A, B, and C are incorrect because they do not describe arterial ulcers.

105. **Answer B is correct.** Applying a fetal heart monitor is the correct action at this time. There is no need to prepare for a Caesarean section or to place the client in Genu Pectoral position (knee-chest), so answers A and C are incorrect. Answer D is incorrect because there is no need for an ultrasound based on the finding.

106. **Answer B is correct.** The nurse decides to apply an external monitor because the membranes are intact. Answers A, C, and D are incorrect. The cervix is dilated enough to use an internal monitor, if necessary. An internal monitor can be applied if the client is at 0-station. Contraction intensity has no bearing on the application of the fetal monitor.

107. **Answer D is correct.** Clients admitted in labor are told not to eat during labor, to avoid nausea and vomiting. Ice chips may be allowed, but this amount of fluid might not be sufficient to prevent fluid volume deficit. In answer A, impaired gas exchange related to hyperventilation would be indicated during the transition phase. Answers B and C are not correct in relation to the stem.

108. **Answer D is correct.** This information indicates a late deceleration. This type of deceleration is caused by uteroplacental lack of oxygen. Answer A has no relation to the readings, so it's incorrect; answer B results in a variable deceleration; and answer C is indicative of an early deceleration.

109. **Answer C is correct.** The initial action by the nurse observing a late deceleration should turn the client to the side—preferably, the left side. Administering oxygen is also indicated. Answer A might be necessary but not before turning the client to her side. Answer B is not necessary at this time. Answer D is incorrect because there is no data to indicate that the monitor has been applied incorrectly.

110. **Answer D is correct.** A deceleration to 90–100bpm at the end of contractions are late decelerations. This finding is ominous (bad) and should be reported. A, B, and D are normal findings and are therefore incorrect.

111. **Answer C is correct.** Epidural anesthesia decreases the urge to void and sensation of a full bladder. A full bladder will decrease the progression of labor. Answers A, B, and D are incorrect for the stem.

112. **Answer B is correct.** Lutenizing hormone released by the pituitary is responsible for ovulation. At about day 14, the continued increase in estrogen stimulates the release of lutenizing hormone from the anterior pituitary. The LH surge is responsible for ovulation, or the release of the dominant follicle in preparation for conception, which occurs within the next 10–12 hours after the LH levels peak. Answers A, C, and D are incorrect because estrogen levels are high at the beginning of ovulation, the endometrial lining is thick, not thin, and the progesterone levels are high, not low.

113. **Answer C is correct.** The success of the rhythm method of birth control is dependent on the client's menses being regular. It is not dependent on the age of the client, frequency of intercourse, or range of the client's temperature; therefore, answers A, B, and D are incorrect.

114. **Answer C is correct.** The best method of birth control for the client with diabetes is the diaphragm. A permanent intrauterine device can cause a continuing inflammatory response in diabetics that should be avoided, oral contraceptives tend to elevate blood glucose levels, and contraceptive sponges are not good at preventing pregnancy. Therefore, answers A, B, and D are incorrect.

115. **Answer D is correct.** The signs of an ectopic pregnancy are vague until the fallopian tube ruptures. The client will complain of sudden, stabbing pain in the lower quadrant that radiates down the leg or up into the chest. Painless vaginal bleeding is a sign of placenta previa, abdominal cramping is a sign of labor, and throbbing pain in the upper quadrant is not a sign of an ectopic pregnancy, making answers A, B, and C incorrect.

116. **Answer C is correct.** All of the choices are tasty, but the pregnant client needs a diet that is balanced and has increased amounts of calcium. Answer A is lacking in fruits and milk. Answer B contains the potato chips, which contain a large amount of sodium. Answer C contains meat, fruit, potato salad, and yogurt, which has about 360mg of calcium. Answer D is not the best diet because it lacks vegetables and milk products.

117. **Answer B is correct.** The client with hyperemesis has persistent nausea and vomiting. With vomiting comes dehydration. When the client is dehydrated, she will have metabolic acidosis. Answers A and C are incorrect because they are respiratory dehydration. Answer D is incorrect because the client will not be in alkalosis with persistent vomiting.

118. **Answer B is correct.** The most definitive diagnosis of pregnancy is the presence of fetal heart tones. The signs in answers A, C, and D are subjective and might be related to other medical conditions. Answers A and C may be related to a hydatidiform mole, and answer D is often present before menses or with the use of oral contraceptives.

119. **Answer C is correct.** The infant of a diabetic mother is usually large for gestational age. After birth, glucose levels fall rapidly due to the absence of glucose from the mother. Answer A is incorrect because the infant will not be small for gestational age. Answer B is incorrect because the infant will not be hyperglycemic. Answer D is incorrect because the infant will be large, not small, and will be hypoglycemic, not hyperglycemic.

120. **Answer B is correct.** When the client is taking oral contraceptives and begins antibiotics, another method of birth control should be used. Antibiotics decrease the effectiveness of oral contraceptives. Approximately 5–10 pounds of weight gain is not unusual, so answer A is incorrect. If the client misses a birth control pill, she should be instructed to take the pill as soon as she remembers the pill. Answer C is incorrect. If she misses two, she should take two; if she misses more than two, she should take the missed pills but use another method of birth control for the remainder of the cycle. Answer D is incorrect because changes in menstrual flow are expected in clients using oral contraceptives. Often these clients have lighter menses.

121. **Answer B is correct.** Clients with HIV should not breastfeed because the infection can be transmitted to the baby through breast milk. The clients in answers A, C, and D— those with diabetes, hypertension, and thyroid disease—can be allowed to breastfeed.

122. **Answer A is correct.** The symptoms of painless vaginal bleeding are consistent with placenta previa. Answers B, C, and D are incorrect. Cervical check for dilation is contraindicated because this can increase the bleeding. Checking for firmness of the uterus can be done, but the first action should be to check the fetal heart tones. A detailed history can be done later.

123. **Answer D is correct.** The client should be advised to come to the labor and delivery unit when the contractions are every 5 minutes and consistent. She should also be told to report to the hospital if she experiences rupture of membranes or extreme bleeding. She should not wait until the contractions are every 2 minutes or until she has bloody discharge, so answers A and B are incorrect. Answer C is a vague answer and can be related to a urinary tract infection.

124. **Answer A is correct.** Infants of mothers who smoke are often low in birth weight. Infants who are large for gestational age are associated with diabetic mothers, so answer B is incorrect. Preterm births are associated with smoking, but not with appropriate size for gestation, making answer C incorrect. Growth retardation is associated with smoking, but this does not affect the infant length; therefore, answer D is incorrect.

125. **Answer A is correct.** To provide protection against antibody production, RhoGam should be given within 72 hours. The answers in B, C, and D are too late to provide antibody protection. RhoGam can also be given during pregnancy.

126. **Answer B is correct.** When the membranes rupture, there is often a transient drop in the fetal heart tones. The heart tones should return to baseline quickly. Any alteration in fetal heart tones, such as bradycardia or tachycardia, should be reported. After the fetal heart tones are assessed, the nurse should evaluate the cervical dilation, vital signs, and level of discomfort, making answers A, C, and D incorrect.

127. **Answer A is correct.** The active phase of labor occurs when the client is dilated 4–7cm. The latent or early phase of labor is from 1cm to 3cm in dilation, so answers B and D are incorrect. The transition phase of labor is 8–10cm in dilation, making answer C incorrect.

128. **Answer B is correct.** The infant of an addicted mother will undergo withdrawal. Snugly wrapping the infant in a blanket will help prevent the muscle irritability that these babies often experience. Teaching the mother to provide tactile stimulation or provide for early infant stimulation are incorrect because he is irritable and needs quiet and little stimulation at this time, so answers A and D are incorrect. Placing the infant in an infant seat in answer C is incorrect because this will also cause movement that can increase muscle irritability.

129. **Answer C is correct.** Following epidural anesthesia, the client should be checked for hypotension and signs of shock every 5 minutes for 15 minutes. The client can be checked for cervical dilation later after she is stable. The client should not be positioned supine because the anesthesia can move above the respiratory center and the client can stop breathing. Fetal heart tones should be assessed after the blood pressure is checked. Therefore, answers A, B, and D are incorrect.

130. **Answer B is correct.** The best way to prevent post-operative wound infection is hand washing. Use of prescribed antibiotics will treat infection, not prevent infections, making answer A incorrect. Wearing a mask and asking the client to cover her mouth are good practices but will not prevent wound infections; therefore, answers C and D are incorrect.

131. **Answer B is correct.** The client with a hip fracture will most likely have disalignment. Answers A, C, and D are incorrect because all fractures cause pain, and coolness of the extremities and absence of pulses are indicative of compartment syndrome or peripheral vascular disease.

132. **Answer B is correct.** After menopause, women lack hormones necessary to absorb and utilize calcium. Doing weight-bearing exercises and taking calcium supplements can help to prevent osteoporosis but are not causes, so answers A and C are incorrect. Body types that frequently experience osteoporosis are thin Caucasian females, but they are not most likely related to osteoporosis, so answer D is incorrect.

133. **Answer B is correct.** The infant's hips should be off the bed approximately 15° in Bryant's traction. Answer A is incorrect because this does not indicate that the traction is working correctly, nor does C. Answer D is incorrect because Bryant's traction is a skin traction, not a skeletal traction.

134. **Answer A is correct.** Balanced skeletal traction uses pins and screws. A Steinman pin goes through large bones and is used to stabilize large bones such as the femur. Answer B is incorrect because only the affected leg is in traction. Kirschner wires are used to stabilize small bones such as fingers and toes, as in answer C. Answer D is incorrect because this type of traction is not used for fractured hips.

135. **Answer A is correct.** Bleeding is a common complication of orthopedic surgery. The blood-collection device should be checked frequently to ensure that the client is not hemorrhaging. The client's pain should be assessed, but this is not life-threatening. When the client is in less danger, the nutritional status should be assessed and an immobilizer is not used; thus, answers B, C, and D are incorrect.

136. **Answer A is correct.** The client's family member should be taught to flush the tube after each feeding and clamp the tube. The placement should be checked before feedings, and indigestion can occur with the PEG tube, just as it can occur with any client, so answers B and C are incorrect. Medications can be ordered for indigestion, but it is not a reason for alarm. A percutaneous endoscopy gastrostomy tube is used for clients who have experienced difficulty swallowing. The tube is inserted directly into the stomach and does not require swallowing; therefore, answer D is incorrect.

137. **Answer C is correct.** The client with a total knee replacement should be assessed for anemia. An hgb of 7 is extremely low and might require a blood transfusion. Scant bleeding on the dressing is not extreme. Circle and date and time the bleeding and monitor for changes in the client's status. A low-grade temperature is not unusual after surgery. Ensure that the client is well hydrated, and recheck the temperature in one hour. Voiding after surgery is also not uncommon and no need for concern; therefore, answers A, B, and D are incorrect.

138. **Answer B is correct.** The parents make stained glass as a hobby. Stained glass is put together with lead, which can drop on the work area, where the child can consume the lead beads. Answers A, C, and D do not pose a threat to the child.

139. **Answer A is correct.** The equipment that can help with activities of daily living is the high-seat commode. The hip should be kept higher than the knee. The recliner is good because it prevents 90° flexion but not daily activities. A TENS (Transcutaneous Electrical Nerve Stimulation) unit helps with pain management and an abduction pillow is used to prevent adduction of the hip and possibly dislocation of the prosthesis; therefore, answers B, C, and D are incorrect.

140. **Answer B is correct.** Narcan is the antidote for narcotic overdose. If hypoxia occurs, the client should have oxygen administered by mask, not cannula. There is no data to support the administration of blood products or cardioresuscitation, so answers A, C, and D are incorrect.

141. **Answer B is correct.** The 6-year-old should have a roommate as close to the same age as possible, so the 12-year-old is the best match. The 10-year-old with sarcoma has cancer and will be treated with chemotherapy that makes him immune suppressed, the 6-year-old with osteomyelitis is infected, and the client in answer A is too old and is female; therefore, answers A, C, and D are incorrect.

142. **Answer B is correct.** Cox II inhibitors have been associated with heart attacks and strokes. Any changes in cardiac status or signs of a stroke should be reported immediately, along with any changes in bowel or bladder habits because bleeding has been linked to use of Cox II inhibitors. The client does not have to take the medication with milk, remain upright, or allow 6 weeks for optimal effect, so answers A, C, and D are incorrect.

143. **Answer D is correct.** A plaster-of-Paris cast takes 24 hours to dry, and the client should not bear weight for 24 hours. The cast should be handled with the palms, not the fingertips, so answer A is incorrect. Petaling a cast is covering the end of the cast with cast batting or a sock, to prevent skin irritation and flaking of the skin under the cast. B is incorrect because petaling the cast is done by the health care provider who applied the cast. The client should be told not to dry the cast with a hair dryer because this causes hot spots and could burn the client. This also causes unequal drying; thus, answer C is incorrect.

144. **Answer A is correct.** There is no reason that the client's friends should not be allowed to autograph the cast; it will not harm the cast in any way, so answers B, C, and D are incorrect.

145. **Answer A is correct.** The nurse is performing the pin care correctly when she uses sterile gloves and Q-tips. Clean gloves are not acceptable. A licensed practical nurse can perform pin care, there is no need to clean the weights; therefore, answers B, C, and D are incorrect.

146. **Answer A is correct.** A body cast or spica cast extends from the upper abdomen to the knees or below. Bowel sounds should be checked to ensure that the client is not experiencing a paralytic illeus. Checking the blood
pressure is a treatment for any client, offering pain medication is not called for, and checking for swelling isn't specific to the stem, so answers B, C, and D are incorrect.

147. **Answer C is correct.** Halo traction will be ordered for the client with a cervical fracture. Russell's traction is used for bones of the lower extremities, as is Buck's traction. Cruchfield tongs are used while in the hospital and the client is immobile; therefore, answers A, B, and D are incorrect.

148. **Answer B is correct.** The controller for the continuous passive-motion device should be placed away from the client. Many clients complain of pain while having treatments with the CPM, so they might turn off the machine. The CPM flexes and extends the leg. The client is in the bed during CPM therapy, so answer A is incorrect. Answer C is incorrect because clients will experience pain with the treatment. Use of the CPM does not alleviate the need for physical therapy, as suggested in answer D.

149. **Answer A is correct.** The client's palms should rest lightly on the handles. The elbows should be flexed no more than 30° but should not be extended. Answer B is incorrect because 0° is not a relaxed angle for the elbows and will not facilitate correct walker use. The client should walk to the middle of the walker, not to the front of the walker, making answer C incorrect. The client should be taught not to carry the walker because this would not provide stability; thus, answer D is incorrect.

150. **Answer C is correct.** The client with a prolapsed cord should be treated by elevating the hips and covering the cord with a moist, sterile saline gauze. The nurse should use her fingers to push up on the presenting part until a cesarean section can be performed. Answers A, B, and D are incorrect. The nurse should not attempt to replace the cord, turn the client on the side, or cover with a dry gauze.

151. **Answer B is correct.** Chest tubes work to reinflate the lung and drain serous fluid. The tube does not equalize expansion of the lungs. Pain is associated with collapse of the lung, and insertion of chest tubes is painful, so answers A and C are incorrect. Answer D is true, but this is not the primary rationale for performing chest tube insertion.

152. **Answer D is correct.** Success with breastfeeding depends on many factors, but the most dependable reason for success is desire and willingness to continue the breastfeeding until the infant and mother have time to adapt. The educational level, the infant's birth weight, and the size of the mother's breast have nothing to do with success, so answers A, B, and C are incorrect.

153. **Answer C is correct.** Green-tinged amniotic fluid is indicative of meconium staining. This finding indicates fetal distress. The presence of scant bloody discharge is normal, as are frequent urination and moderate uterine contractions, making answers A, B, and D incorrect.

154. **Answer C is correct.** Duration is measured from the beginning of one contraction to the end of the same contraction. Answer A refers to frequency. Answer B is incorrect because we do not measure from the end of one contraction to the beginning of the next contraction. Duration is not measured from the peak of the contraction to the end, as stated in D.

155. **Answer B is correct.** The client receiving Pitocin should be monitored for decelerations. There is no association with Pitocin use and hypoglycemia, maternal hyperreflexia, or fetal movement; therefore, answers A, C, and D are incorrect.

156. **Answer D is correct.** Fetal development depends on adequate nutrition and insulin regulation. Insulin needs increase during the second and third trimesters, insulin requirements do not moderate as the pregnancy progresses, and elevated human choronic gonadotrophin elevates insulin needs, not decreases them; therefore, answers A, B, and C are incorrect.

157. **Answer A is correct.** A calm environment is needed to prevent seizure activity. Any stimulation can precipitate seizures. Obtaining a diet history should be done later, and administering an analgesic is not indicated because there is no data in the stem to indicate pain. Therefore, answers B and C are incorrect. Assessing the fetal heart tones is important, but this is not the highest priority in this situation as stated in answer D.

158. **Answer A is correct.** The client who is age 42 is at risk for fetal anomalies such as Down syndrome and other chromosomal aberrations. Answers B, C, and D are incorrect because the client is not at higher risk for respiratory distress syndrome or pathological jaundice, and Turner's syndrome is a genetic disorder.

159. **Answer C is correct.** The client with a missed abortion will have induction of labor. Prostin E. is a form of prostaglandin used to soften the cervix. Magnesium sulfate is used for preterm labor and preeclampsia, calcium gluconate is the antidote for magnesium sulfate, and Parlodel is a dopamine receptor stimulant used to treat Parkinson's disease; therefore, answers A, B, and D are incorrect. Parlodel was used at one time to dry breast milk.

160. **Answer A is correct.** The client's blood pressure and urinary output are within normal limits. The only alteration from normal is the decreased deep tendon reflexes. The nurse should continue to monitor the blood pressure and check the magnesium level. The therapeutic level is 4.8–9.6mg/dL. Answers B, C, and D are incorrect because there is no need to stop the infusion at this time or slow the rate. Calcium gluconate is the antidote for magnesium sulfate, but there is no data to indicate toxicity.

161. **Answer C is correct.** Autosomal recessive disorders can be passed from the parents to the infant. If both parents pass the trait, the child will get two abnormal genes and the disease results. Parents can also pass the trait to the infant. Answer A is incorrect because, to have an affected newborn, the parents must be carriers. Answer B is incorrect because both parents must be carriers. Answer D is incorrect because the parents might have affected children.

162. **Answer D is correct.** Alpha fetoprotein is a screening test done to detect neural tube defects such as spina bifida. The test is not mandatory, as stated in answer A. It does not indicate cardiovascular defects, and the mother's age has no bearing on the need for the test, so answers B and C are incorrect.

163. **Answer B is correct.** During pregnancy, the thyroid gland triples in size. This makes it more difficult to regulate thyroid medication. Answer A is incorrect because there could be a need for thyroid medication during pregnancy. Answer C is incorrect because the thyroid function does not slow. Fetal growth is not arrested if thyroid medication is continued, so answer D is incorrect.

164. **Answer C is correct.** Cyanosis of the feet and hands is acrocyanosis. This is a normal finding 1 minute after birth. An apical pulse should be 120–160, and the baby should have muscle tone, making answers A and B incorrect. Jaundice immediately after birth is pathological jaundice and is abnormal, so answer D is incorrect.

165. **Answer A is correct.** Clients with sickle cell crises are treated with heat, hydration, oxygen, and pain relief. Fluids are increased, not decreased. Blood transfusions are usually not required, and the client can be delivered vaginally; thus, answers B, C, and D are incorrect.

166. **Answer A is correct.** Before ultrasonography, the client should be taught to drink plenty of fluids and not void. The client may ambulate, an enema is not needed, and there is no need to withhold food for 8 hours. Therefore, answers B, C, and D are incorrect.

167. **Answer D is correct.** By 1 year of age, the infant is expected to triple his birth weight. Answers A, B, and C are incorrect because they are too low.

168. **Answer B is correct.** A nonstress test is done to evaluate periodic movement of the fetus. It is not done to evaluate lung maturity as in answer A. An oxytocin challenge test shows the effect of contractions on fetal heart rate and a nonstress test does not measure neurological well-being of the fetus, so answers C and D are incorrect.

169. **Answer D is correct.** Hypospadias is a condition in which there is an opening on the under side of the penis. Answers A, B, and C do not describe hypospadias therefore they are incorrect.

170. **Answer A is correct.** Transition is the time during labor when the client loses concentration due to intense contractions. Potential for injury related to precipitate delivery has nothing to do with the dilation of the cervix, so answer B is incorrect. There is no data to indicate that the client has had anesthesia or fluid volume deficit, making answers C and D incorrect.

171. **Answer C is correct.** Varicella is chicken pox. This herpes virus is treated with antiviral medications. The client is not treated with antibiotics or anticoagulants as stated in answers A and D. The client might have a fever before the rash appears, but when the rash appears, the temperature is usually gone, so answer B is incorrect.

172. **Answer B is correct.** Clients with chest pain can be treated with nitroglycerin, a beta blocker such as propanolol, or Varapamil. There is no indication for an antibiotic such as Ampicillin, so answers A, C, and D are incorrect.

173. **Answer B is correct.** Anti-inflammatory drugs should be taken with meals to avoid stomach upset. Answers A, C, and D are incorrect. Clients with rheumatoid arthritis should exercise, but not to the point of pain. Alternating hot and cold is not necessary, especially because warm, moist soaks are more useful in decreasing pain. Weight-bearing activities such as walking are useful but is not the best answer for the stem.

174. **Answer D is correct.** Morphine is contraindicated in clients with gallbladder disease and pancreatitis because morphine causes spasms of the Sphenter of Oddi. Meperidine, Mylanta, and Cimetadine are ordered for pancreatitis, making answers A, B, and C incorrect.

175. **Answer B is correct.** Hallucinogenic drugs can cause hallucinations. Continuous observation is ordered to prevent the client from harming himself during withdrawal. Answers A, C, and D are incorrect because hallucinogenic drugs don't create both stimulant and depressant effects or produce severe respiratory depression. However, they do produce psychological dependence rather than physical dependence.

176. **Answer B is correct.** Barbiturates create a sedative effect. When the client stops taking barbiturates, he will experience tachycardia, diarrhea, and tachpnea. Answer A is incorrect even though depression and suicidal ideation go along with barbiturate use; it is not the priority. Muscle cramps and abdominal pain are vague symptoms that could be associated with other problems. Tachycardia is associated with stopping barbiturates, but euphoria is not.

177. **Answer A is correct.** If the fetal heart tones are heard in the right upper abdomen, the infant is in a breech presentation. If the infant is positioned in the right occipital anterior presentation, the FHTs will be located in the right lower quadrant, so answer B is incorrect. If the fetus is in the sacral position, the FHTs will be located in the center of the abdomen, so answer C is incorrect. If the FHTs are heard in the left lower abdomen, the infant is most likely in the left occipital transverse position, making answer D incorrect.

178. **Answer D is correct.** Asthma is the presence of bronchiolar spasms. This spasm can be brought on by allergies or anxiety. Answer A is incorrect because the primary physiological alteration is not inflammation. Answer B is incorrect because there is the production of abnormally viscous mucus, not a primary alteration. Answer C is incorrect because infection is not primary to asthma.

179. **Answer A is correct.** The client with mania is seldom sitting long enough to eat and burns many calories for energy. Answer B is incorrect because the client should be treated the same as other clients. Small meals are not a correct option for this client. Allowing her into the kitchen gives her privileges that other clients do not have and should not be allowed, so answer D is incorrect.

180. **Answer B is correct.** Bryant's traction is used for fractured femurs and dislocated hips. The hips should be elevated 15° off the bed. Answer A is incorrect because the hips should not be resting on the bed. Answer C is incorrect because the hips should not be above the level of the body. Answer D is incorrect because the hips and legs should not be flat on the bed.

181. **Answer B is correct.** Herpes zoster is shingles. Clients with shingles should be placed in contact precautions. Wearing gloves during care will prevent transmission of the virus. Covering the lesions with a sterile gauze is not necessary, antibiotics are not prescribed for herpes zoster, and oxygen is not necessary for shingles; therefore, answers A, C, and D are incorrect.

182. **Answer B is correct.** A trough level should be drawn 30 minutes before the third or fourth dose. The times in answers A, C, and D are incorrect times to draw blood levels.

183. **Answer B is correct.** The client using a diaphragm should keep the diaphragm in a cool location. Answers A, C, and D are incorrect. She should refrain from leaving the diaphragm in longer than 8 hours, not 4 hours. She should have the diaphragm resized when she gains or loses 10 pounds or has abdominal surgery.

184. **Answer C is correct.** Mothers who plan to breastfeed should drink plenty of liquids, and four glasses is not enough in a 24-hour period. Wearing a support bra is a good practice for the mother who is breastfeeding as well as the mother who plans to bottle-feed, so answer A is incorrect. Expressing milk from the breast will stimulate milk production, making answer B incorrect. Allowing the water to run over the breast will also facilitate "letdown," when the milk begins to be produced; thus, answer D is incorrect.

185. **Answer A is correct.** The facial nerve is cranial nerve VII. If damage occurs, the client will experience facial pain. The auditory nerve is responsible for hearing loss and tinnitus, eye movement is controlled by the Trochear or C IV, and the olfactory nerve controls smell; therefore, answers B, C, and D are incorrect.

186. **Answer B is correct.** Clients taking Pyridium should be taught that the medication will turn the urine orange or red. It is not associated with diarrhea, mental confusion, or changes in taste; therefore, answers A, C, and D are incorrect. Pyridium can also cause a yellowish color to skin and sclera if taken in large doses.

187. **Answer B is correct.** Accutane is contraindicated for use by pregnant clients because it causes teratogenic effects. Calcium levels, apical pulse, and creatinine levels are not necessary; therefore, answers A, C, and D are incorrect.

188. **Answer D is correct.** Clients taking Acyclovir should be encouraged to drink plenty of fluids because renal impairment can occur. Limiting activity is not necessary, nor is eating a high-carbohydrate diet. Use of an incentive spirometer is not specific to clients taking Acyclovir; therefore, answers A, B, and C are incorrect.

189. **Answer A is correct.** Clients who are pregnant should not have a CAT because radioactive isotopes are used. However, clients with a titanium hip replacement can have an MRI, or CAT scan so answer B is incorrect. No antibiotics are used with this test and the client should remain still only when instructed, so answers C and D are not specific to this test.

190. **Answer D is correct.** Clients taking Amphotericin B should be monitored for liver, renal, and bone marrow function because this drug is toxic to the kidneys and liver, and causes bone marrow suppression. Jaundice is a sign of liver toxicity and is not specific to the use of Amphotericin B. Changes in vision are not related, and nausea is a side effect, not a sign of toxicity; nor is urinary frequency. Thus, answers A, B, and C are incorrect.

191. **Answer C is correct.** The client with chest pain should be seen first because this could indicate a myocardial infarction. The client in answer A has a blood glucose within normal limits. The client in answer B is maintained on blood pressure medication. The client in answer D is in no distress.

192. **Answer B is correct.** Pancreatic enzymes should be given with meals for optimal effects. These enzymes assist the body in digesting needed nutrients. Answers A, C, and D are incorrect methods of administering pancreatic enzymes.

193. **Answer C is correct.** The lens allows light to pass through the pupil and focus light on the retina. The lens does not stimulate the retina, assist with eye movement, or magnify small objects, so answers A, B, and D are incorrect.

194. **Answer C is correct.** Miotic eyedrops constrict the pupil and allow aqueous humor to drain out of the Canal of Schlemm. They do not anesthetize the cornea, dilate the pupil, or paralyze the muscles of the eye, making answers A, B, and D incorrect.

195. **Answer A is correct.** When using eyedrops, allow 5 minutes between the two medications; therefore, answer B is incorrect. These medications can be used by the same client but it is not necessary to use a cyclopegic with these medications, making answers C and D incorrect.

196. **Answer B is correct.** Clients with color blindness will most likely have problems distinguishing violets, blues, and green. The colors in answers A, C, and D are less commonly affected.

197. **Answer D is correct.** The client with a pacemaker should be taught to count and record his pulse rate. Answers A, B, and C are incorrect. Ankle edema is a sign of right-sided congestive heart failure. Although this is not normal, it is often present in clients with heart disease. If the edema is present in the hands and face, it should be reported. Checking the blood pressure daily is not necessary for these clients. The client with a pacemaker can use a microwave oven, but he should stand about 5 feet from the oven while it is operating.

198. **Answer A is correct.** Clients who are being retrained for bladder control should be taught to withhold fluids after about 7 p.m., or 1900. The times in answers B, C, and D are too early in the day.

199. **Answer D is correct.** Cranberry juice is more alkaline and, when metabolized by the body, is excreted with acidic urine. Bacteria does not grow freely in acidic urine. Increasing intake of meats is not associated with urinary tract infections, so answer A is incorrect. The client does not have to avoid citrus fruits and pericare should be done, but hydrogen peroxide is drying, so answers B and C are incorrect.

200. **Answer C is correct.** NPH insulin peaks in 8–12 hours, so a snack should be offered at that time. NPH insulin onsets in 90–120 minutes, so answer A is incorrect. Answer B is untrue because NPH insulin is time released and does not usually cause sudden hypoglycemia. Answer D is incorrect, but the client should eat a bedtime snack.

201. **Answer D is correct.** Methotrexate is a folic acid antagonist. Leucovorin is the drug given for toxicity to this drug. It is not used to treat iron-deficiency anemia, create a synergistic effects, or increase the number of circulating neutrophils. Therefore, answers A, B, and C are incorrect.

202. **Answer B is correct.** The client who is allergic to dogs, eggs, rabbits, and chicken feathers is most likely allergic to the rubella vaccine. The client who is allergic to neomycin is also at risk. There is no danger to the client if he has an order for a TB skin test, ELISA test, or chest x-ray; thus, answers A, C, and D are incorrect.

203. **Answer B is correct.** Zantac (rantidine) is a histamine blocker that should be given with meals for optimal effect, not before meals. However, Tagamet (cimetidine) is a histamine blocker that can be given in one dose at bedtime. Neither of these drugs should be given before or after meals, so answers A and D are incorrect.

204. **Answer C is correct.** The proximal end of the double-barrel colostomy is the end toward the small intestines. This end is on the client's right side. The distal end, as in answers A, B, and D, is on the client's left side.

205. **Answer A is correct.** If the nurse checks the fundus and finds it to be displaced to the right or left, this is an indication of a full bladder. This finding is not associated with hypotension or clots, as stated in answer B. Oxytoxic drugs (Pitocin) are drugs used to contract the uterus, so answer C is incorrect. It has nothing to do with displacement of the uterus. Answer D is incorrect because displacement is associated with a full bladder, not vaginal bleeding.

206. **Answer C is correct.** Clients with an internal defibrillator or a pacemaker should not have an MRI because it can cause dysrhythmias in the client with a pacemaker. If the client has a need for oxygen, is claustrophobic, or is deaf, he can have an MRI, but provisions such as extension tubes for the oxygen, sedatives, or a signal system should be made to accommodate these problems. Therefore, answers A, B, and D are incorrect.

207. **Answer C is correct.** A 6-month-old is too old for the colorful mobile. He is too young to play with the electronic game or the 30-piece jigsaw puzzle. The best toy for this age is the cars in a plastic container, so answers A, B, and D are incorrect.

208. **Answer C is correct.** The client with polio has muscle weakness. Periods of rest throughout the day will conserve the client's energy. A hot bath can cause burns; however, a warm bath would be helpful, so answer A is incorrect. Strenuous exercises are not advisable, making answer B incorrect. Visual disturbances that are directly associated with polio that cannot be corrected with glasses; therefore, answer D is incorrect.

209. **Answer B is correct.** The client with a protoepisiotomy will need stool softeners such as docusate sodium. Suppositories are given only with an order from the doctor, Methergine is a drug used to contract the uterus, and Parlodel is an anti-Parkinsonian drug; therefore, answers A, C, and D are incorrect.

210. **Answer C is correct.** Total Parenteral Nutrition is a high-glucose solution. This therapy often causes the glucose levels to be elevated. Because this is a common complication, insulin might be ordered. Answers A, B, and D are incorrect. TPN is used to treat negative nitrogen balance; it will not lead to negative nitrogen balance. Total Parenteral Nutrition can be managed with oral hypoglycemic drugs, but it is difficult to do so. Total Parenteral Nutrition will not lead to further pancreatic disease.

211. **Answer B is correct.** The client who is 10 weeks pregnant should be assessed to determine how she feels about the pregnancy. It is too early to discuss preterm labor, too late to discuss whether she was using a method of birth control, and after the client delivers, a discussion of future children should be instituted. Thus, answers A, C, and D are incorrect.

212. **Answer A is correct.** The best IV fluid for correction of dehydration is normal saline because it is most like normal serum. Dextrose pulls fluid from the cell, lactated Ringer's contains more electrolytes than the client's serum, and dextrose with normal saline will also alter the intracellular fluid. Therefore, answers B, C, and D are incorrect.

213. **Answer A is correct.** A thyroid scan uses a dye, so the client should be assessed for allergies to iodine. The client will not have a bolus of fluid, will not be asleep, and will not have a urinary catheter inserted, so answers B, C, and D are incorrect.

214. **Answer B is correct.** RhoGam is used to prevent formation of Rh antibodies. It does not provide immunity to Rh isoenzymes, eliminate circulating Rh antibodies, or convert the Rh factor from negative to positive; thus, answers A, C, and D are incorrect.

215. **Answer B is correct.** A client with a fractured foot often has a short leg cast applied to stabilize the fracture. A spica cast is used to stabilize a fractured pelvis or vertebral fracture. Kirschner wires are used to stabilize small bones such as toes and the client will most likely have a cast or immobilizer, so answers A, C, and D are incorrect.

216. **Answer A is correct.** Iridium seeds can be expelled during urination, so the client should be taught to strain his urine and report to the doctor if any of the seeds are expelled. Increasing fluids, reporting urinary frequency, and avoiding prolonged sitting are not necessary; therefore, answers B, C, and D are incorrect.

217. **Answer C is correct.** Immunosuppressants are used to prevent antibody formation. Antivirals, antibiotics, and analgesics are not used to prevent antibody production, so answers A, B, and D are incorrect.

218. **Answer A is correct.** Before cataract removal, the client will have Mydriatic drops instilled to dilate the pupil. This will facilitate removal of the lens. Miotics constrict the pupil and are not used in cataract clients. A laser is not used to smooth and reshape the lens; the diseased lens is removed. Silicone oil is not injected in this client; thus, answers B, C, and D are incorrect.

219. **Answer C is correct.** Placing simple signs that indicate the location of rooms where the client sleeps, eats, and bathes will help the client be more independent. Providing mirrors and pictures is not recommended with the client who has Alzheimer's disease because mirrors and pictures tend to cause agitation, and alternating healthcare workers confuses the client; therefore, answers A, B, and D are incorrect.

220. **Answer C is correct.** A Jackson-Pratt drain is a serum-collection device commonly used in abdominal surgery. A Jackson-Pratt drain will not prevent the need for dressing changes, reduce edema of the incision, or keep the common bile duct open, so answers A, B, and D are incorrect. A t-tube is used to keep the common bile duct open.

221. **Answer C is correct.** The infant who is 32 weeks gestation will not be able to control his head, so head lag will be present. Mongolian spots are common in African American infants, not Caucasian infants; the client at 32 weeks will have scrotal rugae or redness. There is no alteration in the amount of amniotic fluid; therefore, answers A, B, and D are incorrect.

222. **Answer A is correct.** Hematuria in a client with a pelvic fracture can indicate trauma to the bladder or impending bleeding disorders. It is not unusual for the client to complain of muscles spasms with multiple fractures, so answer B is incorrect. Dizziness can be associated with blood loss and is nonspecific, making answer C incorrect. Nausea, as stated in answer D, is also common in the client with multiple traumas.

223. **Answer C is correct.** The client's statement "They are trying to kill me" indicates paranoid delusions. There is no data to indicate that the client is hearing voices or is intoxicated, so answers A and D are incorrect. Delusions of grandeur are fixed beliefs that the client is superior or perhaps a famous person, making answer B incorrect.

224. **Answer B is correct.** Because the nurse is unaware of when the bottle was opened or whether the saline is sterile, it is safest to obtain a new bottle. Answers A, C, and D are not safe practices.

225. **Answer C is correct.** Infants with an Apgar of 9 at 5 minutes most likely have acryocyanosis, a normal physiologic adaptation to birth. It is not related to the infant being hypothermic, experiencing bradycardia, or being lethargic; thus, answers A, B, and D are incorrect.

226. **Answer A is correct.** Rapid continuous rewarming of a frostbite primarily lessens cellular damage. It does not prevent formation of blisters. It does promote movement, but this is not the primary reason for rapid rewarming. It might increase pain for a short period of time as the feeling comes back into the extremity; therefore, answers B, C, and D are incorrect.

227. **Answer D is correct.** Hemodialysis works by using a dialyzing membrane to filter waste that has accumulated in the blood. It does not pass water through a dialyzing membrane nor does it eliminate plasma proteins or lower the pH, so answers A, B, and C are incorrect.

228. **Answer B is correct.** The client who is immune-suppressed and is exposed to measles should be treated with medications to boost his immunity to the virus. An antibiotic or antiviral will not protect the client and it is too late to place the client in isolation, so answers A, C, and D are incorrect.

229. **Answer D is correct.** The client with MRSA should be placed in isolation. Gloves, a gown, and a mask should be used when caring for the client and hand washing is very important. The door should remain closed, but a negative-pressure room is not necessary, so answers A and B are incorrect. MRSA is spread by contact with blood or body fluid or by touching the skin of the client. It is cultured from the nasal passages of the client, so the client should be instructed to cover his nose and mouth when he sneezes or coughs. It is not necessary for the client to wear the mask at all times; the nurse should wear the mask, so answer C is incorrect.

230. **Answer B is correct.** Pain related to phantom limb syndrome is due to peripheral nervous system interruption. Answer A is incorrect because phantom limb pain can last several months or indefinitely. Answer C is incorrect because it is not psychological. It is also not due to infections, as stated in answer D.

231. **Answer A is correct.** During a Whipple procedure the head of the pancreas, which is a part of the stomach, the jejunum, and a portion of the stomach are removed and reanastomosed. Answer B is incorrect because the proximal third of the small intestine is not removed. The entire stomach is not removed, as in answer C, and in answer D, the esophagus is not removed.

232. **Answer C is correct.** Pepper is not processed and contains bacteria. Answers A, B, and D are incorrect because fruits should be cooked or washed and peeled, and salt and ketchup are allowed.

233. **Answer A is correct.** Coumadin is an anticoagulant. One of the tests for bleeding time is a Protime. This test should be done monthly. Eating more fruits and vegetables is not necessary, and dark-green vegetables contain vitamin K, which increases clotting, so answer B is incorrect. Drinking more liquids and avoiding crowds is not necessary, so answers C and D are incorrect.

234. **Answer A is correct.** The client who is having a central venous catheter removed should be told to hold his breath and bear down. This prevents air from entering the line. Answers B, C, and D will not facilitate removal.

235. **Answer B is correct.** Clients with a history of streptococcal infections could have antibodies that render the streptokinase ineffective. There is no reason to assess the client for allergies to pineapples or bananas, there is no correlation to the use of phenytoin and streptokinase, and a history of alcohol abuse is also not a factor in the order for streptokinase; therefore, answers A, C, and D are incorrect.

236. **Answer B is correct.** The client who is immune-suppressed and has bone marrow suppression should be taught not to floss his teeth because platelets are decreased. Using oils and cream-based soaps is allowed, as is eating salt and using an electric razor; therefore, answers A, C, and D are incorrect.

237. **Answer A is correct.** The best method and safest way to change the ties of a tracheotomy is to apply the new ones before removing the old ones. B is incorrect because having a helper is good, but the helper might not prevent the client from coughing out the tracheotomy. Answer C is not the best way to prevent the client from coughing out the tracheotomy. D is incorrect because asking the doctor to suture the tracheotomy in place is not appropriate.

238. **Answer D is correct.** The output of 300mL is indicative of hemorrhage and should be reported immediately. Answer A does nothing to help the client. Milking the tube is done only with an order and will not help in this situation, and slowing the intravenous infusion is not correct; thus, answers B and C are incorrect.

239. **Answer A is correct.** The infant with tetralogy of Fallot has four heart defects. He will be treated with digoxin to slow and strengthen the heart. Epinephrine, aminophyline, and atropine will speed the heart rate and are not used in this client; therefore, answers B, C, and D are incorrect.

240. **The correct answer is marked by an X in the diagram.** The Tail of Spence is located in the upper outer quadrant of the breast.

241. **Answer A is correct.** The toddler with a ventricular septal defect will tire easily. He will not grow normally but will not need more calories. He will be susceptible to bacterial infection, but he will be no more susceptible to viral infections than other children. Therefore, answers B, C, and D are incorrect.

242. **Answer B is correct.** A nonstress test determines periodic movement of the fetus. It does not determine lung maturity, show contractions, or measure neurological well-being, making answers A, C, and D incorrect.

243. **Answer C is correct.** The monitor indicates variable decelerations caused by cord compression. If Pitocin is infusing, the nurse should turn off the Pitocin. Instructing the client to push is incorrect because pushing could increase the decelerations and because the client is 8cm dilated, making answer A incorrect. Performing a vaginal exam should be done after turning off the Pitocin, and placing the client in a semi-Fowler's position is not appropriate for this situation; therefore, answers B and D are incorrect.

244. **Answer C is correct.** The graph indicates ventricular tachycardia. The answers in A, B, and D are not noted on the ECG strip.

245. **Answer B is correct.** Lovenox injections should be given in the abdomen, not in the deltoid muscle. The client should not aspirate after the injection or clear the air from the syringe before injection. Therefore, answers A, C, and D are incorrect.

246. **Answer B is correct.** Valium is not given in the same syringe with other medications, so answer A is incorrect. These medications can be given to the same client, so answer D is incorrect. In answer C, it is not necessary to wait to inject the second medication. Valium is an antianxiety medication, and Phenergan is used as an antiemetic.

247. **Answer B is correct.** Voiding every 3 hours prevents stagnant urine from collecting in the bladder, where bacteria can grow. Douching is not recommended and obtaining a urinalysis monthly is not necessary, making answers A and C incorrect. The client should practice wiping from front to back after voiding and bowel movements, so answer D is incorrect.

248. **Answer C is correct.** Of these clients, the one who should be assigned to the care of the nursing assistant is the client with dementia. Only an RN or the physician can place the client in seclusion, so answer A is incorrect. The nurse should empty the Foley catheter of the preeclamptic client because the client is unstable, making answer B incorrect. A nurse or physical therapist should ambulate the client with a fractured hip, so answer D is incorrect.

249. **Answer A is correct.** The client who has recently had a thyroidectomy is at risk for tracheal edema. A padded tongue blade is used for seizures and not for the client with tracheal edema, so answer B is incorrect. If the client experiences tracheal edema, the endotracheal tube or airway will not correct the problem, so answers C and D are incorrect.

250. **Answer D is correct.** Histoplasmosis is a fungus carried by birds. It is not transmitted to humans by cats, dogs, or turtles. Therefore, answers A, B, and C are incorrect.

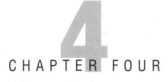

CHAPTER FOUR

Practice Exam 4 and Rationales

1. A client is admitted to the emergency room with a gunshot wound to the right arm. After dressing the wound and administering the prescribed antibiotic, the nurse should:

    ○ **A.** Ask the client if he has any medication allergies

    ○ **B.** Check the client's immunization record

    ○ **C.** Apply a splint to immobilize the arm

    ○ **D.** Administer medication for pain

Quick Answer: **292**
Detailed Answer: **295**

2. The nurse is caring for a client with suspected endometrial cancer. Which symptom is associated with endometrial cancer?

    ○ **A.** Frothy vaginal discharge

    ○ **B.** Thick, white vaginal discharge

    ○ **C.** Purulent vaginal discharge

    ○ **D.** Watery vaginal discharge

Quick Answer: **292**
Detailed Answer: **295**

3. A client with Parkinson's disease is scheduled for stereotactic surgery. Which finding indicates that the surgery had its intended effect?

    ○ **A.** The client no longer has intractable tremors.

    ○ **B.** The client has sufficient production of dopamine.

    ○ **C.** The client no longer requires any medication.

    ○ **D.** The client will have increased production of serotonin.

Quick Answer: **292**
Detailed Answer: **295**

4. A client with AIDS asks the nurse why he cannot have a pitcher of water left at his bedside. The nurse should tell the client that:

    ○ **A.** It would be best for him to drink ice water.

    ○ **B.** He should drink several glasses of juice instead.

    ○ **C.** It makes it easier to keep a record of his intake.

    ○ **D.** He should drink only freshly run water.

Quick Answer: **292**
Detailed Answer: **295**

5. An elderly client is diagnosed with interstitial cystitis. Which finding differentiates interstitial cystitis from other forms of cystitis?

Quick Answer: **292**
Detailed Answer: **295**

- ○ **A.** The client is asymptomatic.
- ○ **B.** The urine is free of bacteria.
- ○ **C.** The urine contains blood.
- ○ **D.** Males are affected more often.

6. The mother of a male child with cystic fibrosis tells the nurse that she hopes her son's children won't have the disease. The nurse is aware that:

Quick Answer: **292**
Detailed Answer: **295**

- ○ **A.** There is a 25% chance that his children will have cystic fibrosis.
- ○ **B.** Most of the males with cystic fibrosis are sterile.
- ○ **C.** There is a 50% chance that his children will be carriers.
- ○ **D.** Most males with cystic fibrosis are capable of having children, so genetic counseling is advised.

7. A 6-month-old is hospitalized with symptoms of botulism. What aspect of the infant's history is associated with *Clostridium botulinum* infection?

Quick Answer: **292**
Detailed Answer: **295**

- ○ **A.** The infant sucks on his fingers and toes.
- ○ **B.** The mother sweetens the infant's cereal with honey.
- ○ **C.** The infant was switched to soy-based formula.
- ○ **D.** The father recently purchased an aquarium.

8. The mother of a 6-year-old with autistic disorder tells the nurse that her son has been much more difficult to care for since the birth of his sister. The best explanation for changes in the child's behavior is:

Quick Answer: **292**
Detailed Answer: **295**

- ○ **A.** The child did not want a sibling.
- ○ **B.** The child was not adequately prepared for the baby's arrival.
- ○ **C.** The child's daily routine has been upset by the birth of his sister.
- ○ **D.** The child is just trying to get the parent's attention.

9. The parents of a child with cystic fibrosis ask what determines the prognosis of the disease. The nurse knows that the greatest determinant of the prognosis is:

Quick Answer: **292**
Detailed Answer: **295**

- ○ **A.** The degree of pulmonary involvement
- ○ **B.** The ability to maintain an ideal weight
- ○ **C.** The secretion of lipase by the pancreas
- ○ **D.** The regulation of sodium and chloride excretion

10. The nurse is assessing a client hospitalized with duodenal ulcer. Which finding should be reported to the doctor immediately?

Quick Answer: **292**
Detailed Answer: **296**

- ○ **A.** BP 82/60, pulse 120
- ○ **B.** Pulse 68, respirations 24
- ○ **C.** BP 110/88, pulse 56
- ○ **D.** Pulse 82, respirations 16

11. While caring for a client in the second stage of labor, the nurse notices a pattern of early decelerations. The nurse should:

Quick Answer: **292**
Detailed Answer: **296**

- ○ **A.** Notify the physician immediately
- ○ **B.** Turn the client on her left side
- ○ **C.** Apply oxygen via a tight face mask
- ○ **D.** Document the finding on the flow sheet

12. The nurse is teaching the client with AIDS regarding needed changes in food preparation. Which statement indicates that the client understands the nurse's teaching?

Quick Answer: **292**
Detailed Answer: **296**

- ○ **A.** "Adding fresh ground pepper to my food will improve the flavor."
- ○ **B.** "Meat should be thoroughly cooked to the proper temperature."
- ○ **C.** "Eating cheese and yogurt will prevent AIDS-related diarrhea."
- ○ **D.** "It is important to eat four to five servings of fresh fruits and vegetables a day."

13. The sputum of a client remains positive for the tubercle bacillus even though the client has been taking Laniazid (isoniazid). The nurse recognizes that the client should have a negative sputum culture within:

Quick Answer: **292**
Detailed Answer: **296**

- ○ **A.** 2 weeks
- ○ **B.** 6 weeks
- ○ **C.** 8 weeks
- ○ **D.** 12 weeks

14. Which person is at greatest risk for developing Lyme's disease?

Quick Answer: **292**
Detailed Answer: **296**

- ○ **A.** Computer programmer
- ○ **B.** Elementary teacher
- ○ **C.** Veterinarian
- ○ **D.** Landscaper

15. The mother of a 1-year-old wants to know when she should begin toilet-training her child. The nurse's response is based on the knowledge that sufficient sphincter control for toilet training is present by:

    ○ **A.** 12–15 months of age

    ○ **B.** 18–24 months of age

    ○ **C.** 26–30 months of age

    ○ **D.** 32–36 months of age

Quick Answer: **292**
Detailed Answer: **296**

16. The nurse is developing a plan of care for a client with an ileostomy. The priority nursing diagnosis is:

    ○ **A.** Fluid volume deficit

    ○ **B.** Alteration in body image

    ○ **C.** Impaired oxygen exchange

    ○ **D.** Alteration in elimination

Quick Answer: **292**
Detailed Answer: **296**

17. The physician has prescribed Cobex (cyanocobalamin) for a client following a gastric resection. Which lab result indicates that the medication is having its intended effect?

    ○ **A.** Neutrophil count of 4500

    ○ **B.** Hgb of 14.2g

    ○ **C.** Platelet count of 250,000

    ○ **D.** Eosinophil count of 200

Quick Answer: **292**
Detailed Answer: **296**

18. A behavior-modification program has been started for an adolescent with oppositional defiant disorder. Which statement describes the use of behavior modification?

    ○ **A.** Distractors are used to interrupt repetitive or unpleasant thoughts.

    ○ **B.** Techniques using stressors and exercise are used to increase awareness of body defenses.

    ○ **C.** A system of tokens and rewards is used as positive reinforcement.

    ○ **D.** Appropriate behavior is learned through observing the action of models.

Quick Answer: **292**
Detailed Answer: **296**

19. Following eruption of the primary teeth, the mother can promote chewing by giving the toddler:

    ○ **A.** Pieces of hot dog

    ○ **B.** Carrot sticks

    ○ **C.** Pieces of cereal

    ○ **D.** Raisins

Quick Answer: **292**
Detailed Answer: **297**

20. The nurse is infusing total parenteral nutrition (TPN). The primary purpose for closely monitoring the client's intake and output is:

Quick Answer: 292
Detailed Answer: 297

○ **A.** To determine how quickly the client is metabolizing the solution

○ **B.** To determine whether the client's oral intake is sufficient

○ **C.** To detect the development of hypovolemia

○ **D.** To decrease the risk of fluid overload

21. An obstetrical client with diabetes has an amniocentesis at 28 weeks gestation. Which test indicates the degree of fetal lung maturity?

Quick Answer: 292
Detailed Answer: 297

○ **A.** Alpha-fetoprotein

○ **B.** Estriol level

○ **C.** Indirect Coomb's

○ **D.** Lecithin sphingomyelin ratio

22. Which nursing assessment indicates that involutional changes have occurred in a client who is 3 days postpartum?

Quick Answer: 292
Detailed Answer: 297

○ **A.** The fundus is firm and 3 finger widths below the umbilicus.

○ **B.** The client has a moderate amount of lochia serosa.

○ **C.** The fundus is firm and even with the umbilicus.

○ **D.** The uterus is approximately the size of a small grapefruit.

23. When administering total parenteral nutrition, the nurse should assess the client for signs of rebound hypoglycemia. The nurse knows that rebound hypoglycemia occurs when:

Quick Answer: 292
Detailed Answer: 297

○ **A.** The infusion rate is too rapid.

○ **B.** The infusion is discontinued without tapering.

○ **C.** The solution is infused through a peripheral line.

○ **D.** The infusion is administered without a filter.

24. A client scheduled for disc surgery tells the nurse that she frequently uses the herbal supplement kava-kava (piper methysticum). The nurse should notify the doctor because kava-kava:

Quick Answer: 292
Detailed Answer: 297

○ **A.** Increases the effects of anesthesia and post-operative analgesia

○ **B.** Eliminates the need for antimicrobial therapy following surgery

○ **C.** Increases urinary output, so a urinary catheter will be needed post-operatively

○ **D.** Depresses the immune system, so infection is more of a problem

25. The physician has ordered 50mEq of potassium chloride for a client with a potassium level of 2.5mEq. The nurse should administer the medication:

Quick Answer: **292**
Detailed Answer: **297**

- ○ **A.** Slow, continuous IV push over 10 minutes
- ○ **B.** Continuous infusion over 30 minutes
- ○ **C.** Controlled infusion over 5 hours
- ○ **D.** Continuous infusion over 24 hours

26. The nurse reviewing the lab results of a client receiving Cytoxan (cyclophasphamide) for Hodgkin's lymphoma finds the following: WBC 4,200, RBC 3,800,000, platelets 25,000, and serum creatinine 1.0mg. The nurse recognizes that the greatest risk for the client at this time is:

Quick Answer: **292**
Detailed Answer: **297**

- ○ **A.** Overwhelming infection
- ○ **B.** Bleeding
- ○ **C.** Anemia
- ○ **D.** Renal failure

27. While administering a chemotherapeutic vesicant, the nurse notes that there is a lack of blood return from the IV catheter. The nurse should:

Quick Answer: **292**
Detailed Answer: **297**

- ○ **A.** Stop the medication from infusing
- ○ **B.** Flush the IV catheter with normal saline
- ○ **C.** Apply a tourniquet and call the doctor
- ○ **D.** Continue the IV and assess the site for edema

28. A client with cervical cancer has a radioactive implant. Which statement indicates that the client understands the nurse's teaching regarding radioactive implants?

Quick Answer: **292**
Detailed Answer: **298**

- ○ **A.** "I won't be able to have visitors while getting radiation therapy."
- ○ **B.** "I will have a urinary catheter while the implant is in place."
- ○ **C.** "I can be up to the bedside commode while the implant is in place."
- ○ **D.** "I won't have any side effects from this type of therapy."

29. The nurse is teaching circumcision care to the mother of a newborn. Which statement indicates that the mother needs further teaching?

Quick Answer: **292**
Detailed Answer: **298**

- ○ **A.** "I will apply a petroleum gauze to the area with each diaper change."
- ○ **B.** "I will clean the area carefully with each diaper change."
- ○ **C.** "I can place a heat lamp to the area to speed up the healing process."
- ○ **D.** I should carefully observe the area for signs of infection."

30. A client admitted for treatment of bacterial pneumonia has an order for intravenous ampicillin. Which specimen should be obtained prior to administering the medication?

Quick Answer: **292**
Detailed Answer: **298**

- ○ **A.** Routine urinalysis
- ○ **B.** Complete blood count
- ○ **C.** Serum electrolytes
- ○ **D.** Sputum for culture and sensitivity

31. While obtaining information about the client's current medication use, the nurse learns that the client takes ginkgo to improve mental alertness. The nurse should tell the client to:

Quick Answer: **292**
Detailed Answer: **298**

- ○ **A.** Report signs of bruising or bleeding to the doctor
- ○ **B.** Avoid sun exposure while using the herbal
- ○ **C.** Purchase only those brands with FDA approval
- ○ **D.** Increase daily intake of vitamin E

32. A client with Hodgkin's lymphoma is receiving Platinol (cisplatin) To help prevent nephrotoxicity, the nurse should:

Quick Answer: **292**
Detailed Answer: **298**

- ○ **A.** Slow the infusion rate
- ○ **B.** Make sure the client is well hydrated
- ○ **C.** Record the intake and output every shift
- ○ **D.** Tell the client to report ringing in the ears

33. The chart of a client hospitalized for a total hip repair reveals that the client is colonized with MRSA. The nurse understands that the client:

Quick Answer: **292**
Detailed Answer: **298**

- ○ **A.** Will not display symptoms of infection
- ○ **B.** Is less likely to have an infection
- ○ **C.** Can be placed in the room with others
- ○ **D.** Cannot colonize others with MRSA

34. A client receiving Vancocin (vancomycin) has a serum level of 20mcg/mL. The nurse knows that the therapeutic range for vancomycin is:

Quick Answer: **292**
Detailed Answer: **298**

- ○ **A.** 5–10mcg/mL
- ○ **B.** 10–25mcg/mL
- ○ **C.** 25–40mcg/mL
- ○ **D.** 40–60mcg/mL

35. A client is admitted with symptoms of pseudomembranous colitis. Which finding is associated with *Clostridium difficile*?

Quick Answer: **292**
Detailed Answer: **298**

   ○ **A.** Diarrhea containing blood and mucus

   ○ **B.** Cough, fever, and shortness of breath

   ○ **C.** Anorexia, weight loss, and fever

   ○ **D.** Development of ulcers on the lower extremities

36. Which vitamin should be administered with INH (isoniazid) in order to prevent possible nervous system side effects?

Quick Answer: **292**
Detailed Answer: **298**

   ○ **A.** Thiamine

   ○ **B.** Niacin

   ○ **C.** Pyridoxine

   ○ **D.** Riboflavin

37. A client is admitted with suspected Legionnaires' disease. Which factor increases the risk of developing Legionnaires' disease?

Quick Answer: **292**
Detailed Answer: **299**

   ○ **A.** Treatment of arthritis with steroids

   ○ **B.** Foreign travel

   ○ **C.** Eating fresh shellfish twice a week

   ○ **D.** Doing volunteer work at the local hospital

38. A client who uses a respiratory inhaler asks the nurse to explain how he can know when half his medication is empty so that he can refill his prescription. The nurse should tell the client to:

Quick Answer: **292**
Detailed Answer: **299**

   ○ **A.** Shake the inhaler and listen for the contents

   ○ **B.** Drop the inhaler in water to see if it floats

   ○ **C.** Check for a hissing sound as the inhaler is used

   ○ **D.** Press the inhaler and watch for the mist

39. The nurse is caring for a client following a right nephrolithotomy. Postoperatively, the client should be positioned:

Quick Answer: **292**
Detailed Answer: **299**

   ○ **A.** On the right side

   ○ **B.** Supine

   ○ **C.** On the left side

   ○ **D.** Prone

40. A client is admitted with sickle cell crises and sequestration. Upon assessing the client, the nurse would expect to find:

Quick Answer: **292**
Detailed Answer: **299**

   ○ **A.** Decreased blood pressure

   ○ **B.** Moist mucus membranes

   ○ **C.** Decreased respirations

   ○ **D.** Increased blood pressure

41. A healthcare worker is referred to the nursing office with a suspected latex allergy. The first symptom of latex allergy is usually:

- ○ **A.** Oral itching after eating bananas
- ○ **B.** Swelling of the eyes and mouth
- ○ **C.** Difficulty in breathing
- ○ **D.** Swelling and itching of the hands

Quick Answer: **292**
Detailed Answer: **299**

42. A client is admitted with disseminated herpes zoster. According to the Centers for Disease Control Guidelines for Infection Control:

- ○ **A.** Airborne precautions will be needed.
- ○ **B.** No special precautions will be needed.
- ○ **C.** Contact precautions will be needed.
- ○ **D.** Droplet precautions will be needed.

Quick Answer: **292**
Detailed Answer: **299**

43. Acticoat (silver nitrate) dressings are applied to the legs of a client with deep partial thickness burns. The nurse should:

- ○ **A.** Change the dressings once per shift
- ○ **B.** Moisten the dressing with sterile water
- ○ **C.** Change the dressings only when they become soiled
- ○ **D.** Moisten the dressing with normal saline

Quick Answer: **292**
Detailed Answer: **299**

44. The nurse is preparing to administer an injection to a 6-month-old when she notices a white dot in the infant's right pupil. The nurse should:

- ○ **A.** Report the finding to the physician immediately
- ○ **B.** Record the finding and give the infant's injection
- ○ **C.** Recognize that the finding is a variation of normal
- ○ **D.** Check both eyes for the presence of the red reflex

Quick Answer: **292**
Detailed Answer: **299**

45. A client is diagnosed with stage II Hodgkin's lymphoma. The nurse recognizes that the client has involvement:

- ○ **A.** In a single lymph node or single site
- ○ **B.** In more than one node or single organ on the same side of the diaphragm
- ○ **C.** In lymph nodes on both sides of the diaphragm
- ○ **D.** In disseminated organs and tissues

Quick Answer: **292**
Detailed Answer: **299**

46. A client has been receiving Rheumatrex (methotrexate) for severe rheumatoid arthritis. The nurse should tell the client to avoid taking:

- ○ **A.** Aspirin
- ○ **B.** Multivitamins
- ○ **C.** Omega 3 fish oils
- ○ **D.** Acetaminophen

47. The physician has ordered a low-residue diet for a client with Crohn's disease. Which food is not permitted in a low-residue diet?

- ○ **A.** Mashed potatoes
- ○ **B.** Smooth peanut butter
- ○ **C.** Fried fish
- ○ **D.** Rice

48. A client hospitalized with cirrhosis has developed abdominal ascites. The nurse should provide the client with snacks that provide additional:

- ○ **A.** Sodium
- ○ **B.** Potassium
- ○ **C.** Protein
- ○ **D.** Fat

49. A diagnosis of multiple sclerosis is often delayed because of the varied symptoms experienced by those affected with the disease. Which symptom is most common in those with multiple sclerosis?

- ○ **A.** Resting tremors
- ○ **B.** Double vision
- ○ **C.** Flaccid paralysis
- ○ **D.** "Pill-rolling" tremors

50. After attending a company picnic, several clients are admitted to the emergency room with *E. coli* food poisoning. The most likely source of infection is:

- ○ **A.** Hamburger
- ○ **B.** Hot dog
- ○ **C.** Potato salad
- ○ **D.** Baked beans

51. A client tells the nurse that she takes St. John's wort (hypericum perfora-tum) three times a day for mild depression. The nurse should tell the client that:

  ○ **A.** St. John's wort seldom relieves depression.

  ○ **B.** She should avoid eating aged cheese.

  ○ **C.** Skin reactions increase with the use of sunscreen.

  ○ **D.** The herbal is safe to use with other antidepressants.

52. The physician has ordered a low-purine diet for a client with gout. Which protein source is high in purine?

  ○ **A.** Dried beans

  ○ **B.** Nuts

  ○ **C.** Cheese

  ○ **D.** Eggs

53. The nurse is observing the ambulation of a client recently fitted for crutch-es. Which observation requires nursing intervention?

  ○ **A.** Two finger widths are noted between the axilla and the top of the crutch.

  ○ **B.** The client bears weight on his hands when ambulating.

  ○ **C.** The crutches and the client's feet move alternately.

  ○ **D.** The client bears weight on his axilla when standing.

54. During the change of shift report, a nurse writes in her notes that she suspects illegal drug use by a client assigned to her care. During the shift, the notes are found by the client's daughter. The nurse could be sued for:

  ○ **A.** Libel

  ○ **B.** Slander

  ○ **C.** Malpractice

  ○ **D.** Negligence

55. The nurse is caring for an adolescent with a 5-year history of bulimia. A common clinical finding in the client with bulimia is:

  ○ **A.** Extreme weight loss

  ○ **B.** Dental caries

  ○ **C.** Hair loss

  ○ **D.** Decreased temperature

56. A client hospitalized for treatment of congestive heart failure is to be discharged with a prescription for Digitek (digoxin) 0.25mg daily. Which of the following statements indicates that the client needs further teaching?

   ○ **A.** "I will need to take the medication at the same time each day."

   ○ **B.** "I can prevent stomach upset by taking the medication with an antacid."

   ○ **C.** "I can help prevent drug toxicity by eating foods containing fiber."

   ○ **D.** "I will need to report visual changes to my doctor."

57. A client with paranoid schizophrenia has an order for Thorazine (chlorpromazine) 400mg orally twice daily.
   Which of the following symptoms should be reported to the physician immediately?

   ○ **A.** Fever, sore throat, weakness

   ○ **B.** Dry mouth, constipation, blurred vision

   ○ **C.** Lethargy, slurred speech, thirst

   ○ **D.** Fatigue, drowsiness, photosensitivity

58. When caring for a client with an anterior cervical discectomy, the nurse should give priority to assessing for post-operative bleeding. The nurse should pay particular attention to:

   ○ **A.** Drainage on the surgical dressing

   ○ **B.** Complaints of neck pain

   ○ **C.** Bleeding from the mouth

   ○ **D.** Swelling in the posterior neck

59. The initial assessment of a newborn reveals a chest circumference of 34cm and an abdominal circumference of 31cm. The chest is asymmetrical and breath sounds are diminished on the left side. The nurse should give priority to:

   ○ **A.** Providing supplemental oxygen by a ventilated mask

   ○ **B.** Performing auscultation of the abdomen for the presence of active bowel sounds

   ○ **C.** Inserting a nasogastric tube to check for esophageal patency

   ○ **D.** Positioning on the left side with head and chest elevated

60. The physician has ordered Eskalith (lithium carbonate) 500mg three times a day and Risperdal (risperidone) 2mg twice daily for a client admitted with bipolar disorder, acute manic episodes. The best explanation for the client's medication regimen is:

Quick Answer: **292**
Detailed Answer: **301**

- ○ **A.** The client's symptoms of acute mania are typical of undiagnosed schizophrenia.
- ○ **B.** Antipsychotic medication is used to manage behavioral excitement until mood stabilization occurs.
- ○ **C.** The client will be more compliant with a medication that allows some feelings of hypomania.
- ○ **D.** Antipsychotic medication prevents psychotic symptoms commonly associated with the use of mood stabilizers.

61. During a unit card game, a client with acute mania begins to sing loudly as she starts to undress. The nurse should:

Quick Answer: **292**
Detailed Answer: **301**

- ○ **A.** Ignore the client's behavior
- ○ **B.** Exchange the cards for a checker board
- ○ **C.** Send the other clients to their rooms
- ○ **D.** Cover the client and walk her to her room

62. A child with Down syndrome has a developmental age of 4 years. According to the Denver Developmental Assessment, the 4-year-old should be able to:

Quick Answer: **292**
Detailed Answer: **301**

- ○ **A.** Draw a man in six parts
- ○ **B.** Give his first and last name
- ○ **C.** Dress without supervision
- ○ **D.** Define a list of words

63. A client with paranoid schizophrenia is brought to the hospital by her elderly parents. During the assessment, the client's mother states, "Sometimes she is more than we can manage." Based on the mother's statement, the most appropriate nursing diagnosis is:

Quick Answer: **292**
Detailed Answer: **301**

- ○ **A.** Ineffective family coping related to parental role conflict
- ○ **B.** Care-giver role strain related to chronic situational stress
- ○ **C.** Altered family process related to impaired social interaction
- ○ **D.** Altered parenting related to impaired growth and development

64. An adolescent client hospitalized with anorexia nervosa is described by her parents as "the perfect child." When planning care for the client, the nurse should:

Quick Answer: **292**
Detailed Answer: **302**

- ○ **A.** Allow her to choose what foods she will eat
- ○ **B.** Provide activities to foster her self-identity
- ○ **C.** Encourage her to participate in morning exercise
- ○ **D.** Provide a private room near the nurse's station

65. The nurse is assigning staff to care for a number of clients with emotional disorders. Which facet of care is suitable to the skills of the nursing assistant?

Quick Answer: **292**
Detailed Answer: **302**

- ○ **A.** Obtaining the vital signs of a client admitted for alcohol withdrawal
- ○ **B.** Helping a client with depression with bathing and grooming
- ○ **C.** Monitoring a client who is receiving electroconvulsive therapy
- ○ **D.** Sitting with a client with mania who is in seclusion

66. A client with angina is being discharged with a prescription for Transderm Nitro (nitroglycerin) patches. The nurse should tell the client to:

Quick Answer: **292**
Detailed Answer: **302**

- ○ **A.** Shave the area before applying the patch
- ○ **B.** Remove the old patch and clean the skin with alcohol
- ○ **C.** Cover the patch with plastic wrap and tape it in place
- ○ **D.** Avoid cutting the patch because it will alter the dose

67. A client with myasthenia gravis is admitted in a cholinergic crisis. Signs of of cholinergic crisis include:

Quick Answer: **292**
Detailed Answer: **302**

- ○ **A.** Decreased blood pressure and constricted pupils
- ○ **B.** Increased heart rate and increased respirations
- ○ **C.** Increased respirations and increased blood pressure
- ○ **D.** Anoxia and absence of the cough reflex

68. The nurse is providing dietary teaching for a client with hypertension. Which food should be avoided by the client on a sodium-restricted diet?

Quick Answer: **292**
Detailed Answer: **302**

- ○ **A.** Dried beans
- ○ **B.** Swiss cheese
- ○ **C.** Peanut butter
- ○ **D.** Colby cheese

69. A client is admitted to the emergency room with partial-thickness burns to his right arm and full-thickness burns to his trunk. According to the Rule of Nines, the nurse calculates that the total body surface area (TBSA) involved is:

- ○ **A.** 20%
- ○ **B.** 35%
- ○ **C.** 45%
- ○ **D.** 60%

Quick Answer: **292**
Detailed Answer: **302**

70. The physician has ordered a paracentesis for a client with severe abdominal ascites. Before the procedure, the nurse should:

- ○ **A.** Provide the client with a urinal
- ○ **B.** Prep the area by shaving the abdomen
- ○ **C.** Encourage the client to drink extra fluids
- ○ **D.** Request an ultrasound of the abdomen

Quick Answer: **292**
Detailed Answer: **302**

71. Which of the following combinations of foods is appropriate for a 6-month-old?

- ○ **A.** Cocoa-flavored cereal, orange juice, and strained meat
- ○ **B.** Graham crackers, strained prunes, and pudding
- ○ **C.** Rice cereal, bananas, and strained carrots
- ○ **D.** Mashed potatoes, strained beets, and boiled egg

Quick Answer: **292**
Detailed Answer: **302**

72. The mother of a 9-year-old with asthma has brought an electric CD player for her son to listen to while he is receiving oxygen therapy. The nurse should:

- ○ **A.** Explain that he does not need the added stimulation
- ○ **B.** Allow the player, but ask him to wear earphones
- ○ **C.** Tell the mother that he cannot have items from home
- ○ **D.** Ask the mother to bring a battery-operated CD instead

Quick Answer: **292**
Detailed Answer: **303**

73. Which one of the following situations represents a maturational crisis for the family?

- ○ **A.** A 4-year-old entering nursery school
- ○ **B.** Development of preeclampsia during pregnancy
- ○ **C.** Loss of employment and health benefits
- ○ **D.** Hospitalization of a grandfather with a stroke

Quick Answer: **292**
Detailed Answer: **303**

74. A client with a history of phenylketonuria is seen at the local family planning clinic. After completing the client's intake history, the nurse provides literature for a healthy pregnancy. Which statement indicates that the client needs further teaching?

    ○ **A.** "I can help control my weight by switching from sugar to Nutrasweet."

    ○ **B.** "I need to resume my old diet before becoming pregnant."

    ○ **C.** "Fresh fruits and raw vegetables will make excellent between-meal snacks."

    ○ **D.** "I need to eliminate most sources of phenylalanine from my diet."

Quick Answer: **292**
Detailed Answer: **303**

75. Parents of a toddler are dismayed when they learn that their child has Duchenne's muscular dystrophy. Which statement describes the inheritance pattern of the disorder?

    ○ **A.** An affected gene is located on 1 of the 21 pairs of autosomes.

    ○ **B.** The disorder is caused by an over-replication of the X chromosome in males.

    ○ **C.** The affected gene is located on the Y chromosome of the father.

    ○ **D.** The affected gene is located on the X chromosome of the mother.

Quick Answer: **292**
Detailed Answer: **303**

76. A client with obsessive compulsive personality disorder annoys his co-workers with his rigid-perfectionistic attitude and his preoccupation with trivial details. An important nursing intervention for this client would be:

    ○ **A.** Helping the client develop a plan for changing his behavior

    ○ **B.** Contracting with him for the time he spends on a task

    ○ **C.** Avoiding a discussion of his annoying behavior because it will only make him worse

    ○ **D.** Encouraging him to set a time schedule and deadlines for himself

Quick Answer: **292**
Detailed Answer: **303**

77. The mother of a child with chickenpox wants to know if there is a medication that will shorten the course of the illness. Which medication is sometimes used to speed healing of the lesions and shorten the duration of fever and itching?

    ○ **A.** Zovirax (acyclovir)

    ○ **B.** Varivax (varicella vaccine)

    ○ **C.** VZIG (varicella-zoster immune globulin)

    ○ **D.** Periactin (cyproheptadine)

Quick Answer: **292**
Detailed Answer: **303**

78. One of the most important criteria for the diagnosis of physical abuse is inconsistency between the appearance of the injury and the history of how the injury occurred. Which one of the following situations should alert the nurse to the possibility of abuse?

 ○ **A.** An 18-month-old with sock and mitten burns from a fall into the bathtub
 ○ **B.** A 6-year-old with a fractured clavicle following a fall from her bike
 ○ **C.** An 8-year-old with a concussion from a skateboarding accident
 ○ **D.** A 2-year-old with burns to the scalp and face from a grease spill

Quick Answer: **292**
Detailed Answer: **303**

79. A patient refuses to take his dose of oral medication. The nurse tells the patient that if he does not take the medication that she will administer it by injection. The nurse's comments can result in a charge of:

 ○ **A.** Malpractice
 ○ **B.** Assault
 ○ **C.** Negligence
 ○ **D.** Battery

Quick Answer: **292**
Detailed Answer: **303**

80. During morning assessments, the nurse finds that a client's nephrostomy tube has been clamped. The nurse's first action should be to:

 ○ **A.** Assess the drainage bag
 ○ **B.** Check for bladder distention
 ○ **C.** Unclamp the tubing
 ○ **D.** Irrigate the tubing

Quick Answer: **292**
Detailed Answer: **304**

81. The nurse caring for a client with chest tubes notes that the Pleuravac's collection chambers are full. The nurse should:

 ○ **A.** Add more water to the suction-control chamber
 ○ **B.** Remove the drainage using a 60mL syringe
 ○ **C.** Milk the tubing to facilitate drainage
 ○ **D.** Prepare a new unit for continuing collection

Quick Answer: **292**
Detailed Answer: **304**

82. A client with severe anemia is to receive a unit of whole blood. In the event of a transfusion reaction, the first action by the nurse should be to:

 ○ **A.** Notify the physician and the nursing supervisor
 ○ **B.** Stop the transfusion and maintain an IV of normal saline
 ○ **C.** Call the lab for verification of type and cross match
 ○ **D.** Prepare an injection of Benadryl (diphenhydramine)

Quick Answer: **292**
Detailed Answer: **304**

83. A new mother tells the nurse that she is getting a new microwave so that her husband can help prepare the baby's feedings. The nurse should:

- ○ **A.** Explain that a microwave should never be used to warm the baby's bottles
- ○ **B.** Tell the mother that microwaving is the best way to prevent bacteria in the formula
- ○ **C.** Tell the mother to shake the bottle vigorously for 1 minute after warming in the microwave
- ○ **D.** Instruct the parents to always leave the top of the bottle open while microwaving so heat can escape

84. A client with HELLP syndrome is admitted to the labor and delivery unit for observation. The nurse knows that the client will have elevated:

- ○ **A.** Serum glucose levels
- ○ **B.** Liver enzymes
- ○ **C.** Pancreatic enzymes
- ○ **D.** Plasma protein levels

85. To reduce the possibility of having a baby with a neural tube defect, the client should be told to increase her intake of folic acid. Dietary sources of folic acid include:

- ○ **A.** Meat, liver, eggs
- ○ **B.** Pork, fish, chicken
- ○ **C.** Spinach, beets, cantaloupe
- ○ **D.** Dried beans, sweet potatoes, Brussels sprouts

86. The nurse is making room assignments for four obstetrical clients. If only one private room is available, it should be assigned to:

- ○ **A.** A multigravida with diabetes mellitus
- ○ **B.** A primigravida with preeclampsia
- ○ **C.** A multigravida with preterm labor
- ○ **D.** A primigravida with hyperemesis gravidarum

87. A client has a tentative diagnosis of myasthenia gravis. The nurse recognizes that myasthenia gravis involves:

- ○ **A.** Loss of the myelin sheath in portions of the brain and spinal cord
- ○ **B.** An interruption in the transmission of impulses from nerve endings to muscles
- ○ **C.** Progressive weakness and loss of sensation that begins in the lower extremities
- ○ **D.** Loss of coordination and stiff "cogwheel" rigidity

88. The physician has ordered an infusion of Osmitrol (mannitol) for a client with increased intracranial pressure. Which finding indicates the direct effectiveness of the drug?

Quick Answer: **292**
Detailed Answer: **304**

- ○ **A.** Increased pulse rate
- ○ **B.** Increased urinary output
- ○ **C.** Decreased diastolic blood pressure
- ○ **D.** Increased pupil size

89. The nurse has just received the change of shift report. Which client should the nurse assess first?

Quick Answer: **292**
Detailed Answer: **304**

- ○ **A.** A client with a supratentorial tumor awaiting surgery
- ○ **B.** A client admitted with a suspected subdural hematoma
- ○ **C.** A client recently diagnosed with akinetic seizures
- ○ **D.** A client transferring to the neuro rehabilitation unit

90. The physician has ordered an IV bolus of Solu-Medrol (methylprednisolone sodium succinate) in normal saline for a client admitted with a spinal cord injury. Solu-Medrol has been shown to be effective in:

Quick Answer: **292**
Detailed Answer: **305**

- ○ **A.** Preventing spasticity associated with cord injury
- ○ **B.** Decreasing the need for mechanical ventilation
- ○ **C.** Improving motor and sensory functioning
- ○ **D.** Treating post injury urinary tract infections

91. The physician has ordered a lumbar puncture for a client with suspected Guillain-Barre syndrome. The spinal fluid of a client with Guillain-Barre syndrome typically shows:

Quick Answer: **292**
Detailed Answer: **305**

- ○ **A.** Decreased protein concentration with a normal cell count
- ○ **B.** Increased protein concentration with a normal cell count
- ○ **C.** Increased protein concentration with an abnormal cell count
- ○ **D.** Decreased protein concentration with an abnormal cell count

92. An 18-month-old is admitted to the hospital with acute laryngotracheobronchitis. When assessing the respiratory status, the nurse should expect to find:

Quick Answer: **292**
Detailed Answer: **305**

- ○ **A.** Inspiratory stridor and harsh cough
- ○ **B.** Strident cough and drooling
- ○ **C.** Wheezing and intercostal retractions
- ○ **D.** Expiratory wheezing and nonproductive cough

93. The school nurse is assessing an elementary student with hemophilia who fell during recess. Which symptoms indicate hemarthrosis?

Quick Answer: **292**
Detailed Answer: **305**

- ○ **A.** Pain, coolness, and blue discoloration in the affected joint
- ○ **B.** Tingling and pain without loss of movement in the affected joint
- ○ **C.** Warmth, redness, and decreased movement in the affected joint
- ○ **D.** Stiffness, aching, and decreased movement in the affected joint

94. The physician has ordered aerosol treatments, chest percussion, and postural drainage for a client with cystic fibrosis. The nurse recognizes that the combination of therapies is to:

Quick Answer: **293**
Detailed Answer: **305**

- ○ **A.** Decrease respiratory effort and mucous production
- ○ **B.** Increase efficiency of the diaphragm and gas exchange
- ○ **C.** Dilate the bronchioles and help remove secretions
- ○ **D.** Stimulate coughing and oxygen consumption

95. The nurse is assessing a 6-year-old following a tonsillectomy. Which one of the following signs is an early indication of hemorrhage?

Quick Answer: **293**
Detailed Answer: **305**

- ○ **A.** Drooling of bright red secretions
- ○ **B.** Pulse rate of 90
- ○ **C.** Vomiting of dark brown liquid
- ○ **D.** Infrequent swallowing while sleeping

96. A client is admitted for suspected bladder cancer. Which one of the following factors is most significant in the client's diagnosis?

Quick Answer: **293**
Detailed Answer: **305**

- ○ **A.** Smoking a pack of cigarettes a day for 30 years
- ○ **B.** Use of nonsteroidal anti-inflammatories
- ○ **C.** Eating foods with preservatives
- ○ **D.** Past employment involving asbestos

97. The nurse is teaching a client with peritoneal dialysis how to manage exchanges at home. The nurse should tell the client to notify the doctor immediately if:

Quick Answer: **293**
Detailed Answer: **305**

- ○ **A.** The dialysate returns become cloudy in appearance.
- ○ **B.** The return of the dialysate is slower than usual.
- ○ **C.** A "tugging" sensation is noted as the dialysate drains.
- ○ **D.** A feeling of fullness is felt when the dialysate is instilled.

98. The physician has prescribed nitroglycerin sublingual tablets as needed for a client with angina. The nurse should tell the client to take the medication:

○ **A.** After engaging in strenuous activity

○ **B.** Every 4 hours to prevent chest pain

○ **C.** As soon as he notices signs of chest pain

○ **D.** At bedtime to prevent nocturnal angina

99. The nurse is caring for a client following a myocardial infarction. Which of the following enzymes are specific to cardiac damage?

○ **A.** SGOT and LDH

○ **B.** SGOT and CK BB

○ **C.** LDH and CK MB

○ **D.** LDH and CK BB

100. Which of the following characterizes peer group relationships in 8- and 9-year-olds?

○ **A.** Activities organized around competitive games

○ **B.** Loyalty and strong same-sex friendships

○ **C.** Informal socialization between boys and girls

○ **D.** Shared activities with one best friend

101. If the school-age child is not given the opportunity to engage in tasks and activities he can carry through to completion, he is likely to develop feelings of:

○ **A.** Guilt

○ **B.** Shame

○ **C.** Stagnation

○ **D.** Inferiority

102. The physician has ordered 2 units of whole blood for a client following surgery. To provide for client safety, the nurse should:

○ **A.** Obtain a signed permit for each unit of blood

○ **B.** Use a new administration set for each unit transfused

○ **C.** Administer the blood using a Y connector

○ **D.** Check the blood type and Rh factor three times before initiating the transfusion

Quick Check

103. A client with B positive blood is scheduled for a transfusion of whole blood. Which finding requires nursing intervention?

Quick Answer: **293**
Detailed Answer: **306**

- ○ **A.** The available blood has been banked for 2 weeks.
- ○ **B.** The blood available for transfusion is Rh negative.
- ○ **C.** The client has a peripheral IV of D5 $\frac{1}{2}$ normal saline.
- ○ **D.** The blood available for transfusion is type O positive.

104. The nurse is reviewing the lab results of a client's arterial blood gases. The $PaCO_2$ indicates effective functioning of the:

Quick Answer: **293**
Detailed Answer: **306**

- ○ **A.** Kidneys
- ○ **B.** Pancreas
- ○ **C.** Lungs
- ○ **D.** Liver

105. The autopsy results in SIDS-related death will show the following consistent findings:

Quick Answer: **293**
Detailed Answer: **306**

- ○ **A.** Abnormal central nervous system development
- ○ **B.** Abnormal cardiovascular development
- ○ **C.** Intraventricular hemorrhage and cerebral edema
- ○ **D.** Pulmonary edema and intrathoracic hemorrhages

106. The nurse is caring for a newborn who is on strict intake and output. The used diaper weighs 73.5gm. The diaper's dry weight was 62gm. The newborn's urine output is:

Quick Answer: **293**
Detailed Answer: **306**

- ○ **A.** 10ml
- ○ **B.** 11.5ml
- ○ **C.** 10gm
- ○ **D.** 12gm

107. The nurse is teaching the parents of an infant with osteogenesis imperfecta. The nurse should explain the need for:

Quick Answer: **293**
Detailed Answer: **306**

- ○ **A.** Additional calcium in the infant's diet
- ○ **B.** Careful handling to prevent fractures
- ○ **C.** Providing extra sensorimotor stimulation
- ○ **D.** Frequent testing of visual function

108. A newborn is diagnosed with respiratory distress syndrome (RDS). Which position is best for maintaining an open airway?

Quick Answer: **293**
Detailed Answer: **306**

- ○ **A.** Prone, with his head turned to one side
- ○ **B.** Side-lying, with a towel beneath his shoulders
- ○ **C.** Supine, with his neck slightly flexed
- ○ **D.** Supine, with his neck slightly extended

109. A client with bipolar disorder is discharged with a prescription for Depakote (divalproex sodium). The nurse should remind the client of the need for:

- ○ **A.** Frequent dental visits
- ○ **B.** Frequent lab work
- ○ **C.** Additional fluids
- ○ **D.** Additional sodium

110. The physician's notes state that a client with cocaine addiction has formication. The nurse recognizes that the client has:

- ○ **A.** Tactile hallucinations
- ○ **B.** Irregular heart rate
- ○ **C.** Paranoid delusions
- ○ **D.** Methadone tolerance

111. The nurse is preparing a client with gastroesophageal reflux disease (GERD) for discharge. The nurse should tell the client to:

- ○ **A.** Eat a small snack before bedtime
- ○ **B.** Sleep on his right side
- ○ **C.** Avoid carbonated beverages
- ○ **D.** Increase his intake of citrus fruits

112. A client with a C3 spinal cord injury experiences autonomic hyperreflexia. After placing the client in high Fowler's position, the nurse's next action should be to:

- ○ **A.** Notify the physician
- ○ **B.** Make sure the catheter is patent
- ○ **C.** Administer an antihypertensive
- ○ **D.** Provide supplemental oxygen

113. A client is to receive Dilantin (phenytoin) via a nasogastric (NG) tube. When giving the medication, the nurse should:

- ○ **A.** Flush the NG tube with 2–4mL of water before giving the medication
- ○ **B.** Administer the medication, flush with 5mL of water, and clamp the NG tube
- ○ **C.** Flush the NG tube with 5mL of normal saline and administer the medication
- ○ **D.** Flush the NG tube with 2–4oz of water before and after giving the medication

114. When assessing the client with acute arterial occlusion, the nurse would expect to find:

Quick Answer: **293**
Detailed Answer: **307**

  ○ **A.** Peripheral edema in the affected extremity

  ○ **B.** Minute blackened areas on the toes

  ○ **C.** Pain above the level of occlusion

  ○ **D.** Redness and warmth over the affected area

115. The nurse is assessing a client following the removal of a pituitary tumor. The nurse notes that the urinary output has increased and that the urine is very dilute. The nurse should give priority to:

Quick Answer: **293**
Detailed Answer: **307**

  ○ **A.** Notifying the doctor immediately

  ○ **B.** Documenting the finding in the chart

  ○ **C.** Decreasing the rate of IV fluids

  ○ **D.** Administering vasopressive medication

116. The physician has ordered Coumadin (sodium warfarin) for a client with a history of clots. The nurse should tell the client to avoid which of the following vegetables?

Quick Answer: **293**
Detailed Answer: **307**

  ○ **A.** Lettuce

  ○ **B.** Cauliflower

  ○ **C.** Beets

  ○ **D.** Carrots

117. The nurse is caring for a child in a plaster-of-Paris hip spica cast. To facilitate drying, the nurse should:

Quick Answer: **293**
Detailed Answer: **307**

  ○ **A.** Use a small hand-held hair dryer set on medium heat

  ○ **B.** Place a small heater near the child's bed

  ○ **C.** Turn the child at least every 2 hours

  ○ **D.** Allow one side to dry before changing positions

118. The local health clinic recommends vaccination against influenza for all its employees. The influenza vaccine is given annually in:

Quick Answer: **293**
Detailed Answer: **307**

  ○ **A.** November

  ○ **B.** December

  ○ **C.** January

  ○ **D.** February

119. A client is admitted with suspected Hodgkin's lymphoma. The diagnosis is confirmed by the:

- ○ **A.** Overproliferation of immature white cells
- ○ **B.** Presence of Reed-Sternberg cells
- ○ **C.** Increased incidence of microcytosis
- ○ **D.** Reduction in the number of platelets

Quick Answer: **293**
Detailed Answer: **307**

120. The nurse is caring for a client following a laryngectomy. The nurse can best help the client with communication by:

- ○ **A.** Providing a pad and pencil
- ○ **B.** Checking on him every 30 minutes
- ○ **C.** Telling him to use the call light
- ○ **D.** Teaching the client simple sign language

Quick Answer: **293**
Detailed Answer: **307**

121. A client has recently been diagnosed with open-angle glaucoma. The nurse should tell the client to avoid taking:

- ○ **A.** Aleve (naprosyn)
- ○ **B.** Benadryl (diphenhydramine)
- ○ **C.** Tylenol (acetaminophen)
- ○ **D.** Robitussin (guaifenesin)

Quick Answer: **293**
Detailed Answer: **308**

122. The nurse is caring for a client with an endemic goiter. The nurse recognizes that the client's condition is related to:

- ○ **A.** Living in an area where the soil is depleted of iodine
- ○ **B.** Eating foods that decrease the thyroxine level
- ○ **C.** Using aluminum cookware to prepare the family's meals
- ○ **D.** Taking medications that decrease the thyroxine level

Quick Answer: **293**
Detailed Answer: **308**

123. A client with a history of schizophrenia is seen in the local health clinic for medication follow-up. To maintain a therapeutic level of medication, the nurse should tell the client to avoid:

- ○ **A.** Taking over-the-counter allergy medication
- ○ **B.** Eating cheese and pickled foods
- ○ **C.** Eating salty foods
- ○ **D.** Taking over-the-counter pain relievers

Quick Answer: **293**
Detailed Answer: **308**

124. The nurse is formulating a plan of care for a client with a goiter. The priority nursing diagnosis for the client with a goiter is:

- ○ **A.** Body image disturbance related to swelling of neck
- ○ **B.** Anxiety-related changes in body image
- ○ **C.** Altered nutrition, less than body requirements, related to difficulty in swallowing
- ○ **D.** Risk for ineffective airway clearance related to pressure on the trachea

125. Upon arrival in the nursery, erythromycin eyedrops are applied to the newborn's eyes. The nurse understands that the medication will:

- ○ **A.** Make the eyes less sensitive to light
- ○ **B.** Help prevent neonatal blindness
- ○ **C.** Strengthen the muscles of the eyes
- ○ **D.** Improve accommodation to near objects

126. A client has a diagnosis of discoid lupus erythematosus (DLE). The nurse recognizes that discoid lupus differs from systemic lupus erythematosus because it:

- ○ **A.** Produces changes in the kidneys
- ○ **B.** Is confined to changes in the skin
- ○ **C.** Results in damage to the heart and lungs
- ○ **D.** Affects both joints and muscles

127. A client sustained a severe head injury to the occipital lobe. The nurse should carefully assess the client for:

- ○ **A.** Changes in vision
- ○ **B.** Difficulty in speaking
- ○ **C.** Impaired judgment
- ○ **D.** Hearing impairment

128. The nurse observes a group of toddlers at daycare. Which of the following play situations exhibits the characteristics of parallel play?

- ○ **A.** Lindie and Laura sharing clay to make cookies
- ○ **B.** Nick and Matt playing beside each other with trucks
- ○ **C.** Adrienne working a puzzle with Meredith and Ryan
- ○ **D.** Ashley playing with a busy box while sitting in her crib

129. Which of the following statements is true regarding language development of young children?

Quick Answer: **293**
Detailed Answer: **308**

- ○ **A.** Infants can discriminate speech from other patterns of sound.
- ○ **B.** Boys are more advanced in language development than girls of the same age.
- ○ **C.** Second-born children develop language earlier than first-born or only children.
- ○ **D.** Using single words for an entire sentence suggests delayed speech development.

130. A mother tells the nurse that her daughter has become quite a collector, filling her room with Beanie babies, dolls, and stuffed animals. The nurse recognizes that the child is developing:

Quick Answer: **293**
Detailed Answer: **308**

- ○ **A.** Object permanence
- ○ **B.** Post-conventional thinking
- ○ **C.** Concrete operational thinking
- ○ **D.** Pre-operational thinking

131. According to Erikson, the developmental task of the infant is to establish trust. Parents and caregivers foster a sense of trust by:

Quick Answer: **293**
Detailed Answer: **308**

- ○ **A.** Holding the infant during feedings
- ○ **B.** Speaking quietly to the infant
- ○ **C.** Providing sensory stimulation
- ○ **D.** Consistently responding to needs

132. The nurse is preparing to walk the postpartum client for the first time since delivery. Before walking the client, the nurse should:

Quick Answer: **293**
Detailed Answer: **309**

- ○ **A.** Give the client pain medication
- ○ **B.** Assist the client in dangling her legs
- ○ **C.** Have the client breathe deeply
- ○ **D.** Provide the client additional fluids

133. To minimize confusion in the elderly hospitalized client, the nurse should:

Quick Answer: **293**
Detailed Answer: **309**

- ○ **A.** Provide sensory stimulation by varying the daily routine
- ○ **B.** Keep the room brightly lit and the television on to provide orientation to time
- ○ **C.** Encourage visitors to limit visitation to phone calls to avoid overstimulation
- ○ **D.** Provide explanations in a calm, caring manner to minimize anxiety

134. A client diagnosed with tuberculosis asks the nurse when he can return to work. The nurse should tell the client that:

Quick Answer: **293**
Detailed Answer: **309**

- ○ **A.** He can return to work when he has three negative sputum cultures.
- ○ **B.** He can return to work as soon as he feels well enough.
- ○ **C.** He can return to work after a week of being on the medication.
- ○ **D.** He should think about applying for disability because he will no longer be able to work.

135. The physician has ordered lab work for a client with suspected disseminated intravascular coagulation (DIC). Which lab finding would provide a definitive diagnosis of DIC?

Quick Answer: **293**
Detailed Answer: **309**

- ○ **A.** Elevated erythrocyte sedimentation rate
- ○ **B.** Prolonged clotting time
- ○ **C.** Presence of fibrin split compound
- ○ **D.** Elevated white cell count

136. The nurse is caring for a client with rheumatoid arthritis. The nurse knows that the client's symptoms will be most improved by:

Quick Answer: **293**
Detailed Answer: **309**

- ○ **A.** Taking a warm shower upon awakening
- ○ **B.** Applying ice packs to the joints
- ○ **C.** Taking two aspirin before going to bed
- ○ **D.** Going for an early morning walk

137. A client with schizophrenia has been taking Clozaril (clozapine) for the past 6 months. This morning the client's temperature was elevated to 102°F. The nurse should give priority to:

Quick Answer: **293**
Detailed Answer: **309**

- ○ **A.** Placing a note in the chart for the doctor
- ○ **B.** Rechecking the temperature in 4 hours
- ○ **C.** Notifying the physician immediately
- ○ **D.** Asking the client if he has been feeling sick

138. Which one of the following clients is most likely to develop acute respiratory distress syndrome?

Quick Answer: **293**
Detailed Answer: **309**

- ○ **A.** A 20-year-old with fractures of the tibia
- ○ **B.** A 36-year-old who is HIV positive
- ○ **C.** A 40-year-old with duodenal ulcers
- ○ **D.** A 32-year-old with barbiturate overdose

139. The complete blood count of a client admitted with anemia reveals that the red blood cells are hypochromic and microcytic. The nurse recognizes that the client has:

- ○ **A.** Aplastic anemia
- ○ **B.** Iron-deficiency anemia
- ○ **C.** Pernicious anemia
- ○ **D.** Hemolytic anemia

Quick Answer: **293**
Detailed Answer: **309**

140. While performing a neurological assessment on a client with a closed head injury, the nurse notes a positive Babinski reflex. The nurse should:

- ○ **A.** Recognize that the client's condition is improving
- ○ **B.** Reposition the client and check reflexes again
- ○ **C.** Do nothing because the finding is an expected one
- ○ **D.** Notify the physician of the finding

Quick Answer: **293**
Detailed Answer: **309**

141. The doctor has ordered neurological checks every 30 minutes for a client injured in a biking accident. Which finding indicates that the client's condition is satisfactory?

- ○ **A.** A score of 13 on the Glascow coma scale
- ○ **B.** The presence of doll's eye movement
- ○ **C.** The absence of deep tendon reflexes
- ○ **D.** Decerebrate posturing

Quick Answer: **293**
Detailed Answer: **310**

142. The nurse is developing a plan for bowel and bladder retraining for a client with paraplegia. The primary goal of a bowel and bladder retraining program is:

- ○ **A.** Optimal restoration of the client's elimination pattern
- ○ **B.** Restoration of the client's neurosensory function
- ○ **C.** Prevention of complications from impaired elimination
- ○ **D.** Promotion of a positive body image

Quick Answer: **293**
Detailed Answer: **310**

143. When checking patellar reflexes, the nurse is unable to elicit a knee-jerk response. To facilitate checking the patellar reflex, the nurse should tell the client to:

- ○ **A.** Pull against her interlocked fingers
- ○ **B.** Shrug her shoulders and hold for a count of five
- ○ **C.** Close her eyes tightly and resist opening
- ○ **D.** Cross her legs at the ankles

Quick Answer: **293**
Detailed Answer: **310**

144. The nurse is performing a physical assessment on a newly admitted client. The last step in the physical assessment is:

- ○ **A.** Inspection
- ○ **B.** Auscultation
- ○ **C.** Percussion
- ○ **D.** Palpation

145. A client with schizophrenia spends much of his time pacing the floor, rocking back and forth, and moving from one foot to another. The client's behaviors are an example of:

- ○ **A.** Dystonia
- ○ **B.** Tardive dyskinesia
- ○ **C.** Akathisia
- ○ **D.** Oculogyric crisis

146. The nurse is assessing a recently admitted newborn. Which finding should be reported to the physician?

- ○ **A.** The umbilical cord contains three vessels.
- ○ **B.** The newborn has a temperature of 98°F.
- ○ **C.** The feet and hands are bluish in color.
- ○ **D.** A large, soft swelling crosses the suture line.

147. Which statement is true regarding the infant's susceptibility to pertussis?

- ○ **A.** If the mother had pertussis, the infant will have passive immunity.
- ○ **B.** Most infants and children are highly susceptible from birth.
- ○ **C.** The newborn will be immune to pertussis for the first few months of life.
- ○ **D.** Infants under 1 year of age seldom get pertussis.

148. A client in labor has been given epidural anesthesia with Marcaine (bupivacaine). To reverse the hypotension associated with epidural anesthesia, the nurse should have which medication available?

- ○ **A.** Narcan (naloxone)
- ○ **B.** Dobutrex (dobutamine)
- ○ **C.** Romazicon (flumazenil)
- ○ **D.** Adrenalin (epinephrine)

149. The physician has prescribed Gantrisin (sulfasoxazole) 1g in divided doses for a client with a urinary tract infection. The nurse should administer the medication:

- ○ **A.** With meals or a snack
- ○ **B.** 30 minutes before meals
- ○ **C.** 30 minutes after meals
- ○ **D.** At bedtime

Quick Answer: **293**
Detailed Answer: **310**

150. A client with a history of depression is treated with Parnate (tranylcypromine), an MAO inhibitor. Ingestion of foods containing tyramine while taking an MAO inhibitor can result in:

- ○ **A.** Extreme elevations in blood pressure
- ○ **B.** Rapidly rising temperature
- ○ **C.** Abnormal movement and muscle spasms
- ○ **D.** Damage to the eighth cranial nerve

Quick Answer: **293**
Detailed Answer: **311**

151. A client is admitted to the emergency room after falling down a flight of stairs. Initial assessment reveals a large bump on the front of the head and a 2-inch laceration above the right eye. Which finding is consistent with injury to the frontal lobe?

- ○ **A.** Complaints of blindness
- ○ **B.** Decreased respiratory rate and depth
- ○ **C.** Failure to recognize touch
- ○ **D.** Inability to identify sweet taste

Quick Answer: **293**
Detailed Answer: **311**

152. The nurse is evaluating the intake and output of a client for the first 12 hours following an abdominal cholecystectomy. Which finding should be reported to the physician?

- ○ **A.** Output of 10mL from the Jackson-Pratt drain
- ○ **B.** Foley catheter output of 285mL
- ○ **C.** Nasogastric tube output of 150mL
- ○ **D.** Absence of stool

Quick Answer: **293**
Detailed Answer: **311**

153. A community health nurse is teaching healthful lifestyles to a group of senior citizens. The nurse knows that the leading cause of death in persons 65 and older is:

- ○ **A.** Chronic pulmonary disease
- ○ **B.** Diabetes mellitus
- ○ **C.** Pneumonia
- ○ **D.** Heart disease

Quick Answer: **293**
Detailed Answer: **311**

154. A client suspected of having Alzheimer's disease is evaluated using the Mini-Mental State Examination. At the beginning of the evaluation, the examiner names three objects. Later in the evaluation, he asks the client to name the same three objects. The examiner is testing the client's:

- ○ **A.** Attention
- ○ **B.** Orientation
- ○ **C.** Recall
- ○ **D.** Registration

155. A client with end stage renal disease is being managed with peritoneal dialysis. If the dialysate return is slowed the nurse should tell the client to:

- ○ **A.** Irrigate the dialyzing catheter with saline
- ○ **B.** Skip the next scheduled infusion
- ○ **C.** Gently retract the dialyzing catheter
- ○ **D.** Change position or turn side to side

156. The nurse is the first person to arrive at the scene of a motor vehicle accident. When rendering aid to the victim, the nurse should give priority to:

- ○ **A.** Establishing a patent airway
- ○ **B.** Checking the quality of respirations
- ○ **C.** Observing for signs of active bleeding
- ○ **D.** Determining the level of consciousness

157. A client hospitalized with renal calculi complains of severe pain in the right flank. In addition to complaints of pain, the nurse can expect to see changes in the client's vital signs that include:

- ○ **A.** Decreased pulse rate
- ○ **B.** Increased blood pressure
- ○ **C.** Decreased respiratory rate
- ○ **D.** Increased temperature

158. The nurse is using the Glascow coma scale to assess the client's motor response. The nurse places pressure at the base of the client's fingernail for 20 seconds. The client's only response is withdrawal of his hand. The nurse interprets the client's response as:

- ○ **A.** A score of 6 because he follows commands
- ○ **B.** A score of 5 because he localizes pain
- ○ **C.** A score of 4 because he uses flexion
- ○ **D.** A score of 3 because he uses extension

159. A 4-year-old is admitted to the hospital for treatment of Kawasaki's disease. The medication commonly prescribed for the treatment of Kawasaki's disease is:

- ○ **A.** Aspirin (acetylsalicylic acid)
- ○ **B.** Benadryl (diphenhydramine)
- ○ **C.** Polycillin (ampicillin)
- ○ **D.** Betaseron (interferon beta)

Quick Answer: **293**
Detailed Answer: **311**

160. The nurse is caring for a client with bulimia nervosa. The nurse recognizes that the major difference in the client with anorexia nervosa and the client with bulimia nervosa is the client with bulimia:

- ○ **A.** Is usually grossly overweight.
- ○ **B.** Has a distorted body image.
- ○ **C.** Recognizes that she has an eating disorder.
- ○ **D.** Struggles with issues of dependence versus independence.

Quick Answer: **293**
Detailed Answer: **312**

161. The Mantoux text is used to determine whether a person has been exposed to tuberculosis. If the test is positive, the nurse will find a:

- ○ **A.** Fluid-filled vesicle
- ○ **B.** Sharply demarcated erythema
- ○ **C.** Central area of induration
- ○ **D.** Circular blanched area

Quick Answer: **293**
Detailed Answer: **312**

162. The physician has ordered continuous bladder irrigation for a client following a prostatectomy. The nurse should:

- ○ **A.** Hang the solution 2–3 feet above the client's abdomen
- ○ **B.** Allow air from the solution tubing to flow into the catheter
- ○ **C.** Use a clean technique when attaching the solution tubing to the catheter
- ○ **D.** Clamp the solution tubing periodically to prevent bladder distention

Quick Answer: **293**
Detailed Answer: **312**

163. A pediatric client is admitted to the hospital for treatment of diarrhea caused by an infection with salmonella. Which of the following most likely contributed to the child's illness?

- ○ **A.** Brushing the family dog
- ○ **B.** Playing with a turtle
- ○ **C.** Taking a pony ride
- ○ **D.** Feeding the family cat

Quick Answer: **293**
Detailed Answer: **312**

164. Which one of the following infants needs a further assessment of growth?

- ○ **A.** 4-month-old: birth weight 7lb, 6oz; current weight 14lb, 4oz
- ○ **B.** 2-week-old: birth weight 6lb, 10oz; current weight 6lb, 12oz
- ○ **C.** 6-month-old: birth weight 8lb, 8oz; current weight 15lb
- ○ **D.** 2-month-old: birth weight 7lb, 2oz; current weight 9lb, 6oz

165. The physician has ordered Pyridium (phenazopyridine) for a client with urinary urgency. The nurse should tell the client that:

- ○ **A.** The urine will have a strong odor of ammonia.
- ○ **B.** The urinary output will increase in amount.
- ○ **C.** The urine will have a red–orange color.
- ○ **D.** The urinary output will decrease in amount.

166. The nurse is teaching the mother of an infant with eczema. Which of the following instructions should be included in the nurse's teaching?

- ○ **A.** Dress the infant warmly to prevent undue chilling
- ○ **B.** Cut the infant's fingernails and toenails regularly
- ○ **C.** Use bubble bath instead of soap for bathing
- ○ **D.** Wash the infant's clothes with mild detergent and fabric softener

167. Skeletal traction is applied to the right femur of a client injured in a fall. The primary purpose of the skeletal traction is to:

- ○ **A.** Realign the tibia and fibula
- ○ **B.** Provide traction on the muscles
- ○ **C.** Provide traction on the ligaments
- ○ **D.** Realign femoral bone fragments

168. The home health nurse is visiting a client with an exacerbation of rheumatoid arthritis. To prevent deformities of the knee joints, the nurse should:

- ○ **A.** Tell the client to walk without bending the knees
- ○ **B.** Encourage movement within the limits of pain
- ○ **C.** Instruct the client to sit only in a recliner
- ○ **D.** Remain in bed as long as the joints are painful

169. The physician has ordered Dextrose 5% in normal saline for an infant admitted with gastroenteritis. The advantage of administering the infant's IV through a scalp vein is:

Quick Answer: **293**
Detailed Answer: **312**

- ○ **A.** The infant can be held and comforted more easily.
- ○ **B.** Dextrose is best absorbed from the scalp veins.
- ○ **C.** Scalp veins do not infiltrate like peripheral veins.
- ○ **D.** There are few pain receptors in the infant's scalp.

170. A newborn diagnosed with bilateral choanal atresia is scheduled for surgery soon after delivery. The nurse recognizes the immediate need for surgery because the newborn:

Quick Answer: **293**
Detailed Answer: **313**

- ○ **A.** Will have difficulty swallowing
- ○ **B.** Will be unable to pass meconium
- ○ **C.** Will regurgitate his feedings
- ○ **D.** Will be unable to breathe through his nose

171. The most appropriate means of rehydration of a 7-month-old with diarrhea and mild dehydration is:

Quick Answer: **293**
Detailed Answer: **313**

- ○ **A.** Oral rehydration therapy with an electrolyte solution
- ○ **B.** Replacing milk-based formula with a lactose-free formula
- ○ **C.** Administering intraveneous Dextrose 5% ¼ normal saline
- ○ **D.** Offering bananas, rice, and applesauce along with oral fluids

172. The nurse is caring for an infant receiving intravenous fluid. Signs of fluid overload in an infant include:

Quick Answer: **293**
Detailed Answer: **313**

- ○ **A.** Swelling of the hands and increased temperature
- ○ **B.** Increased heart rate and increased blood pressure
- ○ **C.** Swelling of the feet and increased temperature
- ○ **D.** Decreased heart rate and decreased blood pressure

173. The nurse is providing care for a 10-month-old diagnosed with Wilms tumor. Most parents of infants with Wilms tumor report finding the mass when:

Quick Answer: **293**
Detailed Answer: **313**

- ○ **A.** The infant is diapered or bathed
- ○ **B.** The infant is unable to use his arms
- ○ **C.** The infant is unable to follow a moving object
- ○ **D.** The infant is unable to vocalize sounds

Quick Check

174. An obstetrical client has just been diagnosed with cardiac disease. The nurse should give priority to:

Quick Answer: **293**
Detailed Answer: **313**

- ○ **A.** Instructing the client to remain on strict bed rest
- ○ **B.** Telling the client to monitor her pulse and respirations
- ○ **C.** Instructing the client to check her temperature in the evening
- ○ **D.** Telling the client to weigh herself monthly

175. The nurse is caring for a client receiving supplemental oxygen. The effectiveness of the oxygen therapy is best determined by:

Quick Answer: **293**
Detailed Answer: **313**

- ○ **A.** The rate of respirations
- ○ **B.** The absence of cyanosis
- ○ **C.** Arterial blood gases
- ○ **D.** The level of consciousness

176. A client having a colonoscopy is medicated with Versed (midazolam). The nurse recognizes that the client:

Quick Answer: **293**
Detailed Answer: **313**

- ○ **A.** Will be able to remember the procedure within 2–3 hours
- ○ **B.** Will not be able to remember having the procedure done
- ○ **C.** Will be able to remember the procedure within 2–3 days
- ○ **D.** Will not be able to remember what occurred before the procedure

177. The nurse is assessing a client with an altered level of consciousness. One of the first signs of altered level of consciousness is:

Quick Answer: **293**
Detailed Answer: **313**

- ○ **A.** Inability to perform motor activities
- ○ **B.** Complaints of double vision
- ○ **C.** Restlessness
- ○ **D.** Unequal pupil size

178. Four clients are to receive medication. Which client should receive medication first?

Quick Answer: **293**
Detailed Answer: **313**

- ○ **A.** A client with an apical pulse of 72 receiving Lanoxin (digoxin) PO daily
- ○ **B.** A client with abdominal surgery receiving Phenergan (promethazine) IM every 4 hours PRN for nausea and vomiting
- ○ **C.** A client with labored respirations receiving a stat dose of IV Lasix (furosemide)
- ○ **D.** A client with pneumonia receiving Polycillin (ampicillin) IVPB every 6 hours

179. The nurse is caring for a cognitively impaired client who begins to pull at the tape securing his IV site. To prevent the client from removing the IV, the nurse should:

  ○ **A.** Place tape completely around the extremity, with tape ends out of the client's vision

  ○ **B.** Tell him that if he pulls out the IV, it will have to be restarted

  ○ **C.** Slap the client's hand when he reaches toward the IV site

  ○ **D.** Apply clove hitch restraints to the client's hands

180. A client is admitted to the emergency room with complaints of substernal chest pain radiating to the left jaw. Which ECG finding is suggestive of acute myocardial infarction?

  ○ **A.** Peaked P wave

  ○ **B.** Changes in ST segment

  ○ **C.** Minimal QRS wave

  ○ **D.** Prominent U wave

181. The nurse is assessing a client with a closed reduction of a fractured femur. Which finding should the nurse report to the physician?

  ○ **A.** Chest pain and shortness of breath.

  ○ **B.** Ecchymosis on the side of the injured leg.

  ○ **C.** Oral temperature of 99.2°F.

  ○ **D.** Complaints of level two pain on a scale of five.

182. According to the American Heart Association (2005) guidelines the compression-to-ventilation ratio for one rescuer cardiopulmonary resuscitation is:

  ○ **A.** 10:1

  ○ **B.** 20:2

  ○ **C.** 30:2

  ○ **D.** 40:1

183. A client is admitted with a diagnosis of renal calculi. The nurse should give priority to:

- ○ **A.** Initiating an intraveneous infusion
- ○ **B.** Encouraging oral fluids
- ○ **C.** Administering pain medication
- ○ **D.** Straining the urine

184. The Joint Commission for Accreditation of Hospital Organizations (JCAHO) specifies that two client identifiers are to be used before administering medication. Which method is best for identifying patients using two patient identifiers?

- ○ **A.** Take the medication administration record (MAR) to the room and compare it with the name and medical number recorded on the armband.
- ○ **B.** Compare the medication administration record (MAR) with the client's room number and name on the armband.
- ○ **C.** Request that a family member identify the client and then ask the client to state his name.
- ○ **D.** Ask the client to state his full name and then to write his full name.

185. A client complains of sharp, stabbing pain in the right lower quadrant that is graded as level 8 on a scale of 10. The nurse knows that pain of this severity can best be managed using:

- ○ **A.** Aleve (naproxen sodium)
- ○ **B.** Tylenol with codeine (acetaminophen with codeine)
- ○ **C.** Toradol (ketorolac)
- ○ **D.** Morphine sulfate (morphine sulfate)

186. A client has had diarrhea for the past 3 days. Which acid/base imbalance would the nurse expect the client to have?

- ○ **A.** Respiratory alkalosis
- ○ **B.** Metabolic acidosis
- ○ **C.** Metabolic alkalosis
- ○ **D.** Respiratory acidosis

187. A home health nurse finds the client lying unconscious in the doorway of her bathroom. The nurse checks for responsiveness by gently shaking the client and calling her name. When it is determined that the client is nonresponsive, the nurse should:

○ **A.** Start cardiac compression

○ **B.** Give two slow, deep breaths

○ **C.** Open the airway using head-tilt, chin-lift maneuver

○ **D.** Call for help

188. The nurse is reviewing the lab reports of a client who is HIV positive. Which lab report provides information regarding the effectiveness of the client's medication regimen?

○ **A.** ELISA

○ **B.** Western Blot

○ **C.** Viral load

○ **D.** CD4 count

189. A client with AIDS-related cytomegalovirus is started on Cytovene (ganciclovir). The nurse should tell the client that the medication will be needed:

○ **A.** Until the infection clears

○ **B.** For 6 months to a year

○ **C.** Until the cultures are normal

○ **D.** For the remainder of life

190. The nurse is caring for a client with suspected AIDS dementia complex. The first sign of dementia in the client with AIDS is:

○ **A.** Changes in gait

○ **B.** Loss of concentration

○ **C.** Problems with speech

○ **D.** Seizures

191. The physician has ordered Activase (alteplase) for a client admitted with a myocardial infarction. The desired effect of Activase is:

○ **A.** Prevention of congestive heart failure

○ **B.** Stabilization of the clot

○ **C.** Increased tissue oxygenation

○ **D.** Destruction of the clot

192. The mother of a 2-year-old asks the nurse when she should schedule her son's first dental visit. The nurse's response is based on the knowledge that most children have all their deciduous teeth by:

- ○ **A.** 15 months
- ○ **B.** 18 months
- ○ **C.** 24 months
- ○ **D.** 30 months

193. The nurse is caring for a child with Down syndrome. Which characteristics are commonly found in the child with Down syndrome?

- ○ **A.** Fragile bones, blue sclera, and brittle teeth
- ○ **B.** Epicanthal folds, broad hands, and transpalmar creases
- ○ **C.** Low posterior hairline, webbed neck, and short stature
- ○ **D.** Developmental regression and cherry-red macula

194. After several hospitalizations for respiratory ailments, a 6-month-old has been diagnosed as having HIV. The infant's respiratory ailments were most likely due to:

- ○ **A.** Pneumocystis carinii
- ○ **B.** Cytomegalovirus
- ○ **C.** Cryptosporidiosis
- ○ **D.** Herpes simplex

195. A client has returned from having a bronchoscopy. Before offering the client sips of water, the nurse should assess the client's:

- ○ **A.** Blood pressure
- ○ **B.** Pupilary response
- ○ **C.** Gag reflex
- ○ **D.** Pulse rate

196. The physician has ordered injections of Neumega (oprellvekin) for a client receiving chemotherapy for prostate cancer. Which finding suggests that the medication is having its desired effect?

- ○ **A.** Hct 12.8g
- ○ **B.** Platelets 250,000mm^3
- ○ **C.** Neutrophils 4,000mm^3
- ○ **D.** RBC 4.7 million

197. A child suspected of having cystic fibrosis is scheduled for a quantitative sweat test. The nurse knows that the quantitative sweat test will be analyzed using:

- ○ **A.** Pilocarpine iontophoresis
- ○ **B.** Choloride iontophoresis
- ○ **C.** Sodium iontophoresis
- ○ **D.** Potassium iontophoresis

Quick Answer: **294**
Detailed Answer: **315**

198. The nurse is caring for a client with a Brown-Sequard spinal cord injury. The nurse should expect the client to have:

- ○ **A.** Total loss of motor, sensory, and reflex activity
- ○ **B.** Incomplete loss of motor function
- ○ **C.** Loss of sensory function with potential for recovery
- ○ **D.** Loss of sensation on the side opposite the injury

Quick Answer: **294**
Detailed Answer: **315**

199. A client with cirrhosis has developed signs of heptorenal syndrome. Which diet is most appropriate for the client at this time?

- ○ **A.** High protein, moderate sodium
- ○ **B.** High carbohydrate, moderate sodium
- ○ **C.** Low protein, low sodium
- ○ **D.** Low carbohydrate, high protein

Quick Answer: **294**
Detailed Answer: **316**

200. The nurse is caring for a client with a basal cell epithelioma. The primary cause of basal cell epithelioma is:

- ○ **A.** Sun exposure
- ○ **B.** Smoking
- ○ **C.** Ingestion of alcohol
- ○ **D.** Food preservatives

Quick Answer: **294**
Detailed Answer: **316**

201. The nurse is teaching a client with an orthotopic bladder replacement. The nurse should tell the client to:

- ○ **A.** Place a gauze pad over the stoma
- ○ **B.** Lie on her side while evacuating the pouch
- ○ **C.** Bear down with each voiding
- ○ **D.** Wear a well-fitting drainage bag

Quick Answer: **294**
Detailed Answer: **316**

202. A client is receiving a blood transfusion following surgery. In the event of a transfusion reaction, any unused blood should be:

- ○ **A.** Sealed and discarded in a red bag
- ○ **B.** Flushed down the client's commode
- ○ **C.** Sealed and discarded in the sharp's container
- ○ **D.** Returned to the blood bank

Quick Answer: **294**
Detailed Answer: **316**

203. The physician has ordered a trivalent botulism antitoxin for a client with botulism poisoning. Before administering the medication, the nurse should assess the client for a history of allergies to:

- ○ **A.** Eggs
- ○ **B.** Horses
- ○ **C.** Shellfish
- ○ **D.** Pork

204. The physician has ordered increased oral hydration for a client with renal calculi. Unless contraindicated, the recommended oral intake for helping with the removal of renal calculi is:

- ○ **A.** 75mL per hour
- ○ **B.** 100mL per hour
- ○ **C.** 150mL per hour
- ○ **D.** 200mL per hour

205. The nurse is caring for a client with acquired immunodeficiency syndrome who has oral candidiasis. The nurse should clean the client's mouth using:

- ○ **A.** A toothbrush
- ○ **B.** A soft gauze pad
- ○ **C.** Antiseptic mouthwash
- ○ **D.** Lemon and glycerin swabs

206. A client taking anticoagulant medication has developed a cardiac tamponade. Which finding is associated with cardiac tamponade?

- ○ **A.** A decrease in systolic blood pressure during inspiration
- ○ **B.** An increase in diastolic blood pressure during expiration
- ○ **C.** An increase in systolic blood pressure during inspiration
- ○ **D.** A decrease in diastolic blood pressure during expiration

207. The nurse is preparing a client for discharge following the removal of a cataract. The nurse should tell the client to:

- ○ **A.** Take aspirin for discomfort
- ○ **B.** Avoid bending over to put on his shoes
- ○ **C.** Remove the eye shield before going to sleep
- ○ **D.** Continue showering as usual

208. The physician has ordered Pentam (pentamidine) IV for a client with pneumocystis carinii. While receiving the medication, the nurse should carefully monitor the client's:

   ○ **A.** Blood pressure
   ○ **B.** Temperature
   ○ **C.** Heart rate
   ○ **D.** Respirations

209. Intra-arterial chemotherapy primarily benefits the client by applying greater concentrations of medication directly to the malignant tumor. An additional benefit of intra-arterial chemotherapy is:

   ○ **A.** Prevention of nausea and vomiting
   ○ **B.** Treatment of micro-metastasis
   ○ **C.** Eradication of bone pain
   ○ **D.** Prevention of therapy-induced anemia

210. A client with rheumatoid arthritis is receiving injections of Myochrysine (gold sodium thiomalate). Before administering the client's medication, the nurse should:

   ○ **A.** Check the lab work
   ○ **B.** Administer an antiemetic
   ○ **C.** Obtain the blood pressure
   ○ **D.** Administer a sedative

211. The nurse is caring for a client following a Whipple procedure. The nurse notes that the drainage from the nasogastric tube is bile tinged in appearance and has increased in the past hour. The nurse should:

   ○ **A.** Document the finding and continue to monitor the client
   ○ **B.** Irrigate the drainage tube with 10mL of normal saline
   ○ **C.** Decrease the amount of intermittent suction
   ○ **D.** Notify the physician of the findings

212. A client with AIDS tells the nurse that he regularly takes echinacea to boost his immune system. The nurse should tell the client that:

   ○ **A.** Herbals can interfere with the action of antiviral medication
   ○ **B.** Supplements have proven effective in prolonging life
   ○ **C.** Herbals have been shown to decrease the viral load
   ○ **D.** Supplements appear to prevent replication of the virus

213. A client with rheumatoid arthritis has Sjogren's syndrome. The nurse can help relieve the symptoms of Sjogren's syndrome by:

- ○ **A.** Providing heat to the joints
- ○ **B.** Instilling eyedrops
- ○ **C.** Administering pain medication
- ○ **D.** Providing small, frequent meals

214. Which one of the following symptoms is common in the client with duodenal ulcers?

- ○ **A.** Vomiting shortly after eating
- ○ **B.** Epigastric pain following meals
- ○ **C.** Frequent bouts of diarrhea
- ○ **D.** Presence of blood in the stools

215. A client with end-stage renal failure receives hemodialysis via an arteriovenous fistula (AV) placed in the right arm. When caring for the client, the nurse should:

- ○ **A.** Take the blood pressure in the right arm above the AV fistula
- ○ **B.** Flush the AV fistula with IV normal saline to keep it patent
- ○ **C.** Auscultate the AV fistula for the presence of a bruit
- ○ **D.** Perform needed venopunctures distal to the AV fistula

216. The nurse is reviewing the lab results of four clients. Which finding should be reported to the physician?

- ○ **A.** A client with chronic renal failure with a serum creatinine of 5.6mg/dL
- ○ **B.** A client with rheumatic fever with a positive C reactive protein
- ○ **C.** A client with gastroenteritis with a hematocrit of 52%
- ○ **D.** A client with epilepsy with a white cell count of 3,800mm^3

217. The physician has prescribed a Becloforte (beclomethasone) inhaler two puffs twice a day for a client with asthma. The nurse should tell the client to report:

- ○ **A.** Increased weight
- ○ **B.** A sore throat
- ○ **C.** Difficulty in sleeping
- ○ **D.** Changes in mood

218. A client treated for depression has developed signs of serotonin syndrome. The nurse recognizes that serotonin syndrome is caused by:

   ○ **A.** Concurrent use of an MAO inhibitor and a SSRI

   ○ **B.** Eating foods that are high in tyramine

   ○ **C.** Drastic decreases in the dopamine level

   ○ **D.** Use of medications containing pseudoephedrine

Quick Answer: **294**
Detailed Answer: **318**

219. The nurse is caring for a client following a transphenoidal hypophysectomy. Post-operatively, the nurse should:

   ○ **A.** Provide the client a toothbrush for mouth care

   ○ **B.** Check the nasal dressing for the "halo sign"

   ○ **C.** Tell the client to cough forcibly every 2 hours

   ○ **D.** Ambulate the client when he is fully awake

Quick Answer: **294**
Detailed Answer: **318**

220. The physician has inserted an esophageal balloon tamponade in a client with bleeding esophageal varices. The nurse should maintain the esophageal balloon at a pressure of:

   ○ **A.** 5–10mmHg

   ○ **B.** 10–15mmHg

   ○ **C.** 15–20mmHg

   ○ **D.** 20–25mmHg

Quick Answer: **294**
Detailed Answer: **318**

221. The nurse is caring for a client with Lyme's disease. The nurse should carefully monitor the client for signs of neurological complications, which include:

   ○ **A.** Complaints of a "drawing" sensation and paralysis on one side of the face

   ○ **B.** Presence of an unsteady gait, intention tremor, and facial weakness

   ○ **C.** Complaints of excruciating facial pain brought on by talking, smiling, or eating

   ○ **D.** Presence of fatigue when talking, dysphagia, and involuntary facial twitching

Quick Answer: **294**
Detailed Answer: **318**

222. When caring for the child with autistic disorder, the nurse should:

   ○ **A.** Take the child to the playroom to be with peers

   ○ **B.** Assign a consistent caregiver

   ○ **C.** Place the child in a ward with other children

   ○ **D.** Assign several staff members to provide care

Quick Answer: **294**
Detailed Answer: **318**

223. A client is admitted with suspected pernicious anemia. Which findings support the diagnosis of pernicious anemia?

Quick Answer: **294**
Detailed Answer: **318**

- ○ **A.** The client complains of feeling tired and listless.
- ○ **B.** The client has waxy, pale skin.
- ○ **C.** The client exhibits loss of coordination and position sense.
- ○ **D.** The client has a rapid pulse rate and a detectable heart murmur.

224. The physician has prescribed Cyclogel (cyclopentolate hydrochloride) drops for a client following a scleral buckling. The nurse knows that the purpose of the medication is to:

Quick Answer: **294**
Detailed Answer: **318**

- ○ **A.** Rest the muscles of accommodation
- ○ **B.** Prevent post-operative infection
- ○ **C.** Constrict the pupils
- ○ **D.** Reduce the production of aqueous humor

225. Which finding is associated with secondary syphilis?

Quick Answer: **294**
Detailed Answer: **319**

- ○ **A.** Painless, papular lesions on the perineum, fingers, and eyelids
- ○ **B.** Absence of lesions
- ○ **C.** Deep asymmetrical granulomatous lesions
- ○ **D.** Well-defined generalized lesions on the palms, soles, and perineum

226. A client is transferred to the intensive care unit following a conornary artery bypass graft. Which one of the post-surgical assessments should be reported to the physician?

Quick Answer: **294**
Detailed Answer: **319**

- ○ **A.** Urine output of 50ml in the past hour
- ○ **B.** Temperature of 99°F
- ○ **C.** Strong pedal pulses bilaterally
- ○ **D.** Central venous pressure 15mmH$_2$O

227. Which symptom is not associated with glaucoma?

Quick Answer: **294**
Detailed Answer: **319**

- ○ **A.** Veil-like loss of vision
- ○ **B.** Foggy loss of vision
- ○ **C.** Seeing halos around lights
- ○ **D.** Complaints of eye pain

228. When caring for a ventilator-dependent client who is receiving tube feedings, the nurse can help prevent aspiration of gastric secretions by:

Quick Answer: **294**
Detailed Answer: **319**

- ○ **A.** Keeping the head of the bed flat
- ○ **B.** Elevating the head of the bed 30–45°
- ○ **C.** Placing the client on his left side
- ○ **D.** Raising the foot of the bed 10–20°

229. When gathering evidence from a victim of rape, the nurse should place the victim's clothing in a:

Quick Answer: **294**
Detailed Answer: **319**

- ○ **A.** Plastic zip-lock bag
- ○ **B.** Rubber tote
- ○ **C.** Paper bag
- ○ **D.** Padded manila envelope

230. The nurse on an orthopedic unit is assigned to care for four clients with displaced bone fractures. Which client will not be treated with the use of traction?

Quick Answer: **294**
Detailed Answer: **319**

- ○ **A.** A client with fractures of the femur
- ○ **B.** A client with fractures of the cervical spine
- ○ **C.** A client with fractures of the humerus
- ○ **D.** A client with fractures of the ankle

231. A client is hospitalized with an acute myocardial infarction. Which nursing diagnosis reflects an understanding of the cause of acute myocardial infarction?

Quick Answer: **294**
Detailed Answer: **319**

- ○ **A.** Decreased cardiac output related to damage to the myocardium
- ○ **B.** Impaired tissue perfusion related to an occlusion in the coronary vessels
- ○ **C.** Acute pain related to cardiac ischemia
- ○ **D.** Ineffective breathing patterns related to decreased oxygen to the tissues

232. The nurse in the emergency department is responsible for the triage of four recently admitted clients. Which client should the nurse send directly to the treatment room?

Quick Answer: **294**
Detailed Answer: **319**

- ○ **A.** A 23-year-old female complaining of headache and nausea
- ○ **B.** A 76-year-old male complaining of dysuria
- ○ **C.** A 56-year-old male complaining of exertional shortness of breath
- ○ **D.** A 42-year-old female complaining of recent sexual assault

233. The physician has ordered an injection of morphine for a client with post-operative pain. Before administering the medication, it is essential that the nurse assess the client's:

   O **A.** Heart rate

   O **B.** Respirations

   O **C.** Temperature

   O **D.** Blood pressure

234. The nurse is caring for a client with a closed head injury. A late sign of increased intracranial pressure is:

   O **A.** Changes in pupil equality and reactivity

   O **B.** Restlessness and irritability

   O **C.** Complaints of headache

   O **D.** Nausea and vomiting

235. The newly licensed nurse has been asked to perform a procedure that he feels unqualified to perform. The nurse's best response at this time is to:

   O **A.** Attempt to perform the procedure

   O **B.** Refuse to perform the procedure and give a reason for the refusal

   O **C.** Request to observe a similar procedure and then attempt to complete the procedure

   O **D.** Agree to perform the procedure if the client is willing

236. A client admitted to the emergency department with complaints of crushing chest pain that radiates to the left jaw. After obtaining a stat electrocardiogram the nurse should:

   O **A.** Obtain a history of prior cardiac problems

   O **B.** Begin an IV using a large-bore catheter

   O **C.** Administer oxygen at 2L per minute via nasal cannula

   O **D.** Perform pupil checks for size and reaction to light

237. Which of the following techniques is recommended for removing a tick from the skin?

- ○ **A.** Grasping the tick with a tissue and quickly jerking it away from the skin

- ○ **B.** Placing a burning match close the tick and watching for it to release

- ○ **C.** Using tweezers, grasp the tick close to the skin and pull the tick free using a steady, firm motion

- ○ **D.** Covering the tick with petroleum jelly and gently rubbing the area until the tick releases

238. A nurse is observing a local softball game when one of the players is hit in the nose with a ball. The player's nose is visibly deformed and bleeding. The best way for the nurse to control the bleeding is to:

- ○ **A.** Tilt the head back and pinch the nostrils

- ○ **B.** Apply a wrapped ice compress to the nose

- ○ **C.** Pack the nose with soft, clean tissue

- ○ **D.** Tilt the head forward and pinch the nostrils

239. What is the responsibility of the nurse in obtaining an informed consent for surgery?

- ○ **A.** Describing in a clear and simply stated manner what the surgery will involve

- ○ **B.** Explaining the benefits, alternatives, and possible risks and complications of surgery

- ○ **C.** Using the nurse/client relationship to persuade the client to sign the operative permit

- ○ **D.** Providing the informed consent for surgery and witnessing the client's signature

240. During the change of shift report, the nurse states that the client's last pulse strength was a 1+. The oncoming nurse recognizes that the client's pulse was:

- ○ **A.** Bounding

- ○ **B.** Full

- ○ **C.** Normal

- ○ **D.** Weak

241. The RN is making assignments for the day. Which one of the following duties can be assigned to the unlicensed assistive personnel?

- ○ **A.** Notifying the physician of an abnormal lab value
- ○ **B.** Providing routine catheter care with soap and water
- ○ **C.** Administering two aspirin to a client with a headache
- ○ **D.** Setting the rate of an infusion of normal saline

242. The nurse is observing the respirations of a client when she notes that the respiratory cycle is marked by periods of apnea lasting from 10 seconds to 1 minute. The apnea is followed by respirations that gradually increase in depth and frequency. The nurse should document that the client is experiencing:

- ○ **A.** Cheyne-Stokes respirations
- ○ **B.** Kussmaul respirations
- ○ **C.** Biot respirations
- ○ **D.** Diaphragmatic respirations

243. A client seen in the doctor's office for complaints of nausea and vomiting is sent home with directions to follow a clear-liquid diet for the next 24–48 hours. Which of the following is not permitted on a clear-liquid diet?

- ○ **A.** Sweetened tea
- ○ **B.** Chicken broth
- ○ C Ice cream
- ○ **D.** Orange gelatin

244. When administering a tuberculin skin test, the nurse should insert the needle at a:

- ○ **A.** 15° angle
- ○ **B.** 30° angle
- ○ **C.** 45° angle
- ○ **D.** 90° angle

245. The nurse is preparing to discharge a client following a trabeculoplasty for the treatment of glaucoma. The nurse should instruct the client to:

- ○ **A.** Wash her eyes with baby shampoo and water twice a day
- ○ **B.** Take only tub baths for the first month following surgery
- ○ **C.** Begin using her eye makeup again 1 week after surgery
- ○ **D.** Wear eye protection for several months after surgery

246. Which type of endotracheal tube is recommended by the Centers for Disease Control (CDC) for reducing the risk of ventilator-associated pneumonia?

Quick Answer: **294**
Detailed Answer: **321**

- ○ **A.** Uncuffed
- ○ **B.** CASS
- ○ **C.** Fenestrated
- ○ **D.** Nasotracheal

247. Which client is at greatest risk for complications following abdominal surgery?

Quick Answer: **294**
Detailed Answer: **321**

- ○ **A.** A 68-year-old obese client with noninsulin-dependent diabetes
- ○ **B.** A 27-year-old client with a recent history of urinary tract infections
- ○ **C.** A 16-year-old client who smokes a half-pack of cigarettes per day
- ○ **D.** A 40-year-old client who exercises regularly, with no history of medical conditions

248. The nurse is preparing a client for surgery. Which lab finding should be reported to the physician?

Quick Answer: **294**
Detailed Answer: **321**

- ○ **A.** Potassium 2.5mEq/L
- ○ **B.** Hemoglobin 14.5g/dL
- ○ **C.** Blood glucose 75mg/dL
- ○ **D.** White cell count 8,000mm^3

249. A client is diagnosed with bleeding from the upper gastrointestinal system. The nurse would expect the client's stools to be:

Quick Answer: **294**
Detailed Answer: **321**

- ○ **A.** Brown
- ○ **B.** Black
- ○ **C.** Clay colored
- ○ **D.** Green

250. The physician has prescribed Chloromycetin (chloramphenicol) for a client with bacterial meningitis. Which lab report should the nurse monitor most carefully?

Quick Answer: **294**
Detailed Answer: **321**

- ○ **A.** Serum creatinine
- ○ **B.** Urine specific gravity
- ○ **C.** Complete blood count
- ○ **D.** Serum sodium

Quick Check Answer Key

1.	B	32.	B	63.	B
2.	D	33.	A	64.	B
3.	A	34.	B	65.	B
4.	D	35.	A	66.	D
5.	B	36.	C	67.	A
6.	B	37.	A	68.	D
7.	B	38.	B	69.	C
8.	C	39.	C	70.	A
9.	A	40.	A	71.	C
10.	A	41.	D	72.	D
11.	D	42.	A	73.	A
12.	B	43.	B	74.	A
13.	D	44.	A	75.	D
14.	D	45.	B	76.	B
15.	B	46.	B	77.	A
16.	A	47.	C	78.	A
17.	B	48.	C	79.	B
18.	C	49.	B	80.	C
19.	C	50.	A	81.	D
20.	C	51.	B	82.	B
21.	D	52.	A	83.	A
22.	A	53.	D	84.	B
23.	B	54.	A	85.	C
24.	A	55.	B	86.	B
25.	C	56.	B	87.	B
26.	B	57.	A	88.	B
27.	A	58.	C	89.	B
28.	B	59.	D	90.	C
29.	C	60.	B	91.	B
30.	D	61.	D	92.	A
31.	A	62.	B	93.	D

94. C	126. B	158. C
95. A	127. A	159. A
96. A	128. B	160. C
97. A	129. A	161. C
98. C	130. C	162. A
99. C	131. D	163. B
100. A	132. B	164. B
101. D	133. D	165. C
102. D	134. A	166. B
103. C	135. C	167. D
104. C	136. A	168. B
105. D	137. C	169. A
106. B	138. D	170. D
107. B	139. B	171. A
108. D	140. D	172. B
109. B	141. A	173. A
110. A	142. C	174. B
111. C	143. A	175. C
112. B	144. B	176. B
113. D	145. C	177. C
114. B	146. D	178. C
115. A	147. B	179. D
116. B	148. D	180. B
117. C	149. B	181. A
118. A	150. A	182. C
119. B	151. C	183. A
120. A	152. B	184. A
121. B	153. D	185. D
122. A	154. C	186. B
123. A	155. D	187. D
124. D	156. A	188. C
125. B	157. B	189. D

190. B	**211.** D	**232.** D
191. D	**212.** A	**233.** B
192. D	**213.** B	**234.** A
193. B	**214.** D	**235.** B
194. A	**215.** C	**236.** C
195. C	**216.** D	**237.** C
196. B	**217.** B	**238.** B
197. A	**218.** A	**239.** D
198. D	**219.** B	**240.** D
199. C	**220.** D	**241.** B
200. A	**221.** A	**242.** A
201. C	**222.** B	**243.** C
202. D	**223.** C	**244.** A
203. B	**224.** A	**245.** D
204. D	**225.** D	**246.** B
205. B	**226.** D	**247.** A
206. A	**227.** A	**248.** A
207. B	**228.** B	**249.** B
208. A	**229.** C	**250.** C
209. B	**230.** D	
210. A	**231.** B	

Answers and Rationales

1. **Answer B is correct.** The nurse should check the client's immunization record to determine the date of the last tetanus immunization. The nurse should question the client regarding allergies to medications before administering medication; therefore, answer A is incorrect. Answer C is incorrect because a sling, not a spint, should be applied to imimobilize the arm and prevent dependent edema. Answer D is incorrect because pain medication would be given before cleaning and dressing the wound, not afterward.

2. **Answer D is correct.** Watery vaginal discharge and painless bleeding are associated with endometrial cancer. Frothy vaginal discharge describes trichomonas infection; thick, white vaginal discharge describes infection with candida albicans; and purulent vaginal discharge describes pelvic inflammatory disease. Therefore, answers A, B, and C are incorrect.

3. **Answer A is correct.** Stereotactic surgery destroys areas of the brain responsible for intractable tremors. The surgery does not increase production of dopamine, making answer B incorrect. Answer C is incorrect because the client will continue to need medication. Serotonin production is not associated with Parkinson's disease; therefore, answer D Is incorrect.

4. **Answer D is correct.** The client with AIDS should not drink water that has been sitting longer than 15 minutes because of bacterial contamination. Answer A is incorrect because ice water is not better for the client. Answer B is incorrect because juices should not replace water intake. Answer C is not an accurate statement.

5. **Answer B is correct.** The finding that differentiates interstitial cystitis from other forms of cystitis is the absence of bacteria in the urine. Answer A is incorrect because symptoms that include burning and pain on urination characterize all forms of cystitis. Answer C is incorrect because blood in the urine is a characteristic of interstitial as well as other forms of cystitis. Answer D is an incorrect statement because females are affected more often than males.

6. **Answer B is correct.** Approximately 99% of males with cystic fibrosis are sterile due to obstruction of the vas deferens. Answers A, C, and D are incorrect because most males with cystic fibrosis are incapable of reproduction.

7. **Answer B is correct.** Infants under the age of 2 years should not be fed honey because of the danger of infection with *Clostridium botulinum*. Answers A, C, and D are not related to the situation; therefore, they are incorrect.

8. **Answer C is correct.** Children with autistic disorder engage in ritualistic behaviors and are easily upset by changes in daily routine. Changes in the environment are usually met with behaviors that are difficult to control. Answers A, B, and D are incorrect because they do not focus on autistic disorder.

9. **Answer A is correct.** The degree of pulmonary involvement is the greatest determinant in the prognosis of cystic fibrosis. Answers B, C, and D are affected by cystic fibrosis; however, they are not major determinants of the prognosis of the disease.

10. **Answer A is correct.** Decreased blood pressure and increased pulse rate are associated with bleeding and shock. Answers B, C, and D are within normal limits; thus, incorrect.

11. **Answer D is correct.** Early decelerations during the second stage of labor are benign and are the result of fetal head compression that occurs during normal contractions. No action is necessary other than documenting the finding on the flow sheet. Answers A, B, and C are interventions for the client with late decelerations, which reflect ureteroplacental insufficiency.

12. **Answer B is correct.** The client's statement that meat should be thoroughly cooked to the appropriate temperature indicates an understanding of the nurse's teaching regarding food preparation. Undercooked meat is a source of toxoplasmosis cysts. Toxoplasmosis is a major cause of encephalitis in clients with AIDS. Answer A is incorrect because fresh-ground pepper contains bacteria that can cause illness in the client with AIDS. Answer C is an incorrect choice because cheese contains molds and yogurt contains live cultures that the client with AIDS must avoid. Answer D is incorrect because fresh fruit and vegetables contain microscopic organisms that can cause illness in the client with AIDS.

13. **Answer D is correct.** The client taking isoniazid should have a negative sputum culture within 3 months. Continued positive cultures reflect noncompliance with therapy or the development of strains resistant to the medication. Answers A, B, and C are incorrect because there has not been sufficient time for the medication to be effective.

14. **Answer D is correct.** Lyme's disease is transmitted by ticks found on deer and mice in wooded areas. The people in answers A and B have little risk of the disease. Veterinarians are exposed to dog ticks, which carry Rocky Mountain Spotted Fever, so answer C is incorrect.

15. **Answer B is correct.** Children ages 18–24 months normally have sufficient sphincter control necessary for toilet training. Answer A is incorrect because the child is not developmentally capable of toilet training. Answers C and D are incorrect choices because toilet training should already be established.

16. **Answer A is correct.** Large amounts of fluid and electrolytes are lost in the stools of the client with an ileostomy. The priority of nursing care is meeting the client's fluid and electrolyte needs. Answers B and D do apply to clients with an ileostomy, but they are not the priority nursing diagnosis. Answer C does not apply to the client with an ileostomy and is, therefore, incorrect.

17. **Answer B is correct.** Cobex is an injectable form of cyanocobalamin or vitamin B12. Increased Hgb levels reflect the effectiveness of the medication. Answers A, C, and D do not reflect the effectiveness of the medication; therefore, they are incorrect.

18. **Answer C is correct.** Behavior modification relies on the principles of operant conditioning. Tokens or rewards are given for appropriate behavior. Answers A and B are incorrect because they refer to techniques used to reduce anxiety, such as thought stopping and bioenergetic techniques, respectively. Answer D is incorrect because it refers to modeling.

19. **Answer C is correct.** Small pieces of cereal promote chewing and are easily managed by the toddler. Pieces of hot dog, carrot sticks, and raisins are unsuitable for the toddler because of the risk of aspiration.

20. **Answer C is correct.** Complications of TPN therapy are osmotic diuresis and hypovolemia. Answer A is incorrect because the intake and output would not reflect metabolic rate. Answer B is incorrect because the client is most likely receiving no oral fluids. Answer D is incorrect because the complication of TPN therapy is hypovolemia, not hypervolemia.

21. **Answer D is correct.** L/S ratios are an indicator of fetal lung maturity. Answer A is incorrect because it is the diagnostic test for neural tube defects. Answer B is incorrect because it measures fetal well-being. Answer C is incorrect because it detects circulating antibodies against red blood cells.

22. **Answer A is correct.** By the third postpartum day, the fundus should be located 3 finger widths below the umbilicus. Answer B is incorrect because the discharge would be light in amount. Answer C is incorrect because the fundus is not even with the umbilicus at 3 days. Answer D is incorrect because the uterus is not enlarged.

23. **Answer B is correct.** Rapid discontinuation of TPN can result in hypoglycemia. Answer A is incorrect because rapid infusion of TPN results in hyperglycemia. Answer C is incorrect because TPN is administered through a central line. Answer D is incorrect because the infusion is administered with a filter.

24. **Answer A is correct.** Kava-kava can increase the effects of anesthesia and post-operative analgesia. Answers B, C, and D are not related to the use of kava-kava; therefore, they are incorrect.

25. **Answer C is correct.** The maximum recommended rate of an intravenous infusion of potassium chloride is 5–10mEq per hour, never to exceed 20mEq per hour. An intravenous infusion controller is always used to regulate the flow. Answer A is incorrect because potassium chloride is not given IV push. Answer B is incorrect because the infusion time is too brief. Answer D is incorrect because the infusion time is too long.

26. **Answer B is correct.** The normal platelet count is 150,000–400,000; therefore, the client is at high risk for spontaneous bleeding. Answer A is incorrect because the WBC is a low normal; therefore, overwhelming infection is not a risk at this time. The RBC is low, but anemia at this point is not life threatening; therefore, answer C is incorrect. Answer D is incorrect because the serum creatinine is within normal limits.

27. **Answer A is correct.** The nurse should stop the infusion. The medication should be restarted through a new IV access. Answer B is incorrect because IV catheters are not to be flushed. Answer C is incorrect because a tourniquet would not be applied to the area. Answer D is incorrect because the IV should not be allowed to continue infusing because the medication is a vesicant and, in the event of infiltration, the tissue would be damaged or destroyed.

28. **Answer B is correct.** The client will have a urinary catheter inserted to keep the bladder empty during radiation therapy. Answer A is incorrect because visitors are allowed to see the client for short periods of time, as long as they maintain a distance of 6 feet from the client. Answer C is incorrect because the client is on bed rest. Side effects from radiation therapy include pain, nausea, vomiting, and dehydration; therefore, answer D is incorrect.

29. **Answer C is correct.** The mother does not need to place an external heat source near the newborn. It will not promote healing, and there is a chance that the newborn could be burned, so the mother needs further teaching. Answers A, B, and D indicate correct care of the newborn who has been circumcised and are incorrect.

30. **Answer D is correct.** A sputum specimen for culture and sensitivity should be obtained before the antibiotic is administered to determine whether the organism is sensitive to the prescribed medication. A routine urinalysis, complete blood count and serum electrolytes can be obtained after the medication is initiated; therefore, Answers A, B, and C are incorrect.

31. **Answer A is correct.** Ginkgo interacts with many medications to increase the risk of bleeding; therefore, bruising or bleeding should be reported to the doctor. Photosensitivity is not a side effect of ginkgo; therefore, answer B is incorrect. Answer C is incorrect because the FDA does not regulate herbals and natural products. The client does not need to take additional vitamin E, so answer D is incorrect.

32. **Answer B is correct.** The client should be well hydrated before and during treatment to prevent nephrotoxicity. The client should be encouraged to drink 2,000–3,000mL of fluid a day to promote excretion of uric acid. Answer A is incorrect because it does not prevent nephrotoxicity. Answer C is incorrect because the intake and output should be recorded hourly. Answer D is incorrect because it refers to ototoxicity, which is also an adverse side effect of the medication but is not accurate for this stem.

33. **Answer A is correct.** The client who is colonized with MRSA will have no symptoms associated with infection. Answer B is incorrect because the client is more likely to develop an infection with MRSA following invasive procedures. Answer C is incorrect because the client should not be placed in the room with others. Answer D is incorrect because the client can colonize others, including healthcare workers, with MRSA.

34. **Answer B is correct.** The therapeutic range for vancomycin is 10–25mcg/mL. Answer A is incorrect because the range is too low to be therapeutic. Answers C and D are incorrect because they are too high.

35. **Answer A is correct.** Pseudomembranous colitis resulting from infection with *Clostridium difficile* produces diarrhea containing blood, mucus, and white blood cells. Answers B, C, and D are incorrect because they are not specific to infection with *Clostridium difficile*.

36. **Answer C is correct.** Pyridoxine (vitamin B6) is usually administered with INH (isoniazid) in order to prevent nervous system side effects. Answers A, B, and D are not associated with the use of INH; therefore, they are incorrect choices.

37. **Answer A is correct.** Factors associated with the development of Legionnaires' disease include immunosuppression, advanced age, alcoholism, and pulmonary disease. Answer B is incorrect because it is associated with the development of SARS. Answer C is associated with food-borne illness, not Legionnaires' disease, and answer D is not related to the question.

38. **Answer B is correct.** The client can check the inhaler by dropping it into a container of water. If the inhaler is half full, it will float upside down with one-fourth of the container remaining above the water line. Answers A, C, and D do not help determine the amount of medication remaining.

39. **Answer C is correct.** Following a nephrolithotomy, the client should be positioned on the unoperative side. Answers A, B, and D are incorrect positions for the client following a nephrolithotomy.

40. **Answer A is correct.** The client with sickle cell crisis and sequestration can be expected to have signs of hypovolemia, including decreased blood pressure. Answer B is incorrect because the client would have dry mucus membranes. Answer C is incorrect because the client would have increased respirations because of pain associated with sickle cell crisis. Answer D is incorrect because the client's blood pressure would be decreased.

41. **Answer D is correct.** The first sign of latex allergy is usually contact dermatitis, which includes swelling and itching of the hands. Answers A, B, and C can also occur but are not the first signs of latex allergy.

42. **Answer A is correct.** The nurse caring for the client with disseminated herpes zoster (shingles) should use airborne precautions as outlined by the CDC. Answer B is incorrect because precautions are needed to prevent transmission of the disease. Answer C and D are incorrect because airborne precautions are used, not contact or droplet precautions.

43. **Answer B is correct.** Acticoat, a commercially prepared dressing, should be moistened with sterile water. Answers A and C are incorrect because Acticoat dressings remain in place up to 5 days. Answer D is incorrect because normal saline should not be used to moisten the dressing.

44. **Answer A is correct.** The presence of a white or gray dot (a cat's eye reflex) in the pupil is associated with retinoblastoma, a highly malignant tumor of the eye. The nurse should report the finding to the physician immediately so that it can be further evaluated. Simply recording the finding can delay diagnosis and treatment; therefore, answer B is incorrect. Answer C is incorrect because it is not a variation of normal. Answer D is incorrect because the presence of the red reflex is a normal finding.

45. **Answer B is correct.** Stage II indicates that multiple lymph nodes or organs are involved on the same side of the diaphragm. Answer A refers to stage I Hodgkin's lymphoma, answer C refers to stage III Hodgkin's lymphoma, and answer D refers to stage IV Hodgkin's lymphoma.

46. **Answer B is correct.** The client taking methotrexate should avoid multivitamins because multivitamins contain folic acid. Methotrexate is a folic acid antagonist. Answers A and D are incorrect because aspirin and acetaminophen are given to relieve pain and inflammation associated with rheumatoid arthritis. Answer C is incorrect because omega 3 and omega 6 fish oils have proven beneficial for the client with rheumatoid arthritis.

47. **Answer C is correct.** Fried foods are not permitted on a low-residue diet. Answers A, B, and D are all allowed on a low-residue diet and, therefore, are incorrect.

48. **Answer C is correct.** The client with cirrhosis and abdominal ascites requires additional protein and calories. (Note: if the ammonia level increases, protein intake should be restricted or eliminated.) Answer A is incorrect because the client needs a low-sodium diet. Answer B is incorrect because the client does not need to increase his intake of potassium. Answer D is incorrect because the client does not need additional fat.

49. **Answer B is correct.** The most common symptom reported by clients with multiple sclerosis is double vision. Answers A, C, and D are not symptoms commonly reported by clients with multiple sclerosis, so they are wrong.

50. **Answer A is correct.** Common sources of *E. coli* are undercooked beef and shellfish. Answers B, C, and D are incorrect because they are not sources of *E. coli.*

51. **Answer B is correct.** St. John's wort has properties similar to those of monoamine oxidase inhibitors (MAOI). Eating foods high in tryramine (example: aged cheese, chocolate, salami, liver) can result in a hypertensive crisis. Answer A is incorrect because it can relieve mild to moderate depression. Answer C is incorrect because use of a sunscreen prevents skin reactions to sun exposure. Answer D is incorrect because St. John's wort should not be used with MAOI antidepressants.

52. **Answer A is correct.** Foods high in purine include dried beans, peas, spinach, oatmeal, poultry, fish, liver, lobster, and oysters. Answers B, C, and D are incorrect because they are low in purine. Other sources low in purine include most vegetables, milk, and gelatin.

53. **Answer D is correct.** The nurse should tell the client to avoid bearing weight on the axilla when using crutches because it can result in nerve damage. Answer A is incorrect because the finger width between the axilla and the crutch is appropriate. Answer B is incorrect because the client should bear weight on his hands when ambulating with crutches. Answer C is incorrect because it describes the correct use of the four-point gait.

54. **Answer A is correct.** By writing down her suspicions, the nurse leaves herself open for a suit of libel, a defamatory tort that discloses a privileged communication and leads to a lowering of opinion of the client. Defamatory torts include libel and slander. Libel is a written statement, whereas slander is an oral statement. Thus, answer B is incorrect because it involves oral statements. Malpractice is an unreasonable lack of skill in performing professional duties that result in injury or death; therefore, answer C is incorrect. Negligence is an act of omission or commission that results in injury to a person or property, making answer D incorrect.

55. **Answer B is correct.** The client with bulimia is prone to tooth erosion and dental caries caused by frequent bouts of self-induced vomiting. Answers A, C, and D are findings associated with anorexia nervosa, not bulimia, and are incorrect.

56. **Answer B is correct.** Antacids should not be taken within 2 hours of taking digoxin; therefore, the nurse needs to do additional teaching regarding the client's medication. Answers A, C, and D are true statements indicating that the client understands the nurse's teaching, so they are incorrect.

57. **Answer A is correct.** Fever, sore throat, and weakness need to be reported immediately. Adverse reactions to Thorazine include agranulocytosis, which makes the client vulnerable to overwhelming infection. Answers B, C, and D are expected side effects that occur with the use of Thorazine; therefore, it is not necessary to notify the doctor immediately.

58. **Answer C is correct.** The anterior approach for cervical discectomy lends itself to covert bleeding. The nurse should pay particular attention to bleeding coming from the mouth. Answer A is incorrect because bleeding will be obvious on the surgical dressing. Answer B is incorrect because complaints of neck pain are expected and will be managed by the use of analgesics. Answer D is incorrect because swelling in the posterior neck can be expected. The nurse should observe for swelling in the anterior neck as well as changes in voice quality, which can indicate swelling of the airway.

59. **Answer D is correct.** The assessment suggests the presence of a diaphragmatic hernia. The newborn should be positioned on the left side with the head and chest elevated. This position will allow the lung on the right side to fully inflate. Supplemental oxygen for newborns is not provided by mask, therefore Answer A is incorrect. Answer B is incorrect because bowel sounds would not be heard in the abdomen since abdominal contents occupy the chest cavity in the newborn with diaphragmatic hernia. Inserting a nasogastric tube to check for esophageal patency refers to the newborn with esophageal atresia; therefore, answer C is incorrect.

60. **Answer B is correct.** It takes 1–2 weeks for mood stabilizers to achieve a therapeutic effect; therefore, antipsychotic medications can also be used during the first few days or weeks to manage behavioral excitement. Answers A and D are not true statements and, therefore, are incorrect. Answer C is incorrect because the combination of medications will not allow for hypomania.

61. **Answer D is correct.** The nurse should first provide for the client's safety, including protecting her from an embarrassing situation. Answer A is incorrect because it allows the client to continue unacceptable behavior. Answer B is incorrect because it does not stop the client's behavior. Answer C is incorrect because it focuses on the other clients, not the client with inappropriate behavior.

62. **Answer B is correct.** According to the Denver Developmental Assessment, a 4-year-old should be able to state his first and last name. Answers A and C are expected abilities of a 5-year-old, and answer D is an expected ability of a 5- and 6-year-old.

63. **Answer B is correct.** The mother's statement reflects the stress placed on her by her daughter's chronic mental illness. Answer A is incorrect because there is no indication of ineffective family coping. Answer C is incorrect because it is not the most appropriate nursing diagnosis. Answer D is incorrect because there is no indication of altered parenting.

64. **Answer B is correct.** Clients with anorexia nervosa have problems with developing self-identity. They are often described by others as "passive," "perfect," and "introverted." Poor self-identity and low self-esteem lead to feelings of personal ineffectiveness. Answer A is incorrect because she will choose only low-calorie food items. Answer C is incorrect because the client with anorexia is restricted from exercising because it promotes weight loss. Placement in a private room increases the likelihood that the client will continue activities that prevent weight gain; therefore, answer D is incorrect.

65. **Answer B is correct.** The nursing assistant has skills suited to assisting the client with activities of daily living, such as bathing and grooming. Answer A is incorrect because the nurse should monitor the client's vital signs. Answer C is incorrect because the client will have an induced generalized seizure, and the nurse should monitor the client's response before, during, and after the procedure. Answer D is incorrect because staff does not remain in the room with a client in seclusion; only the nurse should monitor clients who are in seclusion.

66. **Answer D is correct.** Transderm Nitro is a reservoir patch that releases the medication via a semipermeable membrane. Cutting the patch allows too much of the drug to be released. Answer A is incorrect because the area should not be shaved; this can cause skin irritation. Answer B is incorrect because the skin is cleaned with soap and water. Answer C is incorrect because the patch should not be covered with plastic wrap because it can cause the medication to absorb too rapidly.

67. **Answer A is correct.** Cholinergic crisis is the result of overmedication with anticholinesterase inhibitors. Symptoms of cholinergic crisis are nausea, vomiting, diarrhea, blurred vision, pallor, decreased blood pressure, and constricted pupils. Answers B, C, and D are incorrect because they are symptoms of myasthenia crisis, which is the result of undermedication with cholinesterase inhibitors.

68. **Answer D is correct.** The client should avoid eating American and processed cheeses, such as Colby and Cheddar, because they are high in sodium. Dried beans, peanut butter, and Swiss cheese are low in sodium; therefore, answers A, B, and C are incorrect.

69. **Answer C is correct.** According to the Rule of Nines, the arm (9%) + the trunk (36%) = 45% TBSA burn injury. Answers A, B, and D are inaccurate calculations for the TBSA.

70. **Answer A is correct.** The client should void before the paracentesis to prevent accidental trauma to the bladder. Answer B is incorrect because the abdomen is not shaved. Answer C is incorrect because the client does not need extra fluids, which would cause bladder distention. Answer D is incorrect because the physician, not the nurse, would request an ultrasound, if needed.

71. **Answer C is correct.** Rice cereal, mashed ripe bananas, and strained carrots are appropriate foods for a 6-month-old infant. Answer A is incorrect because the cocoa-flavored cereal contains chocolate and sugar, orange juice is too acidic for the infant, and strained meat is difficult to digest. Answer B is incorrect because graham crackers contain wheat flour and sugar. Pudding contains sugar and additives unsuitable for the 6-month-old. Answer D is incorrect because the white of the egg contains albumin, which can cause allergic reactions.

72. **Answer D is correct.** A battery-operated CD player is a suitable diversion for the 9-year-old who is receiving oxygen therapy for asthma. He should not have an electric player while receiving oxygen therapy because of the danger of fire. Answer A is incorrect because he does need diversional activity. Answer B is incorrect because there is no need for him to wear earphones while he listening to music. Answer C is incorrect because he can have items from home.

73. **Answer A is correct.** Maturational crises are normal expected changes that face the family. Entering nursery school is a maturational crisis because the child begins to move away from the family and spend more time in the care of others. It is a time of adjustment for both the child and the parents. Answers B, C, and D are incorrect because they represent situational crises.

74. **Answer A is correct.** The client with a history of phenylketonuria should not use Nutrasweet or other sugar substitutes containing aspartame because aspartame is not adequately metabolized by the client with PKU. Answers B and C indicate an understanding of the nurse's teaching; therefore, they are incorrect. The client needs to resume a low-phenylalanine diet, making answer D incorrect.

75. **Answer D is correct.** Duchenne's muscular dystrophy is a sex-linked disorder, with the affected gene located on the X chromosome of the mother. Answer A is incorrect because the affected gene is not located on the autosomes. Over-replication of the X chromosomes in males is known as Klinefelter's syndrome; therefore, answer B is incorrect. Answer C is incorrect because the disorder is not located on the Y chromosome of the father.

76. **Answer B is correct.** The nurse and the client should work together to form a contract that outlines the amount of time he spends on a task. Answer A is incorrect because the client with a personality disorder will see no reason to change. The nurse should discuss his behavior and its effects on others with him, so answer C is incorrect. Answer D is incorrect because the client will not be able to set schedules and deadlines for himself.

77. **Answer A is correct.** Zovirax (acyclovir) shortens the course of chickenpox; however, the American Academy of Pediatrics does not recommend it for healthy children because of the cost. Answer B is incorrect because it is the vaccine used to prevent chickenpox. Answer C is incorrect because it is the immune globulin given to those who have been exposed to chickenpox. Answer D is incorrect because it is an antihistamine used to control itching associated with chickenpox.

78. **Answer A is correct.** Sock and mitten burns, burns confined to the hands and feet, indicate submersion in a hot liquid. Falling into the tub would not have produced sock burns; therefore, the nurse should be alert to the possibility of abuse. Answer B and C are within the realm of possibility, given the active play of the school-aged child; therefore, they are incorrect. Answer D is within the realm of possibility; therefore, it is incorrect.

79. **Answer B is correct.** Assault is the intentional threat to bring about harmful or offensive contact. The nurse's threat to give the medication by injection can be considered as assault. Answers A, C, and D do not relate to the nurse's statement; therefore, they are incorrect.

80. **Answer C is correct.** A nephrostomy tube is placed directly into the kidney and should never be clamped or irrigated because of the damage that can result to the kidney. Answers A and B are incorrect because the first action should be to relieve pressure on the affected kidney. Answer D is incorrect because the tubing should not be irrigated.

81. **Answer D is correct.** When the collection chambers of the Pleuravac are full, the nurse should prepare a new unit for continuing the collection. Answer A is incorrect because the unit is providing suction, so the amount of water does not need to be increased. Answer B is incorrect because the drainage is not to be removed using a syringe. Milking a chest tube requires a doctor's order, and because the tube is draining in this case, there is no need to milk it, so answer C is incorrect.

82. **Answer B is correct.** The first action by the nurse is to stop the transfusion and maintain an IV of normal saline. Answers A, C, and D are incorrect because they are not the first action the nurse would take.

83. **Answer A is correct.** Microwaving can cause uneven heating and "hot spots" in the formula, which can cause burns to the baby's mouth and throat. Answers B, C, and D are incorrect because the infant's formula should never be prepared using a microwave.

84. **Answer B is correct.** HELLP syndrome is characterized by hemolytic anemia, elevated liver enzymes, and low platelet counts. Answers A, C, and D have no connection to HELLP syndrome, so they are incorrect.

85. **Answer C is correct.** Dark green, leafy vegetables; members of the cabbage family; beets; kidney beans; cantaloupe; and oranges are good sources of folic acid (B9). Answers A, B, and D are incorrect because they are not sources of folic acid. Meat, liver, eggs, dried beans, sweet potatoes, and Brussels sprouts are good sources of B12; pork, fish, and chicken are good sources of B6.

86. **Answer B is correct.** The client with preeclampsia should be kept as quiet as possible, to minimize the possibility of seizures. The client should be kept in a dimly lit room with little or no stimulation. The clients in answers A, C, and D do not require a private room; therefore, they are incorrect.

87. **Answer B is correct.** Myasthenia gravis is caused by a loss of acetylcholine receptors, which results in the interruption of the transmission of nerve impulses from nerve endings to muscles. Answer A is incorrect because it refers to multiple sclerosis. Answer C is incorrect because it refers to Guillain-Barre syndrome. Answer D is incorrect because it refers to Parkinson's disease.

88. **Answer B is correct.** Osmitrol (mannitol) is an osmotic diuretic, which inhibits reabsorption of sodium and water. The first indication of its effectiveness is an increased urinary output. Answers A, C, and D do not relate to the effectiveness of the drug, so they are incorrect.

89. **Answer B is correct.** The client with a suspected subdural hematoma is more critical than the other clients and should be assessed first. Answers A, C, and D have more stable conditions; therefore, they are incorrect.

90. **Answer C is correct.** When given within 8 hours of the injury, Solu-Medrol has proven effective in reducing cord swelling, thereby improving motor and sensory function. Answer A is incorrect because Solu-Medrol does not prevent spasticity. Answer B is incorrect because Solu-Medrol does not decrease the need for mechanical ventilation. Answer D is incorrect because Solu-Medrol is used to reduce inflammation, not used to treat infections.

91. **Answer B is correct.** The spinal fluid of a client with Guillain-Barre has an increased protein concentration with normal or near-normal cell counts. Answers A, C, and D are inaccurate statements; therefore, they are incorrect.

92. **Answer A is correct.** The child with laryngotracheobronchitis has inspiratory stridor and a harsh, "brassy" cough. Answer B refers to the child with eppiglotitis, answer C refers to the child with bronchiolitis, and answer D refers to the child with asthma.

93. **Answer D is correct.** Hemarthrosis or bleeding into the joints is characterized by stiffness, aching, tingling, and decreased movement in the affected joint. Answers A, B, and C do not describe hemarthrosis, so they are incorrect.

94. **Answer C is correct.** The objective of therapy using aerosol treatments and chest percussion and postural drainage is to dilate the bronchioles and help loosen secretions. Answers A, B, and D are inaccurate statements, so they are incorrect.

95. **Answer A is correct.** Drooling of bright red secretions indicates active bleeding. Answer B is incorrect because the heart rate is within normal range for a 6-year-old. Answer C is incorrect because it indicates old bleeding. Answer D is incorrect because the child would have frequent, not infrequent, swallowing.

96. **Answer A is correct.** Cigarette smoking is the number one cause of bladder cancer. Answer B is incorrect because it is not associated with bladder cancer. Answer C is a primary cause of gastric cancer, and answer D is a cause of certain types of lung cancer.

97. **Answer A is correct.** Cloudy or whitish dialysate returns should be reported to the doctor immediately because it indicates infection and impending peritonitis. Answers B, C, and D are expected with peritoneal dialysis and do not require the doctor's attention.

98. **Answer C is correct.** Nitroglycerin tablets should be used as soon as the client first notices chest pain or discomfort. Answer A is incorrect because the medication should be used before engaging in activity. Strenuous activity should be avoided. Answer B is incorrect because the medication should be used when pain occurs, not on a regular schedule. Answer D is incorrect because the medication will not prevent nocturnal angina.

99. **Answer C is correct.** The LDH and CK MB are specific for diagnosing cardiac damage. Answers A, B, and D are not specific to cardiac function; therefore, they are incorrect.

100. **Answer A is correct.** The school-age child (8 or 9 years old) engages in cooperative play. These children enjoy competitive games in which there are rules and guidelines for winning. Answers B and D describe peer-group relationships of the preschool child, and answer C describes peer-group relationships of the preteen.

101. **Answer D is correct.** According to Erikson, the school-age child needs the opportunity to be involved in tasks that he can complete so that he can develop a sense of industry. If he is not given these opportunities, he is likely to develop feelings of inferiority. Answers A, B, and C are not associated with the psychosocial development of the school-age child; therefore, they are incorrect.

102. **Answer D is correct.** Before initiating a transfusion, the nurse should check the identifying information, including blood type and Rh, at least three times with another staff member. It is not necessary to obtain a signed permit for each unit of blood; therefore, answer A is incorrect. It is not necessary to use a new administration set for each unit transfused; therefore, answer B is incorrect. Administering the blood using a Y connector is not related to client safety; therefore, answer C is incorrect.

103. **Answer C is correct.** The client should have a peripheral IV of normal saline for initiating the transfusion. Solutions containing dextrose are unsuitable for administering blood. Blood that has been banked for 2 weeks is suitable for transfusion; therefore, answer A is incorrect. The client with B positive blood can receive Rh negative and type O positive blood; therefore, answers B and D are incorrect.

104. **Answer C is correct.** The $PaCO_2$ (partial pressure of alveolar carbon dioxide) indicates the effectiveness of the lungs. Adequate exchange of carbon dioxide is one of the major determinants in acid/base balance. Answers A, B, and D are incorrect because they are not represented by the $PaCO_2$.

105. **Answer D is correct.** Although the cause remains unknown, autopsy results consistently reveal the presence of pulmonary edema and intrathoracic hemorrhages in infants dying with SIDS. Answers A, B, and C have not been linked to SIDS deaths; therefore, they are incorrect.

106. **Answer B is correct.** To obtain the urine output, the weight of the dry diaper (62g) is subtracted from the weight of the used diaper (73.5g), for a urine output of 11.5ml. Answers A, C, and D contain wrong amounts; therefore, they are incorrect.

107. **Answer B is correct.** The infant with osteogenesis imperfecta (ribbon bones) should be handled with care, to prevent fractures. Adding calcium to the infant's diet will not improve the condition; therefore, answer A is incorrect. Answers C and D are not related to the disorder, so they are incorrect.

108. **Answer D is correct.** Placing the infant supine with the neck slightly extended helps to maintain an open airway. Answers A, B, and C are incorrect because they do not help to maintain an open airway.

109. **Answer B is correct.** Adverse reactions to Depakote (divalproex sodium) include thrombocytopenia, leukopenia, bleeding tendencies, and hepatotoxicity; therefore, the client will need frequent lab work. Answer A is associated with the use of Dilantin (phenytoin), and answers C and D are associated with the use of Eskalith (lithium carbonate); therefore, they are incorrect.

110. **Answer A is correct.** The client with cocaine addiction frequently reports formication, or "cocaine bugs," which are tactile hallucinations. Answers B and C occur in those addicted to cocaine but do not refer to formication; therefore, they are incorrect. Answer D is not related to the formication; therefore, it is incorrect.

111. **Answer C is correct.** Carbonated beverages increase the pressure in the stomach and increase the incidence of gastroesophageal reflux. Answer A is incorrect because the client with GERD should not eat 3–4 hours before going to bed. Answer B is incorrect because the client should sleep on his left side to prevent reflux. Answer D is incorrect because spicy, acidic foods and beverages are irritating to the gastric mucosa.

112. **Answer B is correct.** After raising the client's head to lower the blood pressure, the nurse should make sure that the catheter is patent. Answers A and C are not the first or second actions the nurse should take; therefore, they are incorrect. The client with autonomic hyperreflexia has an extreme elevation in blood pressure. The use of supplemental oxygen is not indicated; therefore, answer D is incorrect.

113. **Answer D is correct.** The nurse should flush the NG tube with 2–4oz of water before and after giving the medication. Answers A and B are incorrect because they do not use sufficient amounts of water. Answer C is incorrect because water, not normal saline, is used to flush the NG tube.

114. **Answer B is correct.** Acute arterial occlusion results in blackened or gangrenous areas on the toes. Answer A is incorrect because it describes venous occlusion. Answer C is incorrect because the pain is located below the level of occlusion. Answer D is incorrect because the area is cool, pale, and pulseless.

115. **Answer A is correct.** The client's symptoms suggest the development of diabetes insipidus, which can occur with surgery on or near the pituitary. Although the finding will be documented in the chart, it is not the main priority at this time; therefore, answer B is incorrect. Answers C and D must be ordered by the doctor, making them incorrect.

116. **Answer B is correct.** The client taking Coumadin (sodium warfarin) should limit his intake of vegetables such as cauliflower, cabbage, spinach, turnip greens, and collards because they are high in vitamin K. Answers A, C, and D do not contain large amounts of vitamin K; thus, they are incorrect.

117. **Answer C is correct.** Turning the child every 2 hours will help the cast to dry and help prevent complications related to immobility. Answers A and B are incorrect because the cast will transmit heat to the child, which can result in burns. External heat prevents complete drying of the cast because the outside will feel dry while the inside remains wet. Answer D is incorrect because the child should be turned at least every 2 hours.

118. **Answer A is correct.** The influenza vaccine is usually given in October and November. Answers B, C, and D are inaccurate, so they are incorrect.

119. **Answer B is correct.** The presence of Reed-Sternberg cells, sometimes referred to as "owl's eyes," are diagnostic for Hodgkin's lymphoma. Answers A, C, and D are not associated with Hodgkin's lymphoma and are incorrect.

120. **Answer A is correct.** Providing the client a pad and pencil allows him a way to communicate with the nurse. Answers B and C are important in the client's care; however, they do not provide a means for the client to "talk" with the nurse. Answer D is not realistic and is likely to be frustrating to the client, so it is incorrect.

121. **Answer B is correct.** Antihistamines should not be used by the client with open-angle glaucoma because they dilate the pupil and prevent the outflow of aqueous humor, which raises pressures in the eye. Answers A, C, and D are safe for use in the client with open-angle glaucoma; therefore, they are incorrect.

122. **Answer A is correct.** Persons with endemic goiter live in areas where the soil is depleted of iodine. Answers B and D refer to sporadic goiter, and answer C is not related to the occurrence of goiter.

123. **Answer A is correct.** The client should avoid over-the-counter allergy medications because many of them contain Benadryl (diphenhydramine). Benadryl is used to counteract the effects of antipsychotic medications that are prescribed for schizophrenia. Answer B refers to the client taking an MAO inhibitor, and answer C refers to the client taking lithium; therefore, they are incorrect. Over-the-counter pain relievers are safe for the client taking antipsychotic medication, so answer D is incorrect.

124. **Answer D is correct.** The priority care for the client with a goiter is maintaining an effective airway. Answers A, B, and C apply to the client with a goiter; however, they are not the priority of care.

125. **Answer B is correct.** The purpose of applying Erythromycin eyedrops to the newborn's eyes is to prevent neonatal blindness that can result from contamination with *Neisseria gonorrhoeae*. Answers A, C, and D are inaccurate statements and, therefore, are incorrect.

126. **Answer B is correct.** Discoid lupus produces discoid or "coinlike" lesions on the skin. Answers A, C, and D refer to systemic lupus; therefore, they are incorrect.

127. **Answer A is correct.** The visual center of the brain is located in the occipital lobe, so damage to that region results in changes in vision. Answers B and D are associated with the temporal lobe, and answer C is associated with the frontal lobe.

128. **Answer B is correct.** Parallel play, the form of play used by toddlers, involves playing beside one another with like toys but without interaction. Answer A is incorrect because it describes associative play, typical of the preschooler. Answer C is incorrect because it describes cooperative play, typical play of the school-age child. Answer D is incorrect because it describes solitary play, typical play of the infant.

129. **Answer A is correct.** Infants can discriminate speech and the human voice from other patterns of sound. Answers B, C, and D are inaccurate statements; therefore, they are incorrect.

130. **Answer C is correct.** As the school-age child develops concrete operational thinking, she becomes more selective and discriminating in her collections. Answer A refers to the cognitive development of the infant; answer B refers to moral, not cognitive, development; and answer D refers to the cognitive development of the toddler and preschool child. Therefore, all are incorrect.

131. **Answer D is correct.** Consistently responding to the infant's needs fosters a sense of trust. Failure or inconsistency in meeting the infant's needs results in a sense of mistrust. Answers A, B, and C are important to the development of the infant but do not necessarily foster a sense of trust; therefore, they are incorrect.

132. **Answer B is correct.** Before walking the client for the first time after delivery, the nurse should ask the client to sit on the side of the bed and dangle her legs, to prevent postural hypotension. Pain medication should not be given before walking, making answer A incorrect. Answers C and D have no relationship to walking the client, so they are incorrect.

133. **Answer D is correct.** Hospitalized elderly clients frequently become confused. Providing simple explanations in a calm, caring manner will help minimize anxiety and confusion. Answers A and B will increase the client's confusion, and answer C is incorrect because personal visits from family and friends would benefit the client.

134. **Answer A is correct.** The client can return to work when he has three negative sputum cultures. Answers B, C, and D are inaccurate statements, so they are incorrect.

135. **Answer C is correct.** The presence of fibrin split compound provides a definitive diagnosis of DIC. An elevated erythrocyte sedimentation rate is associated with inflammatory diseases; therefore, answer A is incorrect. Answer B is incorrect because the client with DIC clots too readily, forming microscopic thrombi. Answer D is incorrect because an elevated white cell count is associated with infection.

136. **Answer A is correct.** The symptoms of rheumatoid arthritis are worse upon awakening. Taking a warm shower helps relieve the stiffness and soreness associated with the disease. Answer B is incorrect because heat is the most beneficial way of relieving the symptoms. Large doses of aspirin are given in divided doses throughout the day, making answer C incorrect. Answer D is incorrect because the client has more problems with mobility early in the morning.

137. **Answer C is correct.** Temperature elevations in the client receiving antipsychotics (sometimes referred to as neuroleptics) such as Clozaril (clozapine) should be reported to the physician immediately. Antipsychotics can produce adverse reactions that include dystonia, agranulocytosis, and neuromalignant syndrome (NMS). Answers A and B are incorrect because they jeopardize the safety of the client. Answer D is incorrect because the client with schizophrenia is often unaware of his condition; therefore, the nurse must rely on objective signs of illness.

138. **Answer D is correct.** Drug overdose is a primary cause of acute respiratory distress syndrome. Answers A, B, and C are incorrect because they are not associated with the development of acute respiratory distress syndrome.

139. **Answer B is correct.** With iron-deficiency anemia, the RBCs are described as hypochromic and microcytic. Answer A is incorrect because the RBCs would be normochromic and normocytic but would be reduced in number. Answer C is incorrect because the RBCs would be normochromic and macrocytic. Answer D refers to anemias due to an abnormal shape or shortened life span of the RBCs rather than the color or size of the RBC; therefore, it is incorrect.

140. **Answer D is correct.** A positive Babinski reflex in adults should be reported to the physician because it indicates a lesion of the corticospinal tract. Answer A is incorrect because it does not indicate that the client's condition is improving. Answer B is incorrect because changing the position will not alter the finding. Answer C is incorrect because a positive Babinski reflex is an expected finding in an infant, but not in an adult.

141. **Answer A is correct.** The Glascow coma scale, which measures verbal response, motor response, and eye opening, ranges from 0 to 15. A score of 13 indicates the client's condition is satisfactory. Answer B is incorrect because the presence of doll's eye movement indicates damage to the brainstem or oculomotor nerve. Answer C is incorrect because absent deep tendon reflexes are associated with deep coma. Answer D is incorrect because decerebrate posturing is associated with injury to the brain stem.

142. **Answer C is correct.** The primary goal of a bowel and bladder retraining program is to prevent complications that can result from impaired elimination. Answer A is incorrect because the retraining will not restore the client's preinjury elimination pattern. Answer B is incorrect because the retraining will not restore the client's neurosensory function. The client's body image will improve with retraining; however, it is not the primary goal, so answer D is incorrect.

143. **Answer A is correct.** Pulling against interlocked fingers will focus the client's attention away from the area being examined, thus making it easier to elicit a knee-jerk response. Answer B is incorrect because it is a means of checking the spinal accessory nerve. Answer C is incorrect because it is a means of checking the oculomotor nerve. Answer D is incorrect because it will not facilitate checking the patellar reflex.

144. **Answer B is correct.** Auscultation is the last step performed in a physical assessment. Answers A, C, and D are incorrect because they are performed before auscultation.

145. **Answer C is correct.** Akathesia, an extrapyramidal side effect of antipsychotic medication, results in an inability to sit still or stand still. Dystonia, in answer A, refers to a muscle spasm in any muscle of the body; answer B refers to abnormal, involuntary movements of the face, neck, and jaw; and answer D refers to an involuntary deviation and fixation of the eyes; therefore, they are incorrect.

146. **Answer D is correct.** The large soft swelling that crosses the suture line indicates that the newborn has a caput succedaneum. This finding should be reported to the physician. Answer A is incorrect because the umbilical cord normally contains three vessels (two arteries and one vein). Answer B is incorrect because the temperature is normal for the newborn. Answer C refers to acrocyanosis, which is normal in the newborn.

147. **Answer B is correct.** Infants and children are highly susceptible to infection with pertussis. Answers A, C, and D are inaccurate statements; therefore, they are incorrect.

148. **Answer D is correct.** Epidural anesthesia produces vasodilation and lowers the blood pressure; therefore, adrenalin should be available to reverse hypotension. Answer A is incorrect because it is a narcotic antagonist. Answer B is incorrect because it is an adrenergic that increases cardiac output. Answer C is incorrect because it is a benzodiazepine antagonist.

149. **Answer B is correct.** Gantrisin and other sulfa drugs should be given 30 minutes before meals, to enhance absorption. Answer A is incorrect because the medication should be given before eating. Answer C is incorrect because the medication should be given on an empty stomach. Answer D is incorrect because the medication is to be given in divided doses throughout the day.

150. **Answer A is correct.** The client taking Parnate and other MAO inhibitors should avoid ingesting foods containing tyramine, which can result in extreme elevations in blood pressure. Answers B, C, and D are not associated with the use of MAO inhibitors; therefore, they are incorrect.

151. **Answer C is correct.** The frontal lobe interprets sensation, so the client's failure to recognize touch confirms a frontal lobe injury. Answer A is incorrect because the occipital lobe is the visual center. Answer B is incorrect because the medulla is the respiratory center. Taste impulses are interpreted in the parietal lobe; therefore, answer D is incorrect.

152. **Answer B is correct.** The normal urinary output is 30–50mL per hour. The client's urinary output is below normal, indicating that additional fluids are needed. The amount of output from the Jackson-Pratt drain should be small; therefore, answer A is incorrect. The amount of drainage from the nasogastric tube is not excessive, so answer C is incorrect. Answer D is incorrect because the client would not be expected to have a stool in the first 12 hours following surgery.

153. **Answer D is correct.** According to the National Center for Health Statistics, heart disease is the number one cause of death in persons 65 and older. Chronic pulmonary disease is the fourth-leading cause of death in this age group; therefore, answer A is incorrect. Diabetes mellitus is the sixth-leading cause of death in this age group, and pneumonia is the fifth-leading cause of death in this age group; therefore, answers B and C are incorrect.

154. **Answer C is correct.** Recall is the client's ability to restate items mentioned at the beginning of the evaluation. Attention is evaluated by having the client count backward by 7 beginning at 100, so answer A is incorrect. Orientation is evaluated by having the client state the year, month, date, and day, so answer B is incorrect. Registration is evaluated by having the client immediately repeat the name of three items just named by the examiner; thus, answer D is incorrect.

155. **Answer D is correct.** The nurse should tell the client to change position or turn side to side in order to improve the dialysate return. Answers A, B, and C are incorrect ways of managing peritoneal dialysis; therefore, they are incorrect choices.

156. **Answer A is correct.** The nurse should give priority to maintaining the client's airway. The ABCDs of trauma care are airway with cervical spine immobilization, breathing, circulation, and disabilities (neurological); therefore, answers B, C, and D are incorrect.

157. **Answer B is correct.** The client in pain usually has an increased blood pressure. Answers A and C are incorrect because the client in pain will have an increased pulse rate and increased respiratory rate. Temperature is not affected by pain; therefore, answer D is incorrect.

158. **Answer C is correct.** A score of 4 indicates normal flexion. Normal flexion caused the client to withdraw his whole hand from the stimuli. Answers A, B, and D are incorrect because they do not relate to the client's response to the stimulus.

159. **Answer A is correct.** Management of Kawasaki's disease includes the use of large doses of aspirin. Answers B, C, and D are incorrect because they are not used in the treatment of Kawasaki's disease.

160. **Answer C is correct.** The client with bulimia nervosa recognizes that she has an eating disorder but feels helpless to correct it. Answer A is incorrect because the client with bulimia nervosa is usually of normal weight. Answers B and D are incorrect because they describe both the client with anorexia nervosa and the client with bulimia nervosa.

161. **Answer C is correct.** A positive Mantoux test is indicated by the presence of induration. Answers A, B, and D are incorrect because they do not describe the findings of a positive Mantoux test.

162. **Answer A is correct.** The solution bag should be hung 2–3 feet above the client's abdomen to allow a slow, steady irrigation. Answer B is incorrect because it will distend the bladder and cause trauma. Answer C is incorrect because the nurse should use sterile technique when attaching the tubing. Answer D is incorrect because it would be an intermittent irrigation rather than a continuous one.

163. **Answer B is correct.** Salmonella infection is commonly associated with turtles and reptiles. Answers A, C, and D are incorrect because they are not sources of salmonella infection.

164. **Answer B is correct.** The infant is not gaining weight as he should. Further assessment of feeding patterns as well as organic causes for growth failure should be investigated. Answers A, C, and D are incorrect because they are within the expected range for growth.

165. **Answer C is correct.** Pyridium causes the urine to become red-orange in color, so the client should be informed of this. Answers A, B, and D are not associated with the use of Pyridium; therefore, they are incorrect.

166. **Answer B is correct.** The infant's fingernails and toenails should be kept short to prevent scratching the skin. Answers A, C, and D are incorrect because keeping the infant warm will increase itching; bubble bath and perfumed soaps should not be used because they can cause skin irritations; and the infant's clothes should be washed in mild detergent and rinsed in plain water to reduce skin irritations.

167. **Answer D is correct.** Skeletal traction is used to realign bone fragments. Answer A is incorrect because it does not apply to the fractures of the femur. Answers B and C refer to skin traction, so they are incorrect.

168. **Answer B is correct.** The client with rheumatoid arthritis benefits from activity within the limits of pain because it decreases the likelihood of joints becoming nonfunctional. Answer A is incorrect because the client needs to use the knees to prevent further stiffness and disuse. Answer C is incorrect because the client can sit in chairs other than a recliner. Answer D is incorrect because it predisposes the client to further complications associated with immobility.

169. **Answer A is correct.** Use of a scalp vein for IV infusions allows the infant to be picked up and held more easily. Answers B, C, and D are inaccurate statements; therefore, they are incorrect.

170. **Answer D is correct.** The newborn with choanal atresia will not be able to breathe through his nose because of the presence of a bony obstruction that blocks the passage of air through the nares. Answers A, B, and C are not associated with choanal atresia; therefore, they are incorrect.

171. **Answer A is correct.** The most appropriate means of rehydrating the 7-month-old with diarrhea and mild dehydration is to provide oral electrolyte solutions. Answer B is incorrect because formula feedings should be delayed until symptoms improve. Answer C is incorrect because the 7-month-old has symptoms of mild dehydration, which can be managed with oral fluid replacement. Answer D is incorrect because a BRAT diet (bananas, rice, applesauce, toast, or tea) is no longer recommended.

172. **Answer B is correct.** Signs of fluid overload in an infant include increased heart rate and increased blood pressure. Temperature would not be increased by fluid overload; therefore, answers A and C are incorrect. Heart rate and blood pressure are not decreased by fluid overload; therefore, answer D is incorrect.

173. **Answer A is correct.** Most parents report finding Wilms tumor when the infant is being diapered or bathed. Answers B, C, and D are not associated with Wilms tumor; therefore, they are incorrect.

174. **Answer B is correct.** Monitoring her pulse and respirations will provide information on her cardiac status. Answer A is incorrect because she should not remain on strict bed rest. Answer C is incorrect because it does not provide information on her cardiac status. Answer D is incorrect because she needs to weigh more often to determine unusual gain, which could be related to her cardiac status.

175. **Answer C is correct.** The effectiveness of oxygen therapy is best determined by arterial blood gases. Answers A, B, and D are less helpful in determining the effectiveness of oxygen therapy, so they are incorrect.

176. **Answer B is correct.** Versed produces conscious sedation, so the client will not be able to remember having the procedure. Answers A, C, and D are inaccurate statements.

177. **Answer C is correct.** Early indicators of an altered level of consciousness include restlessness and irritability. Answer A is incorrect because it is a sign of impaired motor function. Answer B is incorrect because it is a sign of damage to the optic chiasm or optic nerve. Answer D is incorrect because it is a sign of increased intracranial pressure.

178. **Answer C is correct.** The client receiving a stat dose of medication should receive his medication first. Answers A, B, and D are incorrect because they are regularly scheduled medications for clients whose conditions are more stable.

179. **Answer D is correct.** Wrapping the IV site with Kerlex removes the area from the client's line of vision, allowing his attention to be directed away from the site. Answer A is incorrect because it impedes circulation at and distal to the IV site. Answer B is incorrect because reasoning is a cognitive function and the client has cognitive impairment. Answer C is incorrect because the use of restraints would require a doctor's order, and only one hand would be restrained.

180. Answer B is correct. Changes in the ST segment are associated with acute myocardia 1 infraction. Peaked P waves, minimal QRS wave, and prominent U wave are not associated with acute myocardial infarction; therefore answers A, C, and D are incorrect.

181. Answer A is correct. Chest pain and shortness of breath following a fracture of the long bones is associated with pulmonary embolus, which requires immediate intervention. Answer B is incorrect because ecchymosis is common following fractures. Answer C is incorrect because a low-grade temperature is expected because of the inflammatory response. Answer D is incorrect because level-two pain is expected in the client with a recent fracture.

182. Answer C is correct. According to the American Heart Association (2005), the compression-to-ventilation ratio for one rescuer is 30:2. Answers A, B, and D are incorrect compression-to-ventilation ratios.

183. Answer A is correct. The nurse should give priority to beginning intravenous fluids. Increasing the client's fluid intake to 3,000mL per day will help prevent the obstruction of urine flow by increasing the frequency and volume of urinary output. Answer B is incorrect because the catheter is in the bladder and will do nothing to affect the flow of urine from the kidney. Answer C is important but has no effect on preventing or alleviating the obstruction of urine flow from the kidney; therefore, it is incorrect. Answer D is incorrect because it will help prevent the formation of some stones but will not prevent the obstruction of urine flow.

184. Answer A is correct. JCAHO guidelines state that at least two client identifiers should be used whenever administering medications or blood products, whenever samples or specimens are taken, and when providing treatments. Neither of the identifiers is to be the client's room number. Answer B is incorrect because the client's room number is not used as an identifier. Answer C and D are incorrect because the best identifiers according to the JCAHO are the client's armband, medical record number, and/or date of birth.

185. Answer D is correct. The client's level of pain is severe and requires narcotic analgesia. Morphine, an opioid, is the strongest medication listed. Answer A is incorrect because it is effective only with mild pain. Answers B and C are incorrect because they are not strong enough to relieve severe pain.

186. Answer B is correct. Persistent diarrhea results in the loss of bicarbonate (base) so that the client develops metabolic acidosis. Answers A and D are incorrect because the problem of diarrhea is metabolic, not respiratory, in nature. Answer C is incorrect because the client is losing bicarbonate (base); therefore, he cannot develop alkalosis, caused by excess base.

187. Answer D is correct. According to the American Heart Association (2005), the nurse should call for help before instituting CPR. Answers A, B, and C are incorrect choices because the nurse should call for help before taking action.

188. Answer C is correct. The viral load or viral burden test provides information on the effectiveness of the client's medication regimen as well as progression of the disease. Answers A and B are incorrect because they are screening tests to detect the presence of HIV. Answer D is incorrect because it is a measure of the number of helper cells.

189. **Answer D is correct.** The medication must be taken for the remainder of the client's life, to prevent the reoccurrence of CMV infection. Answers A, B, and C are inaccurate statements and, therefore, are incorrect.

190. **Answer B is correct.** Loss of memory and loss of concentration are the first signs of AIDS dementia complex. Answers A, C, and D are symptoms associated with toxoplasmosis encephalitis, so they are not correct.

191. **Answer D is correct.** Activase (alteplase) is a thrombolytic agent that destroys the clot. Answer A is incorrect because the medication does not prevent congestive heart failure. Answer B is incorrect because it does not stabilize the clot. Answer C is incorrect because Alteplase does not directly increase oxygenation.

192. **Answer D is correct.** The majority of children have all their deciduous teeth by age 30 months, which should coincide with the child's first visit with the dentist. Answers A, B, and C are incorrect because the deciduous teeth are probably not all erupted.

193. **Answer B is correct.** The child with Down syndrome has epicanthal folds, broad hands, and transpalmar creases. Answer A describes the child with osteogenesis imperfecta, answer C describes the child with Turner's syndrome, and answer D describes the child with Tay Sach's disease; therefore, they are incorrect.

194. **Answer A is correct.** The most common opportunistic infection in infants and children with HIV is *Pneumocystis carinii* pneumonia. Answers B, C, and D are incorrect because they are not the most common cause of opportunistic infection in the infant with HIV.

195. **Answer C is correct.** The nurse should ensure that the client's gag reflex is intact before offering sips of water or other fluids in order to reduce the risk of aspiration. Answers A and D should be assessed because the client has returned from having a diagnostic procedure, but they are not related to the question; therefore, they are incorrect. Answer B is not related to the question, so it is incorrect.

196. **Answer B is correct.** Neumega stimulates the production of platelets, so a finding of 250,000mm^3 suggests that the medication is working. Answers A and D are associated with the use of Epogen, and answer C is associated with the use of Neupogen; therefore, they are incorrect.

197. **Answer A is correct.** Pilocarpine, a substance that stimulates sweating, is used to diagnose cystic fibrosis. Chloride and sodium levels in the sweat are measured by the test, but they do not stimulate sweating; therefore, answers B and C are incorrect. Answer D is incorrect because it is not associated with cystic fibrosis.

198. **Answer D is correct.** The client with a Brown Sequard spinal cord injury will have a loss of sensation on the side opposite the cord injury. Answer A is incorrect because it describes a complete cord lesion. Answer B is incorrect because it describes central cord syndrome. Answer C is incorrect because it describes cauda equina syndromes.

199. **Answer C is correct.** The client with signs of heptorenal syndrome should have a diet that is low in protein and sodium, to decrease serum ammonia levels. Answer A is incorrect because the client will not benefit from a high-protein diet and sodium will be restricted. A high-carbohydrate diet will provide the client with calories; however, sodium intake is restricted, making answer B incorrect. Answer D is incorrect because the client will not benefit from a high-protein diet, which would increase ammonia levels.

200. **Answer A is correct.** Basal cell epithelioma, or skin cancer, is related to sun exposure. Answers B, C, and D are incorrect because they are not associated with the development of basal cell epithelioma.

201. **Answer C is correct.** The client with an orthotopic bladder replacement will have a surgically created bladder. Bearing down with each voiding will help to express the urine. Answer A is incorrect because it refers to a client with an ileal conduit, answer B is incorrect because it refers to a client with an ileal reservoir, and answer D is incorrect because it refers to a client with an ileal conduit.

202. **Answer D is correct.** Any unused blood should be returned to the blood bank. Answers A, B, and C are incorrect because they are improper ways of handling the unused blood.

203. **Answer B is correct.** Trivalent botulism antitoxin is made from horse serum; therefore, the nurse needs to assess the client for allergies to horses. Answers A, C, and D are incorrect because they are not involved in the manufacturing of trivalent botulism antitoxin.

204. **Answer D is correct.** Unless contraindicated, the client with renal calculi should receive 200mL of fluid per hour to help flush the calculi from the kidneys. Answers A, B, and C are incorrect choices because the amounts are inadequate.

205. **Answer B is correct.** A soft gauze pad should be used to clean the oral mucosa of a client with oral candidiasis. Answer A is incorrect because it is too abrasive to the mucosa of a client with oral candidiasis. Answer C is incorrect because the mouthwash contains alcohol, which can burn the client's mouth. Answer D is incorrect because lemon and glycerin will cause burning and drying of the client's oral mucosa.

206. **Answer A is correct.** The client with a cardiac tamponade will exhibit a decrease of 10mmHg or greater in systolic blood pressure during inspirations. This phenomenon, known as pulsus paradoxus, is related to blood pooling in the pulmonary veins during inspiration. Answers B, C, and D are incorrect because they contain inaccurate statements.

207. **Answer B is correct.** Following removal of a cataract, the client should avoid bending over for several days because this increases intraocular pressure. The client should avoid aspirin because it increases the likelihood of bleeding, and the client should keep the eye shield on when sleeping, so answers A and C are incorrect. Answer D is incorrect because the client should not face into the shower stream after having cataract removal because this can cause trauma to the operative eye.

208. **Answer A is correct.** A severe toxic side effect of pentamidine is hypotension. Answers B, C, and D are not related to the administration of pentamidine; therefore, they are incorrect.

209. **Answer B is correct.** A secondary benefit of intra-arterial chemotherapy is that it helps in the treatment of micrometastasis from cancerous tumors. Intra-arterial chemotherapy lessens systemic effects but does not prevent or eradicate them; therefore, answers A, C, and D are incorrect.

210. **Answer A is correct.** Before administering gold salts, the nurse should check the lab work for the complete blood count and urine protein level because gold salts are toxic to the kidneys and the bone marrow. Answer B is incorrect because it is not necessary to give an antiemetic before administering the medication. Changes in vital signs are not associated with the medication, and a sedative is not needed before receiving the medication; therefore, answers C and D are incorrect.

211. **Answer D is correct.** The appearance of increased drainage that is clear, colorless, or bile tinged indicates disruption or leakage at one of the anastamosis sites, requiring the immediate attention of the physician. Answer A is incorrect because the client's condition will worsen without prompt intervention. Answers B and C are incorrect choices because they cannot be performed without a physician's order.

212. **Answer A is correct.** Herbals such as Echinacea can interfere with the action of antiviral medications; therefore, the client should discuss the use of herbals with his physician. Answer B is incorrect because supplements have not been shown to prolong life. Answer C is incorrect because herbals have not been shown to be effective in decreasing the viral load. Answer D is incorrect because supplements do not prevent replication of the virus.

213. **Answer B is correct.** The client with Sjogren's syndrome complains of dryness of the eyes. The nurse can help relieve the client's symptoms by instilling artificial tears. Answers A, C, and D do not relieve the symptoms of Sjogren's syndrome; therefore, they are incorrect.

214. **Answer D is correct.** Melena, or blood in the stool, is common in the client with duodenal ulcers. Answers A and B are symptoms of gastric ulcers, and diarrhea is not a symptom of duodenal ulcers; therefore, answers A, B, and C are incorrect.

215. **Answer C is correct.** The nurse should auscultate the fistula for the presence of a bruit, which indicates that the fistula is patent. Answer A is incorrect because repeated compressions such as obtaining the blood pressure can result in damage to the AV fistula. Answer B is incorrect because the AV fistula is not used for the administration of IV fluids. Answer D is incorrect because venopunctures are not done in the arm with an AV fistula.

216. **Answer D is correct.** A client with epilepsy is managed with anticonvulsant medication. An adverse side effect of anticonvulsant medication is decreased white cell count. Answer A is incorrect because elevations in serum creatinine are expected in the client with chronic renal failure. Answer B is incorrect because a positive C reactive protein is expected in the client with rheumatic fever. Elevations in hematocrit are expected in a client with gastroenteritis because of dehydration; therefore, answer C is incorrect.

217. **Answer B is correct.** Clients who use steroid medications, such as beclomethasone, can develop adverse side effects, including oral infections with candida albicans. Symptoms of candida albicans include sore throat and white patches on the oral mucosa. Increased weight, difficulty sleeping, and changes in mood are expected side effects; therefore, answers A, C, and D are incorrect.

218. **Answer A is correct.** Concurrent use of an MAO inhibitor and an SSRI (example: Parnate and Paxil) can result in serotonin syndrome, a potentially lethal condition. Answer B is incorrect because it refers to the Parnate-cheese reaction or hypertension that results when the client taking an MAO inhibitor ingests sources of tyramine. Answer C is incorrect because it refers to neuroleptic malignant syndrome or elevations in temperature caused by antipsychotic medication. Answer D is incorrect because it refers to the hypertension that results when MAO inhibitors are used with cold and hayfever medications containing pseudoephedrine.

219. **Answer B is correct.** The nurse should check the nasal packing for the presence of the "halo sign," or a light yellow color at the edge of clear drainage on the nasal dressing. The presence of the halo sign indicates leakage of cerebral spinal fluid. Answer A is incorrect because the nurse provides mouth care using oral washes not a toothbrush. Answer C is incorrect because coughing increases pressure in the incisional area and can lead to a cerebral spinal fluid leak. Answer D is incorrect because the client should not be ambulated for 1–3 days after surgery.

220. **Answer D is correct.** The esophageal balloon tamponade should be maintained at a pressure of 20–25mmHg to help decrease bleeding from the esophageal varices. Answers A, B, and C are incorrect because the pressures are too low to be effective.

221. **Answer A is correct.** The most common neurological complication of Lyme's disease is Bell's palsy. Symptoms of Bell's palsy include complaints of a "drawing" sensation and paralysis on one side of the face. Answer B is incorrect because it describes symptoms of multiple sclerosis. Answer C is incorrect because it describes symptoms of trigeminal neuralgia. Answer D is incorrect because it describes symptoms of amyotrophic lateral sclerosis. Multiple sclerosis, trigeminal neuralgia, and amyotrophic lateral sclerosis are not associated with Lyme's disease.

222. **Answer B is correct.** The child with autistic disorder is easily upset by changes in routine; therefore, the nurse should assign a consistent caregiver. Answers A, C, and D are incorrect because they provide too much stimulation and change in routine for the child with autistic disorder.

223. **Answer C is correct.** Pernicious anemia is characterized by changes in neurological function such as loss of coordination and loss of position sense. Answers A, B, and D are applicable to all types of anemia; therefore, they are incorrect.

224. **Answer A is correct.** Cyclogel is a cycloplegic medication that inhibits constriction of the pupil and rests the muscles of accommodation. Answer B is incorrect because the medication does not prevent post-operative infection. Answer C is incorrect because the medication keeps the pupil from constricting. Answer D is incorrect because it does not decrease the production of aqueous humor.

225. **Answer D is correct.** Secondary syphilis is characterized by well-defined generalized lesions on the palms, soles, and perineum. Lesions can enlarge and erode, leaving highly contagious pink or grayish-white lesions. Answer A describes the chancre associated with primary syphilis, answer B describes the latent stage of syphilis, and answer C describes late syphilis.

226. **Answer D is correct.** The central venous pressure of 15mm H_2O indicates fluid overload. Answers A, B, and C are incorrect because they are not a cause for concern; therefore, they do not need to be reported to the physician.

227. **Answer A is correct.** Veil-like loss of vision is a symptom of a detached retina, not glaucoma. Answers B, C, and D are symptoms associated with glaucoma; therefore, they are incorrect.

228. **Answer B is correct.** According to the Centers for Disease Control (CDC), the ventilator-dependent client who is receiving tube feedings should have the head of the bed elevated 30–45° to prevent aspiration of gastric secretions. Keeping the head of the bed flat has been shown to increase aspiration of gastric secretions; therefore, answer A is incorrect. Answer C is incorrect because placing the client on his left side has not been shown to decrease the incidence of aspiration of gastric secretions. Answer D is incorrect because it would increase the incidence of aspiration of gastric secretions.

229. **Answer C is correct.** A paper bag should be used for the victim's clothing because it will allow the clothes to dry without destroying evidence. Answers A and B are incorrect because plastic and rubber retain moisture that can deteriorate evidence. Answer D is incorrect because padded envelopes are plastic lined, and plastic retains moisture that can deteriorate evidence.

230. **Answer D is correct.** Because of the anatomic location, fractures of the ankle are not treated with traction. Answers A, B, and C are incorrect because they are treated by the use of traction.

231. **Answer B is correct.** The cause of acute myocardial infarction is occlusion in the coronary vessels by a clot or atherosclerotic plaque. Answers A and C are incorrect because they are the result, not the cause, of acute myocardial infarction. Answer D is incorrect because it reflects a compensatory action in which the depth and rate of respirations changes to compensate for decreased cardiac output.

232. **Answer D is correct.** The client complaining of sexual assault should be taken immediately to a private area rather than left sitting in the waiting room. Answers A, B, and C require intervention, but the clients can remain in the waiting room.

233. **Answer B is correct.** Morphine is an opiate that can severely depress the client's respirations. The word *essential* implies that this vital sign must be assessed to provide for the client's safety. Answers A, C, and D are incorrect choices because they are not necessarily associated before administering morphine.

234. **Answer A is correct.** Changes in pupil equality and reactivity, including sluggish pupil reaction, are late signs of increased intracranial pressure. Answers B, C, and D are incorrect because they are early signs of increased intracranial pressure.

235. **Answer B is correct.** If the newly licensed nurse thinks he is unqualified to perform a procedure at this time, he should refuse, give a reason for the refusal, and request training. Answers A, C, and D can result in injury to the client and bring legal charges against the nurse; therefore, they are incorrect choices.

236. **Answer C is correct.** The nurse should give priority to administering oxygen via nasal cannula. Answer A is incorrect because the history of prior cardiac problems can be obtained after the client's condition has stabilized. Answer B is incorrect because starting an IV is done after the client's oxygen needs are met. Answer D is incorrect because pupil checks are part of a neurological assessment, which is not indicated for the situation.

237. **Answer C is correct.** The recommended way of removing a tick is to use tweezers. The tick is grasped close to the skin and removed using a steady, firm motion. Quickly jerking the tick away from the skin, placing a burning match close to the tick, and covering the tick with petroleum jelly increases the likelihood that the tick will regurgitate contaminated saliva into the wound therefore Answers A, B, and D are incorrect.

238. **Answer B is correct.** The application of a wrapped ice compress will help decrease bleeding by causing vasoconstriction. Answer A is incorrect because the client's head should be tilted forward, not back. Nothing should be placed inside the nose except by the physician; therefore, answer C is incorrect. Answer D is incorrect because the nostrils should not be pinched due to a visible deformity.

239. **Answer D is correct.** The nurse's responsibility in obtaining an informed consent for surgery is providing the client with the consent form and witnessing the client's signature. Answers A and B are the responsibility of the physician, not the nurse. Answer C is incorrect because the nurse-client relationship should never be used to persuade the client to sign a permit for surgery or other medical treatments.

240. **Answer D is correct.** A pulse strength of 1+ is a weak pulse. Answer A is incorrect because it refers to a pulse strength of 4+. Answer B is incorrect because it refers to a pulse strength of 3+. Answer C is incorrect because it refers to a pulse strength of 2+.

241. **Answer B is correct.** Unlicensed assistive personnel can perform routine catheter care with soap and water. Answers A, C, and D are incorrect because they are actions that must be performed by the licensed nurse.

242. **Answer A is correct.** The client's respiratory pattern is that of Cheyne-Stokes respirations. Answer B is incorrect because Kussmaul respirations, associated with diabetic ketoacidosis, are characterized by an increase in the rate and depth of respirations. Answer C is incorrect because Biot respirations are characterized by several short respirations followed by long, irregular periods of apnea. Answer D is incorrect because diaphragmatic respirations refer to abdominal breathing.

243. **Answer C is correct.** Milk and milk products are not permitted on a clear-liquid diet. Answers A, B, and D are permitted on a clear-liquid diet; therefore, they are incorrect.

244. **Answer A is correct.** The tuberculin skin test is given by intradermal injection. Intradermal injections are administered by inserting the needle at a 5–15° angle. Answers B, C, and D are incorrect because the angle is not used for intradermal injections.

245. **Answer D is correct.** Following a trabeculoplasty, the client is instructed to wear eye protection continuously for several months. Eye protection can be in the form of protective glasses or an eye shield that is worn during sleep. Answer A is not correct because the client is instructed to keep soap and water away from the eyes. Answer B is incorrect because showering is permitted as long as soap and water are kept away from the eyes. Answer C is incorrect because the client should avoid using eye makeup for at least a month after surgery.

246. **Answer B is correct.** The CASS (continuous aspiration of subglottic secretions) tube features an evacuation port above the cuff, making it possible to remove secretions above the cuff. Use of an uncuffed tube increases the incidence of ventilator pneumonia by allowing aspiration of secretions, making answer A incorrect. Answer C is incorrect because the fenestrated tube has openings that increase the risk of pneumonia. Answer D is incorrect because *nasotracheal* refers to one of the routes for inserting an endotracheal tube, not a type of tube.

247. **Answer A is correct.** This client has multiple risk factors for complications following abdominal surgery, including age, weight, and an endocrine disorder. Answer B is incorrect because the client has only one significant factor, the recent urinary tract infection. Answer C is incorrect because the client has only one significant factor, the use of tobacco. Answer D is incorrect because the client has no significant factors for post-operative complications.

248. **Answer A is correct.** The client's potassium level is low. The normal potassium level is 3.5–5.5mEq/L. Answers B, C, and D are within normal range and, therefore, are incorrect.

249. **Answer B is correct.** Black or tarry stools are associated with upper gastrointestinal bleeding. Normal stools are brown in color, clay-colored stools are associated with biliary obstruction, and green stools are associated with infection or large amounts of bile; therefore, answers A, C, and D are incorrect.

250. **Answer C is correct.** An adverse side effect of chloramphenicol is aplastic anemia; therefore, the nurse should pay particular attention to the client's complete blood count. Answers A, B, and D should be noted, but they are not directly affected by the medication and are incorrect.

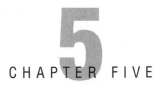

CHAPTER FIVE

Practice Exam 5 and Rationales

1. The nurse is caring for a client who is of the Islam religious group. Which food selection might this client want to avoid?

    ○ **A.** Jello

    ○ **B.** Chicken

    ○ **C.** Milk

    ○ **D.** Broccoli

2. A 65-year-old client is admitted after a stroke. The nurse is concerned about skin breakdown and decubitus ulcer development. Which nursing intervention would best improve tissue perfusion to prevent skin problems?

    ○ **A.** Assessing the skin daily

    ○ **B.** Massaging any erythematous areas on the skin

    ○ **C.** Changing incontinence pads as soon as they become soiled

    ○ **D.** Performing range-of-motion exercises and turning and repositioning the client

3. The nurse is performing discharge diet teaching to a client with a stage 1 decubitus ulcer on the coccyx. Which diet selection by this client would indicate that the client has a clear understanding of the proper diet for healing of a decubitus ulcer?

    ○ **A.** Tossed salad, milk, and a slice of caramel cake

    ○ **B.** Vegetable soup and crackers, and a glass of tea

    ○ **C.** Baked chicken breast, broccoli, wheat roll, and an orange

    ○ **D.** Hamburger, French fries, and corn on the cob

4. The nurse is assessing elderly clients at a community center. Which of the following findings would be the most cause for concern?

Quick Answer: **376**
Detailed Answer: **379**

- ○ **A.** Complaint of dry mouth
- ○ **B.** Loss of 1 inch of height in the last year
- ○ **C.** Stiffened joints
- ○ **D.** Rales bilaterally on chest auscultation

5. A client with chronic pain is being treated with opioid administration via epidural route. Which medication would it be most important to have available due to a possible complication of this pain relief procedure?

Quick Answer: **376**
Detailed Answer: **379**

- ○ **A.** (Ketorolac) Toradol
- ○ **B.** (Naloxone) Narcan
- ○ **C.** (Diphenhydramine) Benadryl
- ○ **D.** (Promethazine) Phenergan

6. The nurse is assessing a client for hypovolemia. Which laboratory result would help the nurse in confirming a volume deficit?

Quick Answer: **376**
Detailed Answer: **379**

- ○ **A.** Hematocrit 55%
- ○ **B.** Potassium 5.0mEq/L
- ○ **C.** Urine specific gravity 1.016
- ○ **D.** BUN 18mg/dL

7. A nurse is triaging in the emergency room when a client enters complaining of muscle cramps and a feeling of exhaustion after a running competition. Which of the following would the nurse suspect?

Quick Answer: **376**
Detailed Answer: **379**

- ○ **A.** Hypernatremia
- ○ **B.** Hyponatremia
- ○ **C.** Syndrome of inappropriate antidiuretic hormone (SIADH)
- ○ **D.** Decreased potassium

8. A client was transferred to the hospital unit as a direct admit from a small community hospital. While the nurse is obtaining part of the admission history information, the client suddenly becomes semiconscious. Assessment reveals a systolic BP of 70, heart rate of 130, and respiratory rate of 24. What is the nurse's initial action?

Quick Answer: **376**
Detailed Answer: **379**

- ○ **A.** Lower the head of the bed
- ○ **B.** Initiate an IV with a large bore needle
- ○ **C.** Notify the physician
- ○ **D.** Call for the cardiopulmonary resuscitation team

9. The nurse is caring for a client post-myocardial infarction on the cardiac unit. The client is exhibiting symptoms of shock. Which clinical manifestation is the best indicator that the shock is cardiogenic rather than anaphylactic?

- ○ **A.** BP 90/60
- ○ **B.** Chest pain
- ○ **C.** Anxiety
- ○ **D.** Temp 98.6°F

10. While reading the progress notes on a client with cancer, the nurse notes a TNM classification of T1, N1, M0. What does this classification indicate?

- ○ **A.** The tumor is in situ, no regional lymph nodes, and no metastasis.
- ○ **B.** No evidence of primary tumor exists, lymph nodes can't be assessed, and metastasis can't be assessed.
- ○ **C.** The tumor is extended, with regional lymph node involvement and distant metastasis.
- ○ **D.** The tumor is extended and regional lymph nodes are involved, but there is no metastasis.

11. The nurse is caring for a client with leukemia who has received the drug (daunorubicin) Cerubidine. Which of the following common side effects would cause the most concern?

- ○ **A.** Nausea
- ○ **B.** Vomiting
- ○ **C.** Cardiotoxicity
- ○ **D.** Alopecia

12. The nurse is caring for an organ donor client with a severe head injury from an MVA. Which of the following is most important when caring for the organ donor client?

- ○ **A.** Maintenance of the BP at 90mmHg or greater
- ○ **B.** Maintenance of a normal temperature
- ○ **C.** Keeping the hematocrit at less than 28%
- ○ **D.** Ensuring a urinary output of at least 300mL/hr

13. The nurse is constructing a nursing care plan for a client post-operative open cholecystectomy. Which nursing diagnosis would be the priority for this client?

- ○ **A.** Risk for ineffective airway clearance
- ○ **B.** Activity intolerance
- ○ **C.** Risk for urinary retention
- ○ **D.** Acute pain

14. A client with a fractured leg is exhibiting shortness of breath, pain upon deep breathing, and hemoptysis. The nurse would determine that these clinical manifestations are indicative of:

○ **A.** Congestive heart failure

○ **B.** Pulmonary embolus

○ **C.** Adult respiratory distress syndrome

○ **D.** Tension pneumothorax

Quick Answer: 376
Detailed Answer: 380

Quick Answer: 376
Detailed Answer: 380

15. A nurse is preparing to mix and administer chemotherapy. What equipment would be unnecessary to obtain?

○ **A.** Surgical gloves

○ **B.** Luer lok fitting IV tubing

○ **C.** Surgical hat cover

○ **D.** Disposable long-sleeve gown

16. The charge nurse is assigning staff for the day. Staff consists of an RN, an LPN, and two certified nursing assistants. Which client assignment should be given to the nursing assistants?

○ **A.** Emergency exploratory laparotomy with a colon resection the previous shift

○ **B.** Client with a stroke who has been hospitalized for 2 days

○ **C.** A client with metastatic cancer on PCA morphine

○ **D.** New admission with diverticulitis

Quick Answer: 376
Detailed Answer: 380

17. The registered nurse is making shift assignments. Which client should be assigned to the licensed practical nurse (LPN)?

○ **A.** A diabetic with a foot ulcer

○ **B.** A client with a deep vein thrombosis receiving intravenous heparin

○ **C.** A client being weaned from a tracheostomy

○ **D.** A post-operative cholecystectomy with a T-tube

Quick Answer: 376
Detailed Answer: 380

18. A client with metastatic cancer of the lung has just been told the prognosis by the oncologist. The nurse hears the client state, "I don't believe the doctor; I think he has me confused with another patient." This is an example of which of Kubler-Ross' stages of dying?

○ **A.** Denial

○ **B.** Anger

○ **C.** Depression

○ **D.** Bargaining

Quick Answer: 376
Detailed Answer: 380

19. The surgical nurse is preparing a patient for surgery on the lower abdomen. In which position would the nurse most likely place the client for surgery on this area?

   ○ **A.** Lithotomy
   ○ **B.** Sim's
   ○ **C.** Prone
   ○ **D.** Trendelenburg

20. The nurse is performing a history on a client admitted for surgery in the morning. Which long-term medication in the client's history would be most important to report to the physician?

   ○ **A.** Prednisone
   ○ **B.** Lisinopril (Zestril)
   ○ **C.** Docusate (Colace)
   ○ **D.** Oscal D

21. A nurse is working in an endoscopy recovery area. Many of the clients are administered midazolam (Versed) to provide conscious sedation. Which medication is important to have available as an antidote for Versed?

   ○ **A.** Diazepam (Valium)
   ○ **B.** Naloxone (Narcan)
   ○ **C.** Flumazenil (Romazicon)
   ○ **D.** Florinef (Fludrocortisone)

22. The nurse is caring for a client with a cerebrovascular accident (CVA) who is complaining of being nauseated and is requesting an emesis basin. Which action would the nurse take first?

   ○ **A.** Administer an ordered antiemetic
   ○ **B.** Obtain an ice bag and apply to the client's throat
   ○ **C.** Turn the client to one side
   ○ **D.** Notify the physician

23. The nurse is assessing a client who had a colon resection 2 days ago. The client states, "I feel like my stitches have burst loose." Upon further assessment, dehiscence of the wound is noted. The nurse should:

   ○ **A.** Place the client in the prone position
   ○ **B.** Apply a sterile, saline-moistened dressing to the wound
   ○ **C.** Administer atropine to decrease abdominal secretions
   ○ **D.** Wrap the abdomen with an ACE bandage

24. A client with hepatitis C is scheduled for a liver biopsy. Which would the nurse include in the teaching plan for this client?

- ○ **A.** The client should lie on the left side after the procedure.
- ○ **B.** Cleansing enemas should be given the morning of the procedure.
- ○ **C.** Blood coagulation studies might be done before the biopsy.
- ○ **D.** The procedure is noninvasive and causes no pain.

Quick Answer: **376**
Detailed Answer: **381**

25. The nurse is caring for a client after a laryngectomy. The client is anxious, with a respiratory rate of 32 and an oxygen saturation of 88. The nurse's first action should be to:

- ○ **A.** Suction the client
- ○ **B.** Increase the oxygen flow rate
- ○ **C.** Notify the physician
- ○ **D.** Recheck the O$_2$ saturation

Quick Answer: **376**
Detailed Answer: **381**

26. The nurse is performing discharge teaching to a client who is on isoniazid (INH). Which diet selection would let the nurse know that the teaching has been ineffective?

- ○ **A.** Tuna casserole
- ○ **B.** Ham salad sandwich
- ○ **C.** Baked potato
- ○ **D.** Broiled beef roast

Quick Answer: **376**
Detailed Answer: **381**

27. A client with a head injury has an intracranial pressure (ICP) monitor in place. Cerebral perfusion pressure calculations are ordered. If the client's ICP is 22 and the mean pressure reading is 70, what is the client's cerebral perfusion pressure?

- ○ **A.** 92
- ○ **B.** 72
- ○ **C.** 58
- ○ **D.** 48

Quick Answer: **376**
Detailed Answer: **381**

28. A student nurse is observing a neurological nurse perform an assessment. When the nurse asks the client to "stick out his tongue," the nurse is assessing the function of which cranial nerve?

- ○ **A.** II optic
- ○ **B.** I olfactory
- ○ **C.** X vagus
- ○ **D.** XII hypoglossal

Quick Answer: **376**
Detailed Answer: **381**

29. Which set of vital signs would best indicate an increase in intracranial pressure?

    ○ **A.** BP 180/70, pulse 50, respirations 16, temperature 101°F

    ○ **B.** BP 100/70, pulse 64, respirations 20, temperature 98.6°F

    ○ **C.** BP 96/70, pulse 132, respirations 20, temperature 98.6°F

    ○ **D.** BP 130/80, pulse 50, respirations 18, temperature 99.6°F

30. The nurse is assessing the laboratory results of a client scheduled to receive phenytoin (Dilantin). The Dilantin level, drawn 2 hours ago, is 30mcg/mL. What is the appropriate nursing action?

    ○ **A.** Administer the Dilantin as scheduled

    ○ **B.** Hold the scheduled dose and notify the physician

    ○ **C.** Decrease the dosage from 100mg to 50mg

    ○ **D.** Increase the dosage to 200mg from 100mg

31. A client with sickle cell disease is admitted in active labor. Which nursing intervention would be most helpful in preventing a sickling crisis?

    ○ **A.** Obtaining blood pressures every 2 hours

    ○ **B.** Administering pain medication every 3–4 hours as ordered

    ○ **C.** Monitoring arterial blood gas results

    ○ **D.** Administering IV fluids at ordered rate of 200mL/hr

32. A client is admitted with a diagnosis of pernicious anemia. Which of the following signs or symptoms would indicate that the client has been noncompliant with ordered B12 injections?

    ○ **A.** Hyperactivity in the evening hours

    ○ **B.** Weight gain of 5 pounds in 1 week

    ○ **C.** Paresthesia of hands and feet

    ○ **D.** Diarrhea stools several times a day

33. The nurse has performed nutritional teaching on a client with gout who is placed on a low-purine diet. Which selection by the client would indicate that teaching has been ineffective?

    ○ **A.** Cabbage

    ○ **B.** Apple

    ○ **C.** Peach cobbler

    ○ **D.** Spinach

34. The nurse is caring for a 70-year-old client with hypovolemia who is receiving a blood transfusion. Assessment findings reveal crackles on chest auscultation and distended neck veins. What is the nurse's initial action?

- ○ **A.** Slow the transfusion
- ○ **B.** Document the finding as the only action
- ○ **C.** Stop the blood transfusion and turn on the normal saline
- ○ **D.** Assess the client's pupils

35. The orthopedic nurse should be particularly alert for a fat embolus in which of the following clients having the greatest risk for this complication after a fracture?

- ○ **A.** A 50-year-old with a fractured fibula
- ○ **B.** A 20-year-old female with a wrist fracture
- ○ **C.** A 21-year-old male with a fractured femur
- ○ **D.** An 8-year-old with a fractured arm

36. The nurse has performed discharge teaching to a client in need of a high-iron diet. The nurse recognizes that teaching has been effective when the client selects which meal plan?

- ○ **A.** Hamburger, French fries, and orange juice
- ○ **B.** Sliced veal, spinach salad, and whole-wheat roll
- ○ **C.** Vegetable lasagna, Caesar salad, and toast
- ○ **D.** Bacon, lettuce, and tomato sandwich; potato chips; and tea

37. An elderly female is admitted with a fractured right femoral neck. Which clinical manifestation would the nurse expect to find?

- ○ **A.** Free movement of the right leg
- ○ **B.** Abduction of the right leg
- ○ **C.** Internal rotation of the right hip
- ○ **D.** Shortening of the right leg

38. The nurse is performing the skill of intramuscular injection by the Z track method. Which technique would the nurse utilize to prevent tracking of the medication?

- ○ **A.** Inject the medication in the deltoid muscle
- ○ **B.** Use a 22-gauge needle
- ○ **C.** Omit aspirating for blood before injecting
- ○ **D.** Draw up 0.2mL of air after the proper medication dose

39. A client is admitted to the surgical unit following a transurethral prostactectomy (TURP). The nurse administers a B&O suppository to help prevent bladder spasms. The nurse would observe the client for:

- ○ **A.** Insomnia and hyperactivity
- ○ **B.** Physiological dependence on the drug
- ○ **C.** Nausea and vomiting
- ○ **D.** Diarrhea and abdominal cramping

Quick Answer: **376**
Detailed Answer: **382**

40. The nurse caring for a client with anemia recognizes which clinical manifestation as the one that is specific for a hemolytic type of anemia?

- ○ **A.** Jaundice
- ○ **B.** Anorexia
- ○ **C.** Tachycardia
- ○ **D.** Fatigue

Quick Answer: **376**
Detailed Answer: **383**

41. A client with cancer who is receiving chemotherapeutic drugs has been given injections of (pegfilgastrin) Neulasta. Which laboratory value reveals that the drug is producing the desired effect?

- ○ **A.** Hemoglobin of 13.5g/dL
- ○ **B.** White blood cells count of 6,000/mm
- ○ **C.** Platelet count of 300,000/mm
- ○ **D.** HCT 39%

Quick Answer: **376**
Detailed Answer: **383**

42. The nurse is performing discharge teaching on a client with polycythemia vera. Which would be included in the teaching plan?

- ○ **A.** Avoid large crowds
- ○ **B.** Keep the head of the bed elevated at night
- ○ **C.** Wear socks and gloves when going outside
- ○ **D.** Recognize clinical manifestations of thrombosis

Quick Answer: **376**
Detailed Answer: **383**

43. A client is being discharged after lithotripsy for removal of a kidney stone. Which statement by the client indicates understanding of the nurse's instructions?

- ○ **A.** "I'll need to strain my urine the first thing in the morning."
- ○ **B.** "I will need to save all urine for the next 2 days and take it to the laboratory to be examined and strained."
- ○ **C.** "I will be careful to strain all the urine and save the stone."
- ○ **D.** "I won't need to strain my urine now that the procedure is complete."

Quick Answer: **376**
Detailed Answer: **383**

44. The nurse is caring for a client with osteoporosis who is being discharged on (alendronate) Fosamax. Which statement would indicate a need for further teaching?

Quick Answer: **376**
Detailed Answer: **383**

- ○ **A.** "I should take the medication immediately before bedtime."
- ○ **B.** "I should remain in an upright position for 30 minutes after taking the medication."
- ○ **C.** "The medication should be taken by mouth with water."
- ○ **D.** "I should not have any food with this medication."

45. A client is being evaluated for carpel tunnel syndrome. The nurse is observed tapping over the median nerve in the wrist and asking the client if there is pain or tingling. Which assessment is the nurse performing?

Quick Answer: **376**
Detailed Answer: **383**

- ○ **A.** Phalen's maneuver
- ○ **B.** Tinel's sign
- ○ **C.** Kernig's sign
- ○ **D.** Brudzinski's sign

46. The nurse is caring for a client who is recovering from a fractured femur. Which diet selection would be best for this client?

Quick Answer: **376**
Detailed Answer: **383**

- ○ **A.** Loaded baked potato, fried chicken, and tea
- ○ **B.** Dressed cheeseburger, French fries, and Coke
- ○ **C.** Tuna fish salad on sourdough bread, potato chips, and skim milk
- ○ **D.** Mandarin orange salad, broiled chicken, and milk

47. The nurse working in the emergency department realizes that it would be contraindicated to induce vomiting if someone had ingested which of the following?

Quick Answer: **376**
Detailed Answer: **383**

- ○ **A.** Ibuprofen
- ○ **B.** Aspirin
- ○ **C.** Vitamins
- ○ **D.** Gasoline

48. A client with AIDS has impaired nutrition because of diarrhea. Which diet selection by the client would indicate a need for further teaching of foods that can worsen the diarrhea?

Quick Answer: **376**
Detailed Answer: **383**

- ○ **A.** Tossed salad
- ○ **B.** Baked chicken
- ○ **C.** Broiled fish
- ○ **D.** Steamed rice

49. The nurse has just received a report from the previous shift. Which of the following clients should the nurse visit first?

Quick Answer: **376**
Detailed Answer: **383**

- ○ **A.** A 50-year-old COPD client with a PCO_2 of 50
- ○ **B.** A 24-year-old admitted after an MVA complaining of shortness of breath
- ○ **C.** A client with cancer requesting pain medication
- ○ **D.** A 1-day post-operative cholecystectomy with a temperature of 100°F

50. The nurse is performing a breast exam on a client when she discovers a mass. Which characteristic of the mass would most indicate a reason for concern?

Quick Answer: **376**
Detailed Answer: **384**

- ○ **A.** Tender to touch
- ○ **B.** Regular shape
- ○ **C.** Moves easily
- ○ **D.** Firm to the touch

51. The nurse is caring for a client after a motor vehicle accident. The client has a fractured tibia, and bone is noted protruding through the skin. Which action is of priority?

Quick Answer: **376**
Detailed Answer: **384**

- ○ **A.** Provide manual traction above and below the leg
- ○ **B.** Cover the bone area with a sterile dressing
- ○ **C.** Apply an ACE bandage around the entire lower limb
- ○ **D.** Place the client in the prone position

52. The RN on the oncology unit is preparing to mix and administer amphoteracin B (Fungizone) to a client. Which action is contraindicated for administering this drug IV?

Quick Answer: **376**
Detailed Answer: **384**

- ○ **A.** Mix the drug with normal saline solution
- ○ **B.** Administer the drug over 4–6 hours
- ○ **C.** Hydrate with IV fluids 2 hours before the infusion
- ○ **D.** Premedicate the client with ordered acetaminophen (Tylenol) and diphenhydramine (Benadryl)

53. A nurse is administering a blood transfusion to a client on the oncology unit. Which clinical manifestation indicates an acute hemolytic reaction to the blood?

Quick Answer: **376**
Detailed Answer: **384**

- ○ **A.** Low back pain
- ○ **B.** A temperature of 101°F
- ○ **C.** Urticaria
- ○ **D.** Neck vein distention

54. The nurse caring for a client diagnosed with metastatic cancer of the bone is exhibiting mental confusion and a BP of 150/100. Which laboratory value would correlate with the client's symptoms reflecting a common complication with this diagnosis?

Quick Answer: **376**
Detailed Answer: **384**

  ○ **A.** Potassium 5.2mEq/L

  ○ **B.** Calcium 13mg/dL

  ○ **C.** Inorganic phosphorus 1.7mEq/L

  ○ **D.** Sodium 138mEq/L

55. A client with a stroke and malnutrition has been placed on Total Parenteral Nutrition (TPN). The nurse notes air entering the client via the central line. Which initial action is most appropriate?

Quick Answer: **376**
Detailed Answer: **384**

  ○ **A.** Notify the physician

  ○ **B.** Elevate the head of the bed

  ○ **C.** Place the client in the left lateral decubitus position

  ○ **D.** Stop the TPN and hang D5 1/2 NS

56. The nurse is preparing a client for cervical uterine radiation implant insertion. Which will be included in the teaching plan?

Quick Answer: **376**
Detailed Answer: **384**

  ○ **A.** TV or telephone use will not be allowed while the implant is in place.

  ○ **B.** A Foley catheter is usually inserted.

  ○ **C.** A high-fiber diet is recommended.

  ○ **D.** Excretions will be considered radioactive.

57. The nurse is caring for a client with a head injury who has an intracranial pressure monitor in place. Assessment reveals an ICP reading of 66. What is the nurse's best action?

Quick Answer: **376**
Detailed Answer: **384**

  ○ **A.** Notify the physician

  ○ **B.** Record the reading as the only action

  ○ **C.** Turn the client and recheck the reading

  ○ **D.** Place the client supine

58. The nurse is caring for a client with leukemia who is receiving the drug doxorubicin (Adriamycin). Which toxic effects of this drug would be reported to the physician immediately?

Quick Answer: **376**
Detailed Answer: **384**

  ○ **A.** Rales and distended neck veins

  ○ **B.** Red discoloration of the urine and output of 75mL the previous hour

  ○ **C.** Nausea and vomiting

  ○ **D.** Elevated BUN and dry, flaky skin

59. A client has developed diabetes insipidous after removal of a pituitary tumor. Which finding would the nurse expect?

Quick Answer: **376**
Detailed Answer: **384**

- ○ **A.** Polyuria
- ○ **B.** Hypertension
- ○ **C.** Polyphagia
- ○ **D.** Hyperkalemia

60. A client with cancer received platelet infusions 24 hours ago. Which of the following assessment findings would indicate the most therapeutic effect from the transfusions?

Quick Answer: **376**
Detailed Answer: **384**

- ○ **A.** Hgb level increase from 8.9 to 10.6
- ○ **B.** Temperature reading of 99.4°F
- ○ **C.** White blood cell count of 11,000
- ○ **D.** Decrease in oozing of blood from IV site

61. A client is admitted with Parkinson's disease who has been taking Carbidopa/levodopa (Sinemet) for 1 year. Which clinical manifestation would be most important to report?

Quick Answer: **376**
Detailed Answer: **385**

- ○ **A.** Dry mouth
- ○ **B.** Spasmodic eye winking
- ○ **C.** Dark urine
- ○ **D.** Dizziness

62. The nurse who is caring for a client with cancer notes a WBC of 500 on the laboratory results. Which intervention would be most appropriate to include in the client's plan of care?

Quick Answer: **376**
Detailed Answer: **385**

- ○ **A.** Assess temperature every 4 hours because of risk for hypothermia
- ○ **B.** Instruct the client to avoid large crowds and people who are sick
- ○ **C.** Instruct in the use of a soft toothbrush
- ○ **D.** Assess for hematuria

63. A client with Crohn's disease requires TPN to provide adequate nutrition. The nurse finds the TPN bag empty. What fluid would the nurse select to hang until another bag is prepared in the pharmacy?

Quick Answer: **376**
Detailed Answer: **385**

- ○ **A.** Lactated Ringers
- ○ **B.** Normal saline
- ○ **C.** D10W
- ○ **D.** Normosol R

64. The nurse is caring for a client with possible cervical cancer. What clinical data would the nurse most likely find in the client's history?

   - ○ **A.** Post-coital vaginal bleeding
   - ○ **B.** Nausea and vomiting
   - ○ **C.** Foul-smelling vaginal discharge
   - ○ **D.** Hyperthermia

Quick Answer: **376**
Detailed Answer: **385**

65. The nurse caring for a client with myasthenias gravis recognizes which of the following as the priority nursing diagnosis?

   - ○ **A.** Risk for injury
   - ○ **B.** Acute pain
   - ○ **C.** Ineffective airway clearance
   - ○ **D.** Impaired mobility

Quick Answer: **376**
Detailed Answer: **385**

66. A client is scheduled to undergo a bone marrow aspiration from the sternum. What position would the nurse assist the client into for this procedure?

   - ○ **A.** Dorsal recumbent
   - ○ **B.** Supine
   - ○ **C.** Fowler's
   - ○ **D.** Lithotomy

Quick Answer: **376**
Detailed Answer: **385**

67. The nurse is caring for a client with a head injury who has increased ICP. The physician plans to reduce the cerebral edema by constricting cerebral blood vessels. Which physician order would serve this purpose?

   - ○ **A.** Hyperventilation per mechanical ventilation
   - ○ **B.** Insertion of a ventricular shunt
   - ○ **C.** Furosemide (Lasix)
   - ○ **D.** Solu medrol

Quick Answer: **376**
Detailed Answer: **385**

68. A client with a T6 injury 6 months ago develops facial flushing and a BP of 210/106. After elevating the head of the bed, which is the most appropriate nursing action?

   - ○ **A.** Notify the physician
   - ○ **B.** Assess the client for a distended bladder
   - ○ **C.** Apply oxygen at 3L/min
   - ○ **D.** Increase the IV fluids

Quick Answer: **376**
Detailed Answer: **385**

69. The nurse is performing an admission history for a client recovering from a stroke. Medication history reveals the drug clopidogrel (Plavix). Which clinical manifestation alerts the nurse to an adverse effect of this drug?

- ○ **A.** Epistaxis
- ○ **B.** Abdominal distention
- ○ **C.** Nausea
- ○ **D.** Hyperactivity

70. The nurse caring for a client with a head injury would recognize which assessment finding as the most indicative of increased ICP?

- ○ **A.** Nausea and vomiting
- ○ **B.** Headache
- ○ **C.** Dizziness
- ○ **D.** Papilledema

71. A client with angina is experiencing migraine headaches. The physician has prescribed Sumatriptan succinate (Imitrex). Which nursing action is most appropriate?

- ○ **A.** Call the physician to question the prescription order
- ○ **B.** Try to obtain samples for the client to take home
- ○ **C.** Perform discharge teaching regarding this drug
- ○ **D.** Consult social services for financial assistance with obtaining the drug

72. A client with COPD is in respiratory failure. Which of the following results would be the most sensitive indicator that the client requires a mechanical ventilator?

- ○ **A.** PCO_2 58
- ○ **B.** SaO_2 90
- ○ **C.** PH 7.23
- ○ **D.** HCO_3 30

73. The nurse in the emergency room is caring for a client with multiple rib fractures and a pulmonary contusion. Assessment reveals a respiratory rate of 38, a heart rate of 136, and restlessness. Which associated assessment finding would require immediate intervention?

- ○ **A.** Occasional hemoptysis
- ○ **B.** Midline trachea with wheezing on auscultation
- ○ **C.** Subcutaneous air and absent breath sounds
- ○ **D.** Pain when breathing deeply, with rales in the upper lobes

Quick Check

74. The nurse is caring for a client with myasthenias gravis who is having trouble breathing. The nurse would encourage which of the following positions for maximal lung expansion?

Quick Answer: 376
Detailed Answer: 386

- ○ **A.** Supine with no pillow, to maintain patent airway
- ○ **B.** Side-lying with back support
- ○ **C.** Prone with head turned to one side
- ○ **D.** Sitting or in high Fowler's

75. The nurse is caring for clients on a respiratory unit. Upon receiving the following client reports, which client should be seen first?

Quick Answer: 376
Detailed Answer: 386

- ○ **A.** Client with emphysema expecting discharge
- ○ **B.** Bronchitis client receiving IV antibiotics
- ○ **C.** Bronchitis client with edema and neck vein distention
- ○ **D.** COPD client with PO_2 of 85

76. A client has sustained a severe head injury and damaged the preoccipital lobe. The nurse should remain particularly alert for which of the following problems?

Quick Answer: 376
Detailed Answer: 386

- ○ **A.** Visual impairment
- ○ **B.** Swallowing difficulty
- ○ **C.** Impaired judgment
- ○ **D.** Hearing impairment

77. The nurse is caring for a client with epilepsy who is to receive Dilantin 100mg IV push. The client has an IV of D51/2NS infusing at 100mL/hr. When administering the Dilantin, the nurse should first:

Quick Answer: 376
Detailed Answer: 386

- ○ **A.** Obtain an ambu bag and put it at bedside
- ○ **B.** Insert a 16g IV catheter
- ○ **C.** Flush the IV line with normal saline
- ○ **D.** Premedicate with phenergan IV push

78. A client with increased intracranial pressure is receiving Mannitol and Lasix. The nurse recognizes that these two drugs are given to reverse which effect?

Quick Answer: 376
Detailed Answer: 386

- ○ **A.** Energy failure
- ○ **B.** Excessive intracellular calcium accumulation
- ○ **C.** Cellular edema
- ○ **D.** Excessive glutamate release

79. The nurse is assessing a client upon arrival to the emergency department. Partial airway obstruction is suspected. Which clinical manifestation is a late sign of airway obstruction?

    Quick Answer: **376**
    Detailed Answer: **386**

    ○ **A.** Rales auscultated in breath sounds

    ○ **B.** Restlessness

    ○ **C.** Cyanotic ear lobes

    ○ **D.** Inspiratory stridor

80. The nurse is working in the trauma unit of the emergency room when a 24-year-old female is admitted after an MVA. The client is bleeding profusely and a blood transfusion is ordered. Which would the nurse be prepared to administer without a type and crossmatch?

    Quick Answer: **376**
    Detailed Answer: **386**

    ○ **A.** AB positive

    ○ **B.** AB negative

    ○ **C.** O positive

    ○ **D.** O negative

81. When preparing a client for magnetic resonance imaging, the nurse should implement which of the following?

    Quick Answer: **376**
    Detailed Answer: **386**

    ○ **A.** Obtain informed consent and administer atropine 0.4mg

    ○ **B.** Scrub the injection site for 15 minutes

    ○ **C.** Remove any jewelry and inquire about metal implants

    ○ **D.** Administer Benadryl 50mg/mL IV

82. Upon admission to the hospital, a client reports having "the worst headache I've ever had." The nurse should give the highest priority to:

    Quick Answer: **376**
    Detailed Answer: **386**

    ○ **A.** Administering pain medication

    ○ **B.** Starting oxygen

    ○ **C.** Performing neuro checks

    ○ **D.** Inserting a Foley catheter

83. The nurse is caring for a client with an acoustic neuroma brain tumor. The location of this tumor warrants which of the following nursing diagnosis as the highest priority?

    Quick Answer: **376**
    Detailed Answer: **386**

    ○ **A.** High risk for constipation

    ○ **B.** Fluid volume deficit

    ○ **C.** Ineffective coping

    ○ **D.** High risk for injury

84. The client is admitted to the ER with multiple rib fractures on the right. The nurse's assessment reveals that an area over the right clavicle is puffy and that there is a "crackling" noise with palpation. The nurse should further assess the client for which of the following problems?

- ○ **A.** Flail chest
- ○ **B.** Subcutaneous emphysema
- ○ **C.** Infiltrated subclavian IV
- ○ **D.** Pneumothorax

85. A client has an order for Demerol 75mg and atropine 0.4mg IM as a pre-operative medication. The Demerol vial contains 50mg/mL, and atropine is available 0.4mg/mL. How many milliliters will the nurse administer in total?

- ○ **A.** 1.0
- ○ **B.** 1.7
- ○ **C.** 2.5
- ○ **D.** 3.0

86. Nimotop (Nimodipine) is ordered for the client with a ruptured cerebral aneurysm. The nurse recognizes that the desired effect of this drug is to:

- ○ **A.** Prevent the influx of calcium into cells
- ○ **B.** Restore the client's blood pressure to a normal reading
- ○ **C.** Prevent the inflammatory process
- ○ **D.** Dissolve the clot that has formed

87. A client is admitted to the hospital with seizures. The client has jerking of the right arm and twitching of the face, but is alert and aware of the seizure. This behavior is characteristic of which type of seizure?

- ○ **A.** Absence
- ○ **B.** Complex partial
- ○ **C.** Simple partial
- ○ **D.** Tonic-clonic

88. The intensive care unit is full and the emergency room just called in a report on a ventilator-dependent client who is being admitted to the medical surgical unit. It would be essential that the nurse have which piece of equipment at the client's bedside?

    ○ **A.** Cardiac monitor

    ○ **B.** Intravenous controller

    ○ **C.** Manual resuscitator

    ○ **D.** Oxygen by nasal cannula

Quick Answer: **376**
Detailed Answer: **387**

89. The nurse is caring for a client on a ventilator that is set on intermittent mandatory ventilation (IMV). Assessment on the ventilator is IMV mode of 8 breaths per minute. The nurse assesses the client's respiratory rate of 13 per minute. These findings indicate that:

    ○ **A.** The client is "fighting" the ventilator.

    ○ **B.** Pressure support ventilation is being used.

    ○ **C.** Additional breaths are being delivered by the ventilator.

    ○ **D.** The client is breathing five additional breaths on his own.

Quick Answer: **376**
Detailed Answer: **387**

90. The nurse has given instructions on pursed-lip breathing to a client with COPD. Which statement by the client would indicate effective teaching?

    ○ **A.** "I should inhale through my mouth."

    ○ **B.** "I should tighten my abdominal muscles with inhalation."

    ○ **C.** "I should contract my abdominal muscles with exhalation."

    ○ **D.** "I should make inhalation twice as long as exhalation."

Quick Answer: **376**
Detailed Answer: **387**

91. A client is receiving aminophylline IV. The nurse monitors the theophylline blood level and assesses that the level is within therapeutic range when it is:

    ○ **A.** 5ug/mL

    ○ **B.** 8ug/mL

    ○ **C.** 15ug/mL

    ○ **D.** 25ug/mL

Quick Answer: **377**
Detailed Answer: **387**

92. The nurse is assessing the arterial blood gases (ABG) of a chest trauma client with the results of pH 7.35, PO_2 85, PCO_2 55, and HCO_3 27. These ABG values indicate that the client is in:

    ○ **A.** Uncompensated respiratory acidosis

    ○ **B.** Uncompensated metabolic acidosis

    ○ **C.** Compensated respiratory acidosis

    ○ **D.** Compensated metabolic acidosis

Quick Answer: **377**
Detailed Answer: **387**

93. A pneumonectomy is performed on a client with lung cancer. Which of the following would probably be omitted from the client's plan of care?

Quick Answer: **377**
Detailed Answer: **387**

   ○ **A.** Closed chest drainage
   ○ **B.** Pain-control measures
   ○ **C.** Supplemental oxygen
   ○ **D.** Coughing and deep-breathing exercises

94. When planning the care for a client after a posterior fossa (infratentorial) craniotomy, which action is contraindicated?

Quick Answer: **377**
Detailed Answer: **387**

   ○ **A.** Keeping the client flat on one side
   ○ **B.** Elevating the head of the bed 30°
   ○ **C.** Log-rolling or turning as a unit
   ○ **D.** Keeping the neck in a neutral position

95. The nurse is performing discharge teaching on a client with ulcerative colitis who has been placed on a low-residue diet. Which food would need to be eliminated from this client's diet?

Quick Answer: **377**
Detailed Answer: **387**

   ○ **A.** Roasted chicken
   ○ **B.** Noodles
   ○ **C.** Cooked broccoli
   ○ **D.** Roast beef

96. The nurse is assisting a client with diverticulitis to select appropriate foods. Which food should be avoided?

Quick Answer: **377**
Detailed Answer: **388**

   ○ **A.** Bran
   ○ **B.** Fresh peach
   ○ **C.** Tomato and cucumber salad
   ○ **D.** Dinner roll

97. A client is admitted with a possible bowel obstruction. Which question during the nursing history is least helpful in obtaining information regarding this diagnosis?

Quick Answer: **377**
Detailed Answer: **388**

   ○ **A.** "Tell me about your pain."
   ○ **B.** "What does your vomit look like?"
   ○ **C.** "Describe your usual diet."
   ○ **D.** "Have you noticed an increase in abdominal size?"

98. The nurse is caring for a client with epilepsy who is being treated with carbamazepine (Tegretol). Which laboratory value might indicate a serious side effect of this drug?

   ○ **A.** BUN 10mg/dL
   ○ **B.** Hemoglobin 13.0gm/dL
   ○ **C.** WBC 4,000/mm³
   ○ **D.** Platelets 200,000/mm³

Quick Answer: **377**
Detailed Answer: **388**

99. A client is admitted with a tumor in the parietal lobe. Which symptoms would be expected due to this tumor's location?

   ○ **A.** Hemiplegia
   ○ **B.** Aphasia
   ○ **C.** Paresthesia
   ○ **D.** Nausea

Quick Answer: **377**
Detailed Answer: **388**

100. A client weighing 150 pounds has received burns over 50% of his body at 1200 hours. Using the Parkland formula, calculate the expected amount of fluid that the client should receive by 2000 hours.

   ○ **A.** 3,400
   ○ **B.** 6,800
   ○ **C.** 10,200
   ○ **D.** 13,600

Quick Answer: **377**
Detailed Answer: **388**

101. The nurse is caring for a client post-op femoral popliteal bypass graft. Which post-operative assessment finding would require immediate physician notification?

   ○ **A.** Edema of the extremity and pain at the incision site
   ○ **B.** A temperature of 99.6°F and redness of the incision
   ○ **C.** Serous drainage noted at the surgical area
   ○ **D.** A loss of posterior tibial and dorsalis pedis pulses

Quick Answer: **377**
Detailed Answer: **388**

102. A client admitted with gastroenteritis and a potassium level of 2.9mEq/dL has been placed on telemetry. Which ECG finding would the nurse expect to find due to the client's potassium results?

   ○ **A.** A depressed ST segment
   ○ **B.** An elevated T wave
   ○ **C.** An absent P wave
   ○ **D.** A flattened QRS

Quick Answer: **377**
Detailed Answer: **388**

103. A client is experiencing acute abdominal pain. Which abdominal assessment sequence is appropriate for the nurse to use for examination of the abdomen?

- ○ **A.** Inspect, palpate, auscultate, percuss
- ○ **B.** Inspect, auscultate, palpate, percuss
- ○ **C.** Auscultate, inspect, palpate, percuss
- ○ **D.** Percuss, palpate, auscultate, inspect

Quick Answer: **377**
Detailed Answer: **388**

104. The nurse is to administer a cleansing enema to a client scheduled for colon surgery. Which client position would be appropriate?

- ○ **A.** Prone
- ○ **B.** Supine
- ○ **C.** Left Sim's
- ○ **D.** Dorsal recumbent

Quick Answer: **377**
Detailed Answer: **388**

105. The nurse is caring for a client following a crushing injury to the chest. Which finding would be most indicative of a tension pneumothorax?

- ○ **A.** Frothy hemoptysis
- ○ **B.** Trachea shift toward the unaffected side of the chest
- ○ **C.** Subcutaneous emphysema noted at the anterior chest
- ○ **D.** Opening chest wound with a whistle sound emitting from the area

Quick Answer: **377**
Detailed Answer: **389**

106. The nurse receives a report from the paramedic on four trauma victims. Which client would need to be treated first? A client with:

- ○ **A.** Lower rib fractures and a stable chest wall
- ○ **B.** Bruising on the anterior chest wall and a possible pulmonary contusion
- ○ **C.** Gun shot wound with open pneumothorax unstabilized
- ○ **D.** Dyspnea, stabilized with intubation and manual resuscitator

Quick Answer: **377**
Detailed Answer: **389**

107. The nurse is discharging a client with asthma who has a prescription for zafirlukast (Accolate). Which comment by the client would indicate a need for further teaching?

- ○ **A.** "I should take this medication with meals."
- ○ **B.** "I need to report flulike symptoms to my doctor."
- ○ **C.** "My doctor might order liver tests while I'm on this drug."
- ○ **D.** "If I'm already having an asthma attack, this drug will not stop it."

Quick Answer: **377**
Detailed Answer: **389**

108. A client is 4 hours post-op left carotid endarterectomy. Which assessment finding would cause the nurse the most concern?

Quick Answer: **377**
Detailed Answer: **389**

- ○ **A.** Temperature 99.4°F, heart rate 110, respiratory rate 24
- ○ **B.** Drowsiness, urinary output of 50mL the past hour, 1cm blood drainage noted on surgical dressing
- ○ **C.** BP 120/60, lethargic, right-sided weakness
- ○ **D.** Alert and oriented, BP 168/96, heart rate 70

109. The RN is making assignments on a 12-bed unit. Staff consists of one RN and two certified nursing assistants. Which client should be self-assigned?

Quick Answer: **377**
Detailed Answer: **389**

- ○ **A.** A client receiving decadron for emphysema
- ○ **B.** A client with chest trauma and a new onset of hemoptysis
- ○ **C.** A client with rib fractures and an O_2 saturation of 93%
- ○ **D.** A client 2 days post-operative lung surgery with a pulse oximetry of 92%

110. The nurse caring for a client after a suspected CVA recognizes which nursing diagnosis as the priority?

Quick Answer: **377**
Detailed Answer: **389**

- ○ **A.** Impaired communication
- ○ **B.** Sensory perceptual alteration
- ○ **C.** Alteration in cerebral tissue perfusion
- ○ **D.** Impaired mobility

111. A client is being discharged on Coumadin after hospitalization for a deep vein thrombosis. The nurse recognizes that which food would be restricted while the client is on this medication?

Quick Answer: **377**
Detailed Answer: **389**

- ○ **A.** Lettuce
- ○ **B.** Apples
- ○ **C.** Potatoes
- ○ **D.** Macaroni

112. Which assessment finding in a client with COPD indicates to the nurse that the respiratory problem is chronic?

Quick Answer: **377**
Detailed Answer: **389**

- ○ **A.** Wheezing on exhalation
- ○ **B.** Productive cough
- ○ **C.** Clubbing of fingers
- ○ **D.** Cyanosis

113. A client who has just undergone a laparoscopic cholecystectomy complains of "free air pain." What would be your best action?

- ○ **A.** Ambulate the client
- ○ **B.** Instruct the client to breathe deeply and cough
- ○ **C.** Maintain the client on bed rest with his legs elevated
- ○ **D.** Insert an NG tube to low wall suction

Quick Answer: **377**
Detailed Answer: **389**

114. The RN is planning client assignments. Which is the least appropriate task for the nursing assistant?

- ○ **A.** Assisting a COPD client admitted 2 days ago to get up in the chair
- ○ **B.** Feeding a client with bronchitis who is paralyzed on the right side
- ○ **C.** Accompanying a discharged emphysema client to the transportation area
- ○ **D.** Assessing an emphysema client complaining of difficulty breathing

Quick Answer: **377**
Detailed Answer: **389**

115. When providing care for a client with pancreatitis, the nurse would anticipate which of the following orders?

- ○ **A.** Force fluids to 3,000mL/24 hours
- ○ **B.** Insert a nasogastric tube and connect it to low intermittent suction
- ○ **C.** Place the client in reverse Trendelenburg position
- ○ **D.** Place the client in enteric isolation

Quick Answer: **377**
Detailed Answer: **389**

116. The nurse is performing a neurological assessment on a client admitted with TIAs. Assessment findings reveal an absence of the gag reflex. The nurse suspects injury to:

- ○ **A.** XII (hypoglossal)
- ○ **B.** X (vagus)
- ○ **C.** IX (glossopharyngeal)
- ○ **D.** VII (facial)

Quick Answer: **377**
Detailed Answer: **390**

117. The nurse arrives at a motorcycle accident and finds the client unresponsive, apneic, and pulseless. After calling for a spectator to help, what would be the nurse's next action?

- ○ **A.** Ventilate with a mouth-to-mask device
- ○ **B.** Begin chest compressions
- ○ **C.** Administer a precordial thump
- ○ **D.** Open the airway

Quick Answer: **377**
Detailed Answer: **390**

118. A client with gallstones and obstructive jaundice is experiencing severe itching. The physician has prescribed cholestyramine (Questran). The client asks, "How does this drug work?" What is the nurse's best response?

- ○ **A.** "It blocks histamine, reducing the allergic response."
- ○ **B.** "It inhibits the enzyme responsible for bile excretion."
- ○ **C.** "It decreases the amount of bile in the gallbladder."
- ○ **D.** "It binds with bile acids and is excreted in bowel movements with stool."

119. A client with inflammatory bowel disease (IBD) requires an illeostomy. The nurse would instruct the client to do which of the following measures as an essential part of caring for the stoma?

- ○ **A.** Perform massage of the stoma three times a day
- ○ **B.** Include high-fiber foods in the diet, especially nuts
- ○ **C.** Limit fluid intake to prevent loose stools
- ○ **D.** Cleanse the peristomal skin meticulously

120. Diphenoxylate hydrochloride and atropine sulfate (Lomotil) is prescribed for the client with ulcerative colitis. The nurse realizes that the medication is having a therapeutic effect when the following is noted:

- ○ **A.** There is an absence of peristalsis.
- ○ **B.** The number of diarrhea stools decreases.
- ○ **C.** Cramping in the abdomen has increased.
- ○ **D.** Abdominal girth size increases.

121. A nurse is assisting the physician with chest tube removal. To remove the chest tube, the client is instructed to:

- ○ **A.** Take a deep breath, exhale, and bear down
- ○ **B.** Hold the breath for 2 minutes and exhale slowly
- ○ **C.** Exhale upon actual removal of the tube
- ○ **D.** Continually breathe deeply in and out during removal

122. A client with advanced Alzheimer's disease has been prescribed haloperidol (Haldol). What clinical manifestation suggests that the client is experiencing side effects from this medication?

- ○ **A.** Cough
- ○ **B.** Tremors
- ○ **C.** Diarrhea
- ○ **D.** Pitting edema

123. A student in a cardiac unit is performing auscultation of a client's heart. The nurse recognizes that the student is performing pulmonic auscultation correctly when the stethoscope is placed:

- ○ **A.** Between the apex and the sternum
- ○ **B.** At the fifth intercostal space at the left midclavicular line
- ○ **C.** At the second intercostal space, left of the sternum
- ○ **D.** At the manubrium

Quick Answer: **377**
Detailed Answer: **390**

124. A client with Alzheimer's disease has been prescribed donepezil (Aricept). Which information should the nurse include in the teaching plan for a client on Aricept?

- ○ **A.** "Take the medication with meals."
- ○ **B.** "The medicine can cause dizziness, so rise slowly."
- ○ **C.** "If a dose is skipped, take two the next time."
- ○ **D.** "The pill can cause an increase in heart rate."

Quick Answer: **377**
Detailed Answer: **390**

125. A client who had major abdominal surgery is having delayed healing of the wound. Which laboratory test result would most closely correlate with this problem?

- ○ **A.** Decreased albumin
- ○ **B.** Decreased creatinine
- ○ **C.** Increased calcium
- ○ **D.** Increased sodium

Quick Answer: **377**
Detailed Answer: **390**

126. A client is admitted to the medical-surgical unit with a report of severe hematemesis. The nurse should give priority to:

- ○ **A.** Performing an assessment
- ○ **B.** Obtaining a blood permit
- ○ **C.** Initiating an IV with a large-bore needle
- ○ **D.** Inserting an NG tube

Quick Answer: **377**
Detailed Answer: **390**

127. The nurse caring for a client with a suspected peptic ulcer recognizes which exam as the one most reliable in diagnosing the disease?

- ○ **A.** Upper-gastrointestinal x-ray
- ○ **B.** Gastric analysis
- ○ **C.** Endoscopy
- ○ **D.** Barium studies

Quick Answer: **377**
Detailed Answer: **391**

128. On the second post-operative day after a subtotal thyroidectomy, the client tells the nurse, "I feel numbness and my face is twitching." What is the nurse's best initial action?

   ○ **A.** Offer mouth care

   ○ **B.** Loosen the neck dressing

   ○ **C.** Notify the physician

   ○ **D.** Document the finding as the only action

129. A client with adult respiratory distress syndrome has been placed on mechanical ventilation with PEEP. Which finding would indicate to the nurse that the client is experiencing the undesirable effect of an increase in airway and chest pressure?

   ○ **A.** A PO_2 of 88

   ○ **B.** Rales on auscultation

   ○ **C.** Blood pressure decrease to 90/48 from 120/70

   ○ **D.** A decrease in spontaneous respirations

130. A nurse is teaching a group of teenagers the correct technique for applying a condom. Which point would the nurse include in the teaching plan?

   ○ **A.** The condom can be reused one time.

   ○ **B.** Unroll the condom all the way over the erect penis.

   ○ **C.** Apply petroleum jelly to reduce irritation.

   ○ **D.** Place water in the tip of the condom before use.

131. The nurse recognizes which of the following as the priority nursing diagnosis for the client in thyroid crisis?

   ○ **A.** Risk for ineffective breathing pattern

   ○ **B.** Risk for imbalanced body temperature

   ○ **C.** Risk for decreased cerebral tissue perfusion

   ○ **D.** Activity intolerance

132. The nurse in the ER has received report of four clients en route to the emergency department. Which client should the nurse see first? A client with:

   ○ **A.** Third-degree burns to the face and neck area, with singed nasal hairs

   ○ **B.** Second-degree burns to each leg and thigh area, who is alert and oriented

   ○ **C.** A chemical burn that has been removed and liberally flushed before admission

   ○ **D.** An electrical burn entering and leaving on the same side of the body

133. A client with epilepsy has a vagal nerve stimulator in place. Which would indicate that the device is working properly?

- ○ **A.** The client's voice changes when the stimulator is operating.
- ○ **B.** Hiccups occur with each stimulation.
- ○ **C.** The client can feel vibrations in the area of the vagal nerve stimulator when operational.
- ○ **D.** The client's radial pulse obliterates when the stimulator is activated.

134. Which of the following clients has the highest risk for pulmonary complications after surgery?

- ○ **A.** A 24-year-old with open reduction internal fixation of the ulnar
- ○ **B.** A 45-year-old with an open cholecystectomy
- ○ **C.** A 36-year-old after a hysterectomy
- ○ **D.** A 50-year-old after a lumbar laminectomy

135. What clinical manifestation is most indicative of possible carbon monoxide poisoning?

- ○ **A.** Pulse oximetry reading of 80%
- ○ **B.** Expiratory stridor and nasal flaring
- ○ **C.** Cherry red color to the mucous membranes
- ○ **D.** Presence of carbonaceous particles in the sputum

136. A client is admitted with a ruptured spleen following a four-wheeler accident. In preparation for surgery, the nurse suspects that the client is in the compensatory stage of shock because of which clinical manifestation?

- ○ **A.** Blood pressure 120/70, confusion, heart rate 120
- ○ **B.** Crackles on chest auscultation, mottled skin, lethargy
- ○ **C.** Skin color jaundice, urine output less than 30mL the past hour, heart rate 170
- ○ **D.** Rapid shallow respirations, unconscious, petechiae anterior chest

137. A client is post-operative laryngectomy for cancer of the larynx. Which nursing diagnosis would be the priority for this client?

- ○ **A.** Disturbed body image related to major changes in the structure and function of the larynx
- ○ **B.** Ineffective airway clearance related to excess mucus in airway, due to surgical procedure
- ○ **C.** Imbalanced nutrition less than body requirement related to the inability to have food intake, due to dysphagia
- ○ **D.** Impaired verbal communication related to inability to talk, due to removal of larynx

138. A client arrives in the emergency room with severe burns of the hands, right arm, face, and neck. The nurse needs to start an IV. Which site would be most suitable for this client?

- ○ **A.** Top of client's right hand
- ○ **B.** Left antecubital fossa
- ○ **C.** Top of either foot
- ○ **D.** Left forearm

139. Which clinical manifestation during the actual bone marrow transplantation alerts you to the possibility of an adverse reaction?

- ○ **A.** Fever
- ○ **B.** Red urine
- ○ **C.** Hypertension
- ○ **D.** Shortness of breath

140. The nurse is assessing the integumentary system of a dark-skinned individual. Which area would be the most likely to show a skin cancer lesion?

- ○ **A.** Chest
- ○ **B.** Arms
- ○ **C.** Face
- ○ **D.** Palms

141. A client with a gastrointestinal bleed has an NG tube to low continuous wall suction. Which technique is the correct procedure for the nurse to utilize when assessing bowel sounds?

Quick Answer: **377**
Detailed Answer: **392**

- ○ **A.** Insert 10mL of air in the NG tube and listen over the abdomen with a stethoscope
- ○ **B.** Clamp the tube while listening to the abdomen with a stethoscope
- ○ **C.** Irrigate the tube with 30mL of NS while auscultating the abdomen
- ○ **D.** Turn the suction on high and auscultate over the naval area

142. A burn client's care plan reveals an expected outcome of no localized or systemic infection. Which assessment by the nurse supports this outcome?

Quick Answer: **377**
Detailed Answer: **392**

- ○ **A.** Wound culture results that show minimal bacteria
- ○ **B.** Cloudy, foul-smelling urine output
- ○ **C.** White blood cell count of 14,000
- ○ **D.** Temperature of 101°F

143. The nurse is discharging a client with a prescription of eyedrops. Which observation by the nurse would indicate a need for further client teaching?

Quick Answer: **377**
Detailed Answer: **392**

- ○ **A.** Shaking of the suspension to mix the medication
- ○ **B.** Administering a second eyedrop medication immediately after the first one was instilled
- ○ **C.** Washing the hands before and after the administration of the drops
- ○ **D.** Holding the lower lid down without pressing the eyeball to instill the drops

144. The nurse is caring for a client with pneumonia who is allergic to penicillin. Which antibiotic is safest to administer to this client?

Quick Answer: **377**
Detailed Answer: **392**

- ○ **A.** Cefazolin (Ancef)
- ○ **B.** Amoxicillin
- ○ **C.** Erythrocin (Erythromycin)
- ○ **D.** Ceftriaxone (Rocephin)

145. The nurse notes the following laboratory test results on a 24-hour post-burn client. Which abnormality should be reported to the physician immediately?

Quick Answer: **377**
Detailed Answer: **392**

- ○ **A.** Potassium 7.5mEq/L
- ○ **B.** Sodium 131mEq/L
- ○ **C.** Arterial pH 7.34
- ○ **D.** Hematocrit 52%

146. The nurse is observing a student nurse administering ear drops to a 2-year-old. Which observation by the nurse would indicate correct technique?

    ○ **A.** Holds the child's head up and extended

    ○ **B.** Places the head in chin-tuck position

    ○ **C.** Pulls the pinna down and back

    ○ **D.** Irrigates the ear before administering medication

Quick Answer: **377**
Detailed Answer: **392**

147. The nurse is caring for a client with scalding burns across the face, neck, upper half of the anterior chest, and entire right arm. Using the rule of nines, estimate the percentage of body burned.

    ○ **A.** 18%

    ○ **B.** 23%

    ○ **C.** 32%

    ○ **D.** 36%

Quick Answer: **377**
Detailed Answer: **393**

148. The nurse caring for a client in shock recognizes that the glomerular filtration rate of the kidneys will fail if the client's mean arterial pressure falls below:

    ○ **A.** 140

    ○ **B.** 120

    ○ **C.** 100

    ○ **D.** 80

Quick Answer: **377**
Detailed Answer: **393**

149. The nurse is caring for a child with a diagnosis of possible hydrocephalus. Which assessment data on the admission history would be the most objective?

    ○ **A.** Anorexia

    ○ **B.** Vomiting

    ○ **C.** Head measurement

    ○ **D.** Temperature

Quick Answer: **377**
Detailed Answer: **393**

150. Which type of leukemia is more common in older adults?

    ○ **A.** Acute myelocytic leukemia

    ○ **B.** Acute lymphocytic leukemia

    ○ **C.** Chronic lymphocytic leukemia

    ○ **D.** Chronic granulocytic leukemia

Quick Answer: **377**
Detailed Answer: **393**

151. The nurse is caring for a client after a burn. Which assessment finding best indicates that the client's respiratory efforts are currently adequate?

Quick Answer: **377**
Detailed Answer: **393**

- ○ **A.** The client is able to talk.
- ○ **B.** The client is alert and oriented.
- ○ **C.** The client's O_2 saturation is 97%.
- ○ **D.** The client's chest movements are uninhibited.

152. The nurse is performing discharge teaching to the parents of a 7-year-old who has been diagnosed with asthma. Which sports activity would be most appropriate for this client?

Quick Answer: **377**
Detailed Answer: **393**

- ○ **A.** Baseball
- ○ **B.** Swimming
- ○ **C.** Football
- ○ **D.** Track

153. The leukemic client is prescribed a low-bacteria diet. Which does the nurse expect to be included in this diet?

Quick Answer: **377**
Detailed Answer: **394**

- ○ **A.** Cooked spinach and sautéed celery
- ○ **B.** Lettuce and alfalfa sprouts
- ○ **C.** Fresh strawberries and whipped cream
- ○ **D.** Raw cauliflower or broccoli

154. A child is to receive heparin sodium 5 units per kilogram of body weight by subcutaneous route every 4 hours. The child weighs 52.8 lb. How many units should the child receive in a 24-hour period?

Quick Answer: **377**
Detailed Answer: **394**

- ○ **A.** 300
- ○ **B.** 480
- ○ **C.** 720
- ○ **D.** 960

155. A client with cancer is experiencing a common side effect of chemotherapy administration. Which laboratory assessment finding would cause the most concern?

Quick Answer: **377**
Detailed Answer: **394**

- ○ **A.** A sodium level of 50mg/dL
- ○ **B.** A blood glucose of 110mg/dL
- ○ **C.** A platelet count of 100,000/mm³
- ○ **D.** A white cell count of 5,000/mm³

156. A client's admission history reveals complaints of fatigue, chronic sore throat, and enlarged lymph nodes in the axilla and neck. Which exam would assist the physician to make a tentative diagnosis of leukemia?

    ○ **A.** A complete blood count

    ○ **B.** An x-ray of the chest

    ○ **C.** A bone marrow aspiration

    ○ **D.** A CT scan of the abdomen

Quick Answer: **377**
Detailed Answer: **394**

157. A client is admitted with symptoms of vertigo and syncope. Diagnostic tests indicate left subclavian artery obstruction. What additional findings would the nurse expect?

    ○ **A.** Memory loss and disorientation

    ○ **B.** Numbness in the face, mouth, and tongue

    ○ **C.** Radial pulse differences over 10bpm

    ○ **D.** Frontal headache with associated nausea or emesis

Quick Answer: **377**
Detailed Answer: **394**

158. The nurse is performing discharge teaching on a client at high risk for the development of skin cancer. Which instruction should be included in the client teaching?

    ○ **A.** "You should see the doctor every 6 months."

    ○ **B.** "Sunbathing should be done between the hours of noon and 3 p.m."

    ○ **C.** "If you have a mole, it should be removed and biopsied."

    ○ **D.** "You should wear sunscreen when going outside."

Quick Answer: **377**
Detailed Answer: **394**

159. A client with pancreatitis has been transferred to the intensive care unit. The nurse assesses a pulmonary arterial wedge pressure (PAWP) of 14mmHg. Based on this finding, the nurse would want to further assess for:

    ○ **A.** A drop in blood pressure

    ○ **B.** Rales on chest auscultation

    ○ **C.** Complaints of chest pain

    ○ **D.** Dry mucous membranes

Quick Answer: **377**
Detailed Answer: **394**

160. The nurse is caring for a client with a diagnosis of hepatitis who is experiencing pruritis. Which would be the most appropriate nursing intervention?

    ○ **A.** Suggest that the client take warm showers two times a day

    ○ **B.** Add baby oil to the client's bath water

    ○ **C.** Apply powder to the client's skin

    ○ **D.** Suggest a hot-water rinse after bathing

Quick Answer: **377**
Detailed Answer: **394**

161. The school nurse assessed and referred a 14-year-old with scoliosis. An 18° curvature of the spine was diagnosed. Which treatment plan would the nurse expect?

Quick Answer: **377**
Detailed Answer: **394**

- ○ **A.** Application of a Milwaukee brace
- ○ **B.** Electrical stimulation to the outward side of the curve
- ○ **C.** Re-evaluation, with no treatment at this time
- ○ **D.** Surgical realignment of the spine

162. The physician has ordered a homocysteine blood level on a client. The nurse recognizes that the results will be increased in a client with a deficiency in:

Quick Answer: **377**
Detailed Answer: **394**

- ○ **A.** Vitamin B12
- ○ **B.** Vitamin C
- ○ **C.** Vitamin A
- ○ **D.** Vitamin E

163. The registered nurse is assigning staff for four clients on the 3–11 shift. Which client should be assigned to the LPN?

Quick Answer: **377**
Detailed Answer: **394**

- ○ **A.** A client with a diagnosis of adult respiratory distress syndrome (ARDS) who was transferred from the critical care unit at 1400
- ○ **B.** A 1-hour post-operative colon resection
- ○ **C.** A client with pneumonia expecting discharge in the morning
- ○ **D.** A client with cirrhosis of the liver experiencing bleeding from esophageal varices

164. A client with multiple sclerosis has an order to receive Solu Medrol 200mg IV push. The available dose is Solu Medrol 250mg per mL. How much medication will the nurse administer?

Quick Answer: **377**
Detailed Answer: **394**

- ○ **A.** 0.5 mL
- ○ **B.** 0.8 mL
- ○ **C.** 1.1 mL
- ○ **D.** 1.4 mL

165. The nurse is obtaining a history on a 74-year-old client. Which statement made by the client would alert the nurse to a possible fluid and electrolyte imbalance?

Quick Answer: **377**
Detailed Answer: **395**

- ○ **A.** "My skin is always so dry."
- ○ **B.** "I often use a laxative for constipation."
- ○ **C.** "I have always liked to drink a lot of water."
- ○ **D.** "I sometimes have a problem with dribbling urine."

166. The nurse is caring for a client in the acute care unit. Initial laboratory values reveal serum sodium of 156mEq/L. What behavior changes would the nurse expect the client to exhibit?

   ○ **A.** Hyporeflexia

   ○ **B.** Manic behavior

   ○ **C.** Depression

   ○ **D.** Muscle cramps

Quick Answer: **377**
Detailed Answer: **395**

167. The nurse is completing the preoperative checklist on a client scheduled for surgery and finds that the consent form has been signed, but the client is unclear about the surgery and possible complications. Which is the most appropriate action?

   ○ **A.** Call the surgeon and ask him to come see the client to clarify the information

   ○ **B.** Explain the procedure and complications to the client

   ○ **C.** Check in the physician's progress notes to see if understanding has been documented

   ○ **D.** Check with the client's family to see if they understand the procedure fully

Quick Answer: **377**
Detailed Answer: **395**

168. When preparing a client for admission to the surgical suite, the nurse recognizes that which one of the following items is most important to remove before sending the client to surgery?

   ○ **A.** Hearing aid

   ○ **B.** Contact lenses

   ○ **C.** Wedding ring

   ○ **D.** Dentures

Quick Answer: **377**
Detailed Answer: **395**

169. A client with cancer is to undergo a bone scan. The nurse should:

   ○ **A.** Force fluids 24 hours before the procedure

   ○ **B.** Ask the client to void immediately before the study

   ○ **C.** Hold medication that affects the central nervous system for 12 hours pre- and post-test

   ○ **D.** Cover the client's reproductive organs with an x-ray shield

Quick Answer: **377**
Detailed Answer: **395**

170. A client with suspected leukemia is to undergo a bone marrow aspiration. The nurse plans to include which statement in the teaching session?

Quick Answer: **377**
Detailed Answer: **395**

- ○ **A.** "You will be lying on your abdomen for the examination procedure."
- ○ **B.** "Portions of the procedure will cause pain or discomfort."
- ○ **C.** "You will be given some medication to cause amnesia of the test."
- ○ **D.** "You will not be able to drink fluids for 24 hours before the study."

171. The nurse is caring for a client scheduled for a surgical repair of an abdominal aortic aneurysm. Which assessment is most crucial during the preoperative period?

Quick Answer: **377**
Detailed Answer: **395**

- ○ **A.** Assessment of the client's level of anxiety
- ○ **B.** Evaluation of the client's exercise tolerance
- ○ **C.** Identification of peripheral pulses
- ○ **D.** Assessment of bowel sounds and activity

172. The nurse should carefully monitor the client for which common dysrhythmia that can occur during suctioning?

Quick Answer: **377**
Detailed Answer: **395**

- ○ **A.** Bradycardia
- ○ **B.** Tachycardia
- ○ **C.** Ventricular ectopic beats
- ○ **D.** Sick sinus syndrome

173. The nurse is performing discharge instruction for a client with an implantable permanent pacemaker. What discharge instruction is an essential part of the plan?

Quick Answer: **377**
Detailed Answer: **395**

- ○ **A.** "You cannot eat food prepared in a microwave."
- ○ **B.** "You should avoid moving the shoulder on the side of the pacemaker site for 6 weeks."
- ○ **C.** "You will have to learn to take your own pulse."
- ○ **D.** "You will not be able to fly on a commercial airliner with the pacemaker in place."

174. The nurse is completing admission on a client with possible esophageal cancer. Which finding would not be common for this diagnosis?

Quick Answer: **377**
Detailed Answer: **395**

- ○ **A.** Foul breath
- ○ **B.** Dysphagia
- ○ **C.** Diarrhea
- ○ **D.** Chronic hiccups

175. A client arrives from surgery following an abdominal perineal resection with a permanent illeostomy. What should be the priority nursing care during the post-op period?

    ○ **A.** Teaching how to irrigate the illeostomy

    ○ **B.** Stopping electrolyte loss through the stoma

    ○ **C.** Encouraging a high-fiber diet

    ○ **D.** Facilitating perineal wound drainage

176. The nurse is making initial rounds on a client with a C5 fracture. The client is in a halo vest and is receiving O_2 at 40% via mask to a tracheostomy. Assessment reveals a respiratory rate of 40 and O_2 saturation of 88. The client is restless. Which initial nursing action is most indicated?

    ○ **A.** Notifying the physician

    ○ **B.** Performing tracheal suctioning

    ○ **C.** Repositioning the client to the left side

    ○ **D.** Rechecking the client's O_2 saturation

177. A client has just finished her lunch, consisting of shrimp with rice, fruit salad, and a roll. The client calls for the nurse, stating, "My throat feels thick and I'm having trouble breathing." What action should the nurse implement first?

    ○ **A.** Place the bed in Trendelenburg position and call the physician

    ○ **B.** Take the client's vital signs and administer Benadryl 50mg PO

    ○ **C.** Place the bed in high Fowler's position and call the physician

    ○ **D.** Start an Aminophylline drip and call the physician

178. The nurse is caring for a client with cirrhosis of the liver. Which is the best method to use for determining that the client has ascites?

    ○ **A.** Inspection of the abdomen for enlargement

    ○ **B.** Bimanual palpation for hepatomegaly

    ○ **C.** Daily measurement of abdominal girth

    ○ **D.** Assessment for a fluid wave

179. A client arrives in the emergency room after a motor vehicle accident. Witnesses tell the nurse that they observed the client's head hit the side of the car door. Nursing assessment findings include BP 70/34, heart rate 130, and respirations 22. Which is the client's most appropriate priority nursing diagnosis?

- ○ **A.** Alteration in cerebral tissue perfusion
- ○ **B.** Fluid volume deficit
- ○ **C.** Ineffective airway clearance
- ○ **D.** Alteration in sensory perception

180. The home health nurse is visiting a 30-year-old with sickle cell disease. Assessment findings include splenomegaly. What information obtained on the visit would cause the most concern? The client:

- ○ **A.** Eats fast food daily for lunch
- ○ **B.** Drinks a beer occasionally
- ○ **C.** Sometimes feels fatigued
- ○ **D.** Works as a furniture mover

181. The nurse on the oncology unit is caring for a client with a WBC of 1500. During evening visitation, a visitor brings in a fruit basket. What action should the nurse take?

- ○ **A.** Encourage the client to eat small snacks of the fruit
- ○ **B.** Remove fruits that are not high in vitamin C
- ○ **C.** Instruct the client to avoid the high-fiber fruits
- ○ **D.** Remove the fruits from the client's room

182. The nurse is giving an end-of-shift report when a client with a chest tube is noted in the hallway with the tube disconnected. What is the most appropriate action?

- ○ **A.** Clamp the chest tube immediately
- ○ **B.** Put the end of the chest tube into a cup of sterile normal saline
- ○ **C.** Assist the client back to the room and place him on his left side
- ○ **D.** Reconnect the chest tube to the chest tube system

183. A client with deep vein thrombosis is receiving a continuous heparin infusion and Coumadin PO. INR lab test result is 8.0. Which intervention would be most important to include in the nursing care plan?

- ○ **A.** Assess for signs of abnormal bleeding
- ○ **B.** Anticipate an increase in the heparin drip rate
- ○ **C.** Instruct the client regarding the drug therapy
- ○ **D.** Increase the frequency of vascular assessments

184. Which breakfast selection by a client with osteoporosis indicates that the client understands the dietary management of the disease?

- ○ **A.** Scrambled eggs, toast, and coffee
- ○ **B.** Bran muffin with margarine
- ○ **C.** Granola bar and half of a grapefruit
- ○ **D.** Bagel with jam and skim milk

185. A client with hepatitis C who has cirrhosis changes has just returned from a liver biopsy. The nurse will place the client in which position?

- ○ **A.** Trendelenburg
- ○ **B.** Supine
- ○ **C.** Right side-lying
- ○ **D.** Left Sim's

186. The nurse is caring for a client who was admitted to the burn unit 4 hours after the injury with second-degree burns to the trunk and head. Which finding would the nurse least expect to find during this time period?

- ○ **A.** Hypovolemia
- ○ **B.** Laryngeal edema
- ○ **C.** Hypernatremia
- ○ **D.** Hyperkalemia

187. The nurse is evaluating nutritional outcomes for a client with anorexia nervosa. Which one of the following is the most objective favorable outcome for the client?

- ○ **A.** The client eats all the food on her tray
- ○ **B.** The client requests that family bring special foods
- ○ **C.** The client's weight has increased
- ○ **D.** The client weighs herself each morning

188. The client who is 2 weeks post-burn with a 40% deep partial-thickness injury still has open wounds. The nurse's assessment reveals the following findings: temperature 96.5°F, BP 87/40, and severe diarrhea stools. What problem does the nurse most likely suspect?

- ○ **A.** Findings are normal, not suspicious of a problem
- ○ **B.** Systemic gram—positive infection
- ○ **C.** Systemic gram—negative infection
- ○ **D.** Systemic fungal infection

Quick Answer: **378**
Detailed Answer: **397**

189. The nurse assesses a new order for a blood transfusion. The order is to transfuse 1 unit of packed red blood cells (contains 250mL) in a 2-hour period. What will be the hourly rate of infusion?

- ○ **A.** 50mL/hr
- ○ **B.** 62mL/hr
- ○ **C.** 125mL/hr
- ○ **D.** 137mL/hr

Quick Answer: **378**
Detailed Answer: **397**

190. A client has signs of increased intracranial pressure. Which one of the following is an early indicator of deterioration in the client's condition?

- ○ **A.** Widening pulse pressure
- ○ **B.** Decrease in the pulse rate
- ○ **C.** Dilated, fixed pupils
- ○ **D.** Decrease in level of consciousness

Quick Answer: **378**
Detailed Answer: **397**

191. Which of the following statements by a client with a seizure disorder who is taking topiramate (Topamax) indicates that the client has understood the nurse's instruction?

- ○ **A.** "I will take the medicine before going to bed."
- ○ **B.** "I will drink 8 to 10 ten-ounce glasses of water a day."
- ○ **C.** "I will eat plenty of fresh fruits."
- ○ **D.** "I must take the medicine with a meal or snack."

Quick Answer: **378**
Detailed Answer: **397**

192. A client with terminal lung cancer is admitted to the unit. A family member asks the nurse, "How much longer will it be?" Which response by the nurse is most appropriate?

- ○ **A.** "This must be a terrible situation for you."
- ○ **B.** "I don't know. I'll call the doctor."
- ○ **C.** "I cannot say exactly. What are your concerns at this time?"
- ○ **D.** "Don't worry, it will be very soon."

Quick Answer: **378**
Detailed Answer: **397**

193. The nurse is administering a mantoux test. Which is a part of the correct technique for administering this test?

Quick Answer: 378
Detailed Answer: 397

- ○ **A.** Administer IM in the deltoid muscle
- ○ **B.** Deposit the PPD subcutaneously in the upper arm
- ○ **C.** Deposit the PPD subcutaneously with the needle bevel up
- ○ **D.** Give the test subcutaneously in the inner aspect of the forearm using a 1¹/₂-inch needle

194. The nurse is caring for a client with a closed head injury. Fluid is assessed leaking from the ear. The nurse's first action will be to:

Quick Answer: 378
Detailed Answer: 397

- ○ **A.** Irrigate the ear canal gently
- ○ **B.** Notify the physician
- ○ **C.** Test the drainage for glucose
- ○ **D.** Apply an occlusive dressing

195. The nurse has inserted an NG tube for enteral feedings. Which assessment result is the best indicator of the tube's stomach placement?

Quick Answer: 378
Detailed Answer: 397

- ○ **A.** Aspiration of tan-colored mucus
- ○ **B.** Green aspirate with a pH of 3
- ○ **C.** A swish auscultated with the injection of air
- ○ **D.** Bubbling in a cup of NS when the end of the tube is placed in the cup

196. The nurse would identify which one of the following assessment findings as a normal response in a craniotomy client post-operatively?

Quick Answer: 378
Detailed Answer: 397

- ○ **A.** A decrease in responsiveness the third post-op day
- ○ **B.** Sluggish pupil reaction the first 24–48 hours
- ○ **C.** Dressing changes 3 to 4 times a day for the first 3 days
- ○ **D.** Temperature range of 98.8°F to 99.6°F the first 2–3 days

197. A client with alcoholism has been instructed to increase his intake of thiamine. The nurse knows the client understands the instructions when he selects which food?

Quick Answer: 378
Detailed Answer: 397

- ○ **A.** Roast beef
- ○ **B.** Broiled fish
- ○ **C.** Baked chicken
- ○ **D.** Sliced pork

198. The nurse is caring for a client who abuses narcotics. The client is exhibiting a respiratory rate of 10 and dilated pupils. Which drug would the nurse expect to administer?

- ○ **A.** Meperidine (Demerol)
- ○ **B.** Naloxone (Narcan)
- ○ **C.** Chlordiazepoxide (Librium)
- ○ **D.** Haloperidol (Haldol)

199. A client has a CVP monitor in place. Which would be included in the nursing care plan for this client?

- ○ **A.** Notify the physician of readings less than 3cm or more than 8cm of water
- ○ **B.** Use the clean technique to change the dressing at the insertion site
- ○ **C.** Elevate the head of the bed to 90° to obtain CVP readings
- ○ **D.** The 0 mark on the manometer should align with the client's right clavicle for the readings

200. A client is admitted to the chemical dependency unit for poly-drug abuse. The client states, "I don't know why you are all so worried; I am in control. I don't have a problem." Which defense mechanism is being utilized?

- ○ **A.** Rationalization
- ○ **B.** Projection
- ○ **C.** Dissociation
- ○ **D.** Denial

201. A client scheduled for a carotid endarterectomy requires insertion of an intra-arterial blood pressure-monitoring device. The nurse plans to perform the Allen test. Which observation indicates patency of the ulnar artery?

- ○ **A.** Blanching of the hand on compression and release of the ulnar artery
- ○ **B.** Muscular twitching of the bicep muscle with use of a tourniquet at the wrist
- ○ **C.** Hand turning pink after the nurse releases the pressure on the ulnar artery
- ○ **D.** Flexion of the wrist when tapping the ulnar artery with a reflex hammer

202. The chest tube drainage system has continuous bubbling in the water seal chamber. When the nurse clamps different areas of the tube to find out where the bubbling stops, he is checking for:

- ○ **A.** An air leak
- ○ **B.** The suction being too high
- ○ **C.** The suction being too low
- ○ **D.** A tension pneumothorax

Quick Answer: **378**
Detailed Answer: **398**

203. The nurse should be particularly alert for which one of the following problems in a client with barbiturate overdose?

- ○ **A.** Oliguria
- ○ **B.** Cardiac tamponade
- ○ **C.** Apnea
- ○ **D.** Hemorrhage

Quick Answer: **378**
Detailed Answer: **398**

204. A client taking the drug disulfiram (Antabuse) is admitted to the ER. Which clinical manifestations are most indicative of recent alcohol ingestion?

- ○ **A.** Vomiting, heart rate 120, chest pain
- ○ **B.** Nausea, mild headache, bradycardia
- ○ **C.** Respirations 16, heart rate 62, diarrhea
- ○ **D.** Temp 101°F, tachycardia, respirations 20

Quick Answer: **378**
Detailed Answer: **398**

205. The nurse caring for clients with coronary artery disease recognizes which one of the following as a modifiable risk factor?

- ○ **A.** History of heart disease in family
- ○ **B.** African American race
- ○ **C.** An LDL blood level of 180mg/dL
- ○ **D.** Gender

Quick Answer: **378**
Detailed Answer: **398**

206. A client with cocaine addiction would most likely be placed on which medication?

- ○ **A.** Amantidine (Symmetrel)
- ○ **B.** Methadone
- ○ **C.** THC
- ○ **D.** Disulfiram (Antabuse)

Quick Answer: **378**
Detailed Answer: **398**

207. Which laboratory test is used to identify injury to the myocardium and can remain elevated for up to 3 weeks?

- ○ **A.** Total CK
- ○ **B.** CK-MB
- ○ **C.** Myoglobulin
- ○ **D.** Troponin T or I

208. A client with newly diagnosed epilepsy tells the nurse, "If I keep having seizures, I'm scared my husband will feel differently toward me." Which response by the nurse would be most appropriate?

- ○ **A.** "You don't know if you'll ever have another seizure. Why don't you wait and see what happens?"
- ○ **B.** "You seem to be concerned that there could be a change in the relationship with your husband."
- ○ **C.** "You should focus on your children. They need you."
- ○ **D.** "Let's see how your husband reacts before getting upset."

209. While interviewing a client who abuses alcohol, the nurse learns that the client has experienced "blackouts." The wife asks what this means. The best response at this time is:

- ○ **A.** "Your husband has experienced short-term memory amnesia."
- ○ **B.** "Your husband has experienced loss of remote memory."
- ○ **C.** "Your husband has experienced loss of consciousness due to drinking alcohol."
- ○ **D.** "Your husband has experienced a fainting spell."

210. Which would be included in the nursing care plan of a client experiencing severe delirium tremens?

- ○ **A.** Placing the client in a darkened room
- ○ **B.** Keeping the closet and bathroom doors closed
- ○ **C.** Administering a diuretic to decrease fluid excess
- ○ **D.** Checking vital signs every 8 hours

211. The nurse is caring for a client admitted with a diagnosis of epilepsy. The client begins to have a seizure. Which action by the nurse is contraindicated?

- ○ **A.** Turning the client to the side-lying position
- ○ **B.** Inserting a padded tongue blade and oral airway
- ○ **C.** Loosening restrictive clothing
- ○ **D.** Removing the pillow and raising padded side rails

212. A client has been placed on the drug valproic acid (Depakene). Which would indicate to the nurse that the client is experiencing an adverse reaction to this medication?

Quick Answer: **378**
Detailed Answer: **399**

- ○ **A.** Photophobia
- ○ **B.** Poor skin turgor
- ○ **C.** Lethargy
- ○ **D.** Visual disturbances

213. The nurse is caring for a 16-year-old female with second- and third-degree burns to the face, neck, chest, and arms. The client's wounds are almost healed. The nurse would expect rehabilitation to focus on problems related to:

Quick Answer: **378**
Detailed Answer: **399**

- ○ **A.** Body image disturbance
- ○ **B.** Risk for infection
- ○ **C.** Sensory perceptual alterations
- ○ **D.** Activity intolerance

214. The nurse is performing fluid resuscitation on a burn client. Which piece of assessment data is the best indicator that it is effective?

Quick Answer: **378**
Detailed Answer: **399**

- ○ **A.** Respirations 24, unlabored
- ○ **B.** Urine output of 30ml/hr
- ○ **C.** Capillary refill < 4 seconds
- ○ **D.** Apical pulse of 110/min

215. A client diagnosed with COPD is receiving theophylline. Morning laboratory values reveal a theophylline level of 38mcg/mL. The most appropriate action by the nurse would be to:

Quick Answer: **378**
Detailed Answer: **399**

- ○ **A.** Take no action; this is within normal range
- ○ **B.** Notify the physician of the level results
- ○ **C.** Administer Narcan 2mg IV push stat
- ○ **D.** Give the client a double dose of Theodur at the next time due

216. A client has suffered a severe electrical burn. Which medication would the nurse expect to have ordered for application to the burned area?

Quick Answer: **378**
Detailed Answer: **399**

- ○ **A.** Mafenide acetate (Sulfamylon)
- ○ **B.** Silver nitrate
- ○ **C.** Providone-iodine ointment
- ○ **D.** Silver sulfadiazine (Silvadene)

217. A client with a head injury develops syndrome of inappropriate antidiuretic hormone (SIADH). Which physician prescription would the nurse question?

- ○ **A.** D5W at 200mL/hr
- ○ **B.** Demeclocycline (Declomycin) 150mg Q6h
- ○ **C.** Daily weights
- ○ **D.** Intake and output Q4h

218. The nurse is caring for a postpartum client. Which of the following assessment findings would be a reason for concern during the client's postpartum stay?

- ○ **A.** Pulse rate of 70–90 the third postpartum day
- ○ **B.** Diuresis her second and third postpartum days
- ○ **C.** Vaginal discharge of rubra, serosa, then rubra
- ○ **D.** Diaphoresis her third postpartum day

219. The nurse is caring for a postpartum client 2 hours post-delivery who is unable to void. Which of the following nursing interventions should be considered initially?

- ○ **A.** Insert a straight catheter for residual
- ○ **B.** Encourage oral intake of fluids
- ○ **C.** Check perineum for swelling or hematoma
- ○ **D.** Palpate bladder for distention and position

220. A client is admitted to the intensive care unit after falling on an icy sidewalk and striking the right side of the head. An MRI revealed a right-sided epidural hematoma. Which physical force explains the location of the client's injury?

- ○ **A.** Coup
- ○ **B.** Contrecoup
- ○ **C.** Deceleration
- ○ **D.** Acceleration

221. The nurse is preparing to teach a client about phenytoin sodium (Dilantin). Which fact would be most important to teach the client regarding why the drug should not be stopped suddenly?

- ○ **A.** Physical dependence can develop over time.
- ○ **B.** Status epilepticus can develop.
- ○ **C.** A hypoglycemic reaction can develop.
- ○ **D.** Heart block can develop.

222. One week after discharge of a postpartum client, the client's husband calls the postpartum unit and asks the nurse, "Is it normal for my wife to cry at the drop of a hat? I'm worried I've done something to upset her." The nurse's best initial response would be:

- ○ **A.** "Have you noticed any pattern to her periods of crying?"
- ○ **B.** "Try not to worry about it. I'm sure it's just the postpartum blues."
- ○ **C.** "Can you think of something you might have done to upset her?"
- ○ **D.** "Let's consider some of the ways you can decrease her depression."

223. A client is admitted with suspected Guillain-Barre syndrome. The nurse would expect the cerebrospinal fluid (CSF) analysis to reveal which of the following to confirm the diagnosis?

- ○ **A.** CSF protein 10mg/dL and WBC 2 cells/mm^3
- ○ **B.** CSF protein of 60mg/dL and WBC 0 cells/mm^3
- ○ **C.** CSF protein of 50mg/dL and WBC 20 cells/mm^3
- ○ **D.** CSF protein of 5mg/dL and WBC 20 cells/mm^3

224. A client with burns is admitted and fluid resuscitation has begun. Central venous pressure (CVP) readings are ordered every 4 hours; the client's CVP reading is 14cm/H_2O. Which evaluation by the nurse would be most accurate?

- ○ **A.** The client has received enough fluid.
- ○ **B.** The client's fluid status is unaltered.
- ○ **C.** The client has inadequate fluids.
- ○ **D.** The client has a volume excess.

225. The nurse is working on a neurological unit. If the following events occur simultaneously, which would receive RN priority?

- ○ **A.** A client with a cerebral aneurysm complains of sudden weakness on the right side.
- ○ **B.** A client with a suspected brain tumor complains of a headache.
- ○ **C.** A client post-op lumbar laminectomy vomits.
- ○ **D.** A client with Guillain-Barre syndrome has a temp of 99.6°F.

226. The nurse assesses a client's fundal height every 15 minutes during the first hour postpartum. The height of the fundus during this hour should be:

Quick Answer: 378
Detailed Answer: 400

- ○ **A.** 1–2 fingerbreadths under the umbilicus
- ○ **B.** 4 fingerbreadths under the umbilicus
- ○ **C.** 1 fingerbreadth above the umbilicus
- ○ **D.** 4 fingerbreadths above the umbilicus

227. The nurse assesses a client complaining of a headache. When the nurse shines a light on the frontal and maxillary sinuses, the light does not penetrate the tissues. What is the best interpretation of this finding?

Quick Answer: 378
Detailed Answer: 400

- ○ **A.** This is a normal finding indicating no problem in the sinuses.
- ○ **B.** Inflammation is present in the sinuses.
- ○ **C.** The cavity likely contains fluid or pus.
- ○ **D.** The client has a sinus infection.

228. A client with chronic obstructive pulmonary disease (COPD) is admitted to the respiratory unit. Which physician prescription should the nurse question?

Quick Answer: 378
Detailed Answer: 400

- ○ **A.** O_2 at 5L/min by nasal cannula
- ○ **B.** Solu Medrol 125mg IV push every 6 hours
- ○ **C.** Ceftriaxone (Rocephin) 1gram IVPB daily
- ○ **D.** Darvocet N 100 po prn pain

229. A burn client begins treatments with silver sulfadiazine (Silvadene) applied to the wounds. The nurse should carefully monitor for which adverse affect associated with this drug?

Quick Answer: 378
Detailed Answer: 400

- ○ **A.** Hypokalemia
- ○ **B.** Leukopenia
- ○ **C.** Hyponatremia
- ○ **D.** Thrombocytopenia

230. The nurse is caring for clients on the postpartum unit. Which of the following should the nurse assess first?

Quick Answer: 378
Detailed Answer: 400

- ○ **A.** A primapara who has delivered an 8-pound baby boy
- ○ **B.** A gravida IV para IV who experienced 1 hour of labor
- ○ **C.** A gravida II para II whose placenta was delivered 10 minutes after the infant
- ○ **D.** A primapara receiving 100mg of meperidine (Demerol) during her labor

231. The nurse is assessing a client for tactile fremitus. Which client would most likely exhibit a decrease in tactile fremitus? A client with:

Quick Answer: **378**
Detailed Answer: **401**

- ○ **A.** Emphysema
- ○ **B.** Pneumonia
- ○ **C.** Tuberculosis
- ○ **D.** A lung tumor

232. A client who has been diagnosed with lung cancer is starting a smoking-cessation program. Which of the following drugs would the nurse expect to be included in the program's plan?

Quick Answer: **378**
Detailed Answer: **401**

- ○ **A.** Bupropion SR (Zyban)
- ○ **B.** Metoproterenol (Alupent)
- ○ **C.** Oxitropuim (Oxivent)
- ○ **D.** Alprazolam (Xanax)

233. A client delivered a 9-pound infant 2 hours ago. The client has an IV of D5W with oxytocin. The nurse determines that the medication is achieving the desired effect when she observes:

Quick Answer: **378**
Detailed Answer: **401**

- ○ **A.** A rise in blood pressure
- ○ **B.** A decrease in pain
- ○ **C.** An increase in lochia rubra
- ○ **D.** A firm uterine fundus

234. The nurse is evaluating cerebral perfusion outcomes for a client with a subdural hematoma. The nurse evaluates which of the following as a favorable outcome for this client?

Quick Answer: **378**
Detailed Answer: **401**

- ○ **A.** Arterial blood gas PO_2 of 98
- ○ **B.** Increase in lethargy
- ○ **C.** Pupils slow to react to light
- ○ **D.** Temperature of 101°F

235. The nurse is caring for a client with COPD. Which of the associated disorders has changes that are reversible?

Quick Answer: **378**
Detailed Answer: **401**

- ○ **A.** Bronchiectasis
- ○ **B.** Emphysema
- ○ **C.** Asthma
- ○ **D.** Chronic bronchitis

236. A client experienced a major burn over 55% of his body 36 hours ago. The client is restless and anxious, and states, "I am in pain." There is a physician prescription for intravenous morphine. The nurse's first action would be to:

- ○ **A.** Administer the morphine
- ○ **B.** Assess respirations
- ○ **C.** Assess urine output
- ○ **D.** Check serum potassium levels

237. The nurse is caring for a client 7 days post-burn injury with 60% body surface area involved. The nursing care of this client would primarily focus on:

- ○ **A.** Meticulous infection-control measures
- ○ **B.** Fluid-replacement evaluation
- ○ **C.** Psychological adjustment to the wound
- ○ **D.** Measurement and application of a pressure garment

238. The nurse is caring for a child 4 days after a tracheostomy tube insertion. The child's mother calls the desk and states, "He pulled out his trach tube and threw it on the floor; it's closing—come quick, he can't breathe." What is the best action for the nurse to take?

- ○ **A.** Cover the stoma with a sterile 4×4
- ○ **B.** Keep the stoma open using sterile technique, and call for help
- ○ **C.** Retrieve the tracheostomy tube and reinsert it
- ○ **D.** Apply O_2 at 4L/min by nasal cannula

239. The nurse is performing discharge teaching for a client after a cardiac catheterization. Which statement by the client indicates a need for further teaching?

- ○ **A.** "I should not bend, strain, or lift heavy objects for 1 day."
- ○ **B.** "If bleeding occurs, I should place an ice bag on the site for 10 minutes."
- ○ **C.** "I need to call the doctor if my temperature goes above 101°F."
- ○ **D.** "I should talk to the doctor to find out when I can go back to work."

240. A burn client is in the acute phase of burn care. The nurse assesses jugular vein distention, edema, urine output of 20cc in 2 hours, and crackles on auscultation. Which order would the nurse anticipate from the physician?

- ○ **A.** Furosemide (Lasix) IV push
- ○ **B.** Irrigate the Foley catheter
- ○ **C.** Increase the IV fluids to 200mL/hr
- ○ **D.** Place the client in Trendelenburg position

241. When performing suctioning of a tracheostomy, the nurse would know that the suction pressure should not exceed:

- ○ **A.** 120mmHg
- ○ **B.** 145mmHg
- ○ **C.** 160mmHg
- ○ **D.** 185mmHg

242. A client admitted with transient ischemia attacks has returned from a cerebral arteriogram. The nurse performs an assessment and finds a newly formed hematoma in the right groin area. What is the nurse's initial action?

- ○ **A.** Apply direct pressure to the site
- ○ **B.** Check the pedal pulses on the right leg
- ○ **C.** Notify the physician
- ○ **D.** Turn the client to the prone position

243. The nurse is assessing an ECG strip of a 42-year-old client and finds a regular rate greater than 100, a normal QRS complex, a normal P wave in front of each QRS, a PR interval between 0.12 and 0.20 seconds, and a P: QRS ratio of 1:1. What is the nurse's interpretation of this rhythm?

- ○ **A.** Premature atrial complex
- ○ **B.** Sinus tachycardia
- ○ **C.** Atrial flutter
- ○ **D.** Supraventricular tachycardia

244. A client is complaining of chest pain. Nursing assessment reveals a BP of 78/40, shortness of breath, and third-degree AV block on the heart monitor. What medication would the nurse prepare for initial administration?

- ○ **A.** Atropine
- ○ **B.** Verapamil (Calan)
- ○ **C.** Lidocaine (Xylocaine)
- ○ **D.** Procainamide (Pronestyl)

245. The nurse is discussing cigarette smoking with an emphysema client. The client states, "I don't know why I should worry about cancer." The nurse's response is based on the fact that the most important reason for a client with emphysema to avoid smoking is that it:

- ○ **A.** Affects peripheral blood vessels
- ○ **B.** Causes vasoconstriction
- ○ **C.** Destroys the lung parenchyma
- ○ **D.** Paralyzes ciliary activity

246. The nurse is caring for a client admitted with congestive heart failure. Which finding would the nurse expect if the failure was on the right side of the heart?

- ○ **A.** Jugular vein distention
- ○ **B.** Dry, nonproductive cough
- ○ **C.** Orthopnea
- ○ **D.** Crackles on chest auscultation

247. A client with chest pain is scheduled for a heart catheterization. Which of the following would the nurse include in the client's care plan?

- ○ **A.** Keep the client NPO for 12 hours after the procedure
- ○ **B.** Inform the client that general anesthesia will be administered
- ○ **C.** Assess the site for bleeding or hematoma once per shift
- ○ **D.** Instruct the client that he might be asked to cough and breathe deeply during the procedure

248. The nurse is caring for a COPD client who is discharged on p.o. Theophylline. Which of the following statements by the client would indicate a correct understanding of discharge instructions?

- ○ **A.** "A slow, regular pulse could be a side effect."
- ○ **B.** "Take the pill with antacid or milk and crackers."
- ○ **C.** "The doctor might order it intravenously if symptoms worsen."
- ○ **D.** "Hold the drug if symptoms decrease."

249. The nurse has just admitted a client with emphysema. Arterial blood gas results indicate hypoxia. Which physician prescription would the nurse implement for the best improvement in the client's hypoxia?

Quick Answer: **378**
Detailed Answer: **402**

- ○ **A.** Elevate the head of the bed 45°
- ○ **B.** Encourage diaphragmatic breathing
- ○ **C.** Initiate an Alupent nebulizer treatment
- ○ **D.** Start O_2 at 2L/min

250. The nurse is assessing the chart of a client with a stroke. MRI results reveal a hemorrhagic stroke to the brain. Which physician prescription would the nurse question?

Quick Answer: **378**
Detailed Answer: **402**

- ○ **A.** Normal saline IV at 50mL/hr
- ○ **B.** O_2 at 3L/min by nasal cannula
- ○ **C.** Heparin infusion per pharmacist protocol
- ○ **D.** Insert a Foley catheter

Quick Check Answer Key

1. A	31. D	61. B
2. D	32. C	62. B
3. C	33. D	63. C
4. D	34. A	64. A
5. B	35. C	65. C
6. A	36. B	66. C
7. B	37. D	67. A
8. A	38. D	68. B
9. B	39. C	69. A
10. D	40. A	70. D
11. C	41. B	71. A
12. A	42. D	72. C
13. A	43. C	73. C
14. B	44. A	74. D
15. C	45. B	75. C
16. B	46. D	76. A
17. A	47. D	77. C
18. A	48. A	78. C
19. D	49. B	79. C
20. A	50. D	80. D
21. C	51. B	81. C
22. C	52. A	82. C
23. B	53. A	83. D
24. C	54. B	84. D
25. A	55. C	85. C
26. A	56. B	86. A
27. D	57. A	87. C
28. D	58. A	88. C
29. A	59. A	89. D
30. B	60. D	90. C

91. C	123. C	155. A
92. C	124. B	156. A
93. A	125. A	157. C
94. B	126. A	158. D
95. C	127. C	159. B
96. C	128. C	160. B
97. C	129. C	161. C
98. C	130. B	162. A
99. C	131. B	163. C
100. B	132. A	164. B
101. D	133. A	165. B
102. A	134. B	166. B
103. B	135. C	167. A
104. C	136. A	168. D
105. B	137. B	169. B
106. C	138. B	170. B
107. A	139. D	171. C
108. C	140. D	172. A
109. B	141. B	173. C
110. C	142. A	174. C
111. A	143. B	175. D
112. C	144. C	176. B
113. A	145. A	177. C
114. D	146. C	178. C
115. B	147. B	179. B
116. B	148. D	180. D
117. D	149. C	181. D
118. D	150. C	182. B
119. D	151. C	183. A
120. B	152. B	184. D
121. A	153. A	185. C
122. B	154. C	186. C

187. C	**209.** A	**231.** A
188. C	**210.** B	**232.** A
189. C	**211.** B	**233.** D
190. D	**212.** C	**234.** A
191. B	**213.** A	**235.** C
192. C	**214.** B	**236.** B
193. C	**215.** B	**237.** A
194. C	**216.** A	**238.** B
195. B	**217.** A	**239.** B
196. D	**218.** C	**240.** A
197. D	**219.** D	**241.** A
198. B	**220.** A	**242.** A
199. A	**221.** B	**243.** B
200. D	**222.** A	**244.** A
201. C	**223.** B	**245.** D
202. A	**224.** D	**246.** A
203. C	**225.** A	**247.** D
204. A	**226.** C	**248.** B
205. C	**227.** C	**249.** D
206. A	**228.** A	**250.** C
207. D	**229.** B	
208. B	**230.** B	

Answers and Rationales

1. **Answer A is correct.** People of the Islam religion are prohibited from eating some gelatins. They also must avoid pork, alcohol products and beverages, and some lard products. Answers B, C, and D would all be appropriate foods for people of the Islamic faith.

2. **Answer D is correct.** Activity, exercise, and repositioning the client will increase circulation and improve tissue perfusion. Answer A will help to identify problem areas but will not improve the perfusion of the tissue. Answer B should be avoided because it could increase the damage if trauma was present. Answer C should be done to prevent irritation of the skin, but this action does not improve perfusion.

3. **Answer C is correct.** This client needs a balanced nutritional diet with protein and vitamin C. Answers A and B both lack protein, which is very important in maintaining a positive nitrogen balance. Answer D has protein but is lacking in vitamin C.

4. **Answer D is correct.** Rales would indicate lung congestion and the need for follow-up. Answers A, B, and C are all normal health-related changes associated with aging.

5. **Answer B is correct.** Respiratory depression can occur from the administration of opioids. Naloxone should be available as an antagonist for these drugs. Answers A, C, and D might also be needed, but the most important problem that could occur would be the respiratory depression. These clients might also develop itching and nausea, and would likely use Benadryl and Phenergan, respectively, for treatment. Toradol is classified as an NSAID and is useful for its anti-inflammatory properties.

6. **Answer A is correct.** Hematocrit levels are elevated with hypovolemia. Answers B, C, and D are all normal levels. Potassium (normal 3.5–5.3mEq/L) levels can be either increased or decreased with hypovolemia; BUN (normal 5–20mg/dL) and specific gravity (1.016–1.022) levels would be elevated with hypovolemia.

7. **Answer B is correct.** Athletes can sometimes consume large amounts of water when competing. This can lead to decreased sodium levels. Symptoms of hyponatremia include an altered mental status, anorexia, muscle cramps, and exhaustion. Answers A, C, and D do not correlate with the history or the symptoms given.

8. **Answer A is correct.** If the nurse suspects a leaking or a ruptured abdominal aortic aneurysm, the first action is to improve blood flow to the brain and elevate the blood pressure. This can be accomplished quickly with the change in position. Answers B and C would be appropriate, but not before answer A. Answer D would not be required at this time.

9. **Answer B is correct.** Clients with cardiogenic shock often have chest pain. This symptom is not related to anaphylactic shock. Answers A and C can occur with both types of shock, but are not specific to the cardiogenic type. Answer D is a normal temperature reading.

10. **Answer D is correct.** This is the correct classification for the primary tumor of T1, N1, and M0. The letter T denotes the extent of the primary tumor, N indicates the absence or presence and extent of regional lymph nodes, and M denotes the absence or presence of distant metastasis. Answer A is correct for T1, N0, and M0. Answer B is correct for the classification of TX, NX, MX. Answer C is the correct classification for T1, N1, M1.

11. **Answer C is correct.** Daunorubicin can damage the heart muscle and is the most serious of the ones listed. It can also cause bone marrow suppression. Answers A, B, and D are all common, but not as life-threatening as answer C.

12. **Answer A is correct.** The organ donor must have a BP of 90 or greater to ensure tissue perfusion. Answers B, C, and D are not required for adequate tissue maintenance.

13. **Answer A is correct.** Airway clearance is the priority. After gallbladder surgery, clients can have respiratory problems because the location of the incision is in the proximity of the diaphragm. Answers B, C, and D can also occur but are not the priority.

14. **Answer B is correct.** Hemoptysis is a hallmark symptom of a pulmonary embolus, and this client's fracture history and other clinical manifestations lead to this conclusion. The clinical manifestations do not correlate with the diagnoses in answers A, C, and D.

15. **Answer C is correct.** A surgical hat cover is not necessary to mix or administer chemotherapy. OSHA (Occupational Safety and Health Administration) and ONS (Oncology Nurse Society) recommend answers A, B, and D when mixing or administering chemotherapy. The nurse should dispose of all equipment used in chemotherapy preparation and administration as hazardous waste in leak-proof, puncture-proof containers.

16. **Answer B is correct.** The client who had a stroke is the most stable client of the ones listed. The client in answer A needs extensive assessment. The client in answer C has a patient-controlled analgesic (PCA) pump and requires an RN because of the intravenous infusion. The client in answer D is a new admission with an infected diverticulum and would be less stable, with more unknowns.

17. **Answer A is correct.** The diabetic with the foot ulcer is the most stable client and should be assigned to the LPN. Answer B requires assessments for clotting and bleeding complications, as well as monitoring of the IV heparin. Weaning from a tracheostomy could constitute an airway problem, making answer C incorrect. A postoperative client would be less stable and require more extensive care, so answer D is incorrect.

18. **Answer A is correct.** Kubler-Ross identified five stages of dying as ways that people cope with death. The stage of denial can be used as a buffer and a way to adapt. When dealing with these clients, the nurse would need to use open-ended statements, such as, "Tell me more." Other examples of statements made by the client in this stage are "This can't be true" and "I want another opinion." Answers B, C, and D are a few of the other stages of dying. In order, the stages are denial, anger, bargaining, depression, and acceptance.

19. **Answer D is correct.** The Trendelenburg position is used for surgeries on the lower abdomen and pelvis. This position helps to displace intestines into the upper abdomen and out of the surgical area. Answer A is reserved for vaginal, perineal, and some rectal surgeries. Answer B is used for renal surgery, and answer C is used for back surgery and some rectal surgeries.

20. **Answer A is correct.** Abrupt withdrawal of steroids can lead to collapse of the cardiovascular system; therefore, the physician should be notified for drug coverage. The medications in answers B, C, and D would not be as important as the maintenance of the steroids. Answer B is an ace inhibitor used as an antihypertensive. Answer C is a stool softener, and answer D is a calcium and vitamin agent.

21. **Answer C is correct.** Versed is used for conscious sedation and is an antianxiety agent. The antidote for this drug is Romazicon, a benzodiazepine. Answers A, B, and D are not utilized as antagonists for Versed; however, answer B is the antagonist for narcotics.

22. **Answer C is correct.** Turning the client to the side will allow any vomit to drain from the mouth and decrease the risk for aspiration. Answers A, B, and D are all appropriate nursing interventions, but a patent airway and prevention of aspiration are priorities.

23. **Answer B is correct.** When dehiscence and/or evisceration of a wound occurs, the nurse should apply a sterile saline dressing before notifying the physician. Answer A is not the appropriate position; the client should be placed in low Fowler's position. Answers C and D will not help in this situation.

24. **Answer C is correct.** There is a risk of bleeding with a liver biopsy; therefore, laboratory tests are done to determine any problems with coagulation before the biopsy. Answers A, B, and D are incorrect statements. The client lies on the right side, not the left; no enemas are given; and the test is invasive and can cause some pain.

25. **Answer A is correct.** Obstruction of the tracheostomy can cause anxiety, increased respiratory rate, and an O_2 saturation decrease. The nurse should first suction the client. If this doesn't work, she should notify the physician, as in answer C. Answer B would not help if the tube was obstructed. Answer D would be done to assess for improvement after the suctioning was performed.

26. **Answer A is correct.** Clients who are taking INH should avoid tuna, red wine, soy sauce, and yeast extracts because of the side effects that can occur, such as headaches and hypotension. Answers B, C, and D are all allowed with this drug.

27. **Answer D is correct.** The cerebral perfusion pressure is obtained by subtracting the ICP from the mean arterial pressure (MAP). A client must have a CPP of 70–100 to have a normal reading and adequate cerebral perfusion. Answers A, B, and C are all incorrect calculations.

28. **Answer D is correct.** The XII hypoglossal cranial nerve deals with the function of the tongue and its movement. Clients can exhibit weakness and deviation with impairment of this cranial nerve. Answers A, B, and C are not tested by this procedure. Cranial nerve I is involved with smelling, cranial nerve II is involved with visual function, and cranial nerve X deals with the gag reflex.

29. **Answer A is correct.** Increased intracranial pressure vital sign changes include an elevated BP with a widening pulse pressure, decreased heart rate, and temperature elevation. Answer C could occur with shock or hypovolemia. Answer B does not correlate with increased ICP. Answer D is not as evident of increased intracranial pressure as answer A.

30. **Answer B is correct.** The normal Dilantin level is 10–20mcg/mL; a level of 30 exceeds the normal. The appropriate action is to notify the physician for orders. Answer A would be inappropriate with a high level, and answers C and D would require changing the physician's prescription.

31. **Answer D is correct.** Hydration is needed to prevent slowing of blood flow and occlusion. It is important to perform assessments in answers A, B, and C, but answer D is the best intervention for preventing the crisis.

32. **Answer C is correct.** B12 is an essential component for proper functioning of the peripheral nervous system. Clients who have a B12 deficit will have symptoms such as paresthesia. Answers A and D do not occur with pernicious anemia; the client in answer B would have weight loss rather than weight gain.

33. **Answer D is correct.** Spinach should be avoided on a low-purine diet; other foods to avoid include poultry, liver, lobster, oysters, peas, fish, and oatmeal. Answers A, B, and C are all foods included on a low-purine diet.

34. **Answer A is correct.** The client is exhibiting symptoms of fluid volume excess; slowing the rate is the proper action. The nurse would not stop the infusion of blood, as in answer C, and answers B and D would not help.

35. **Answer C is correct.** Fat emboli occur more frequently with long bone or pelvic fractures and usually in young adults ages 20–30. Answers A, B, and D are not high-risk groups for this complication.

36. **Answer B is correct.** Sliced veal, a spinach salad, and a whole-wheat roll is the selection with the highest iron content. Other foods high in iron include cream of wheat, oatmeal, liver, collard greens, mustard greens, clams, chili with beans, brown rice, and dried apricots. Answers A, C, and D are not high in iron.

37. **Answer D is correct.** Symptoms of a fractured femoral neck include shortening, adduction, and external rotation of the affected limb. Answer A is incorrect because the patient usually is unable to move the leg because of pain. Answers B and C are incorrect because the leg would be adducted and externally rotated if a fracture was present.

38. **Answer D is correct.** The 0.2mL of air that would be administered after the medication with an intramuscular injection would allow the medication to be dispersed into the muscle. In answer A, the muscle is too small. Answer C is an incorrect procedure, and answer B does not help prevent tracking.

39. **Answer C is correct.** Nausea and vomiting are common side effects of the drug due to the opium. Answer A is incorrect because the drug should promote sleep because it has a sedative effect. The nurse would not be concerned with physical dependence on the drug during this early surgical time period, so answer B is incorrect. The drug has an anticholinergic effect, making answer D incorrect.

40. **Answer A is correct.** Hemolytic anemia involves the destruction of red blood cells that prompt the release of bilirubin, leading to a yellow hue of the skin. Answers C and D occur with several types of anemia but are not specific to hemolytic anemia. Answer B is not related to anemia.

41. **Answer B is correct.** Neulasta is given to increase the white blood cell count in patients with leucopenia. This white blood cell count is within the normal range for showing an improvement. Answers A, C, and D are not specific to the drug's desired effect.

42. **Answer D is correct.** Clients with a diagnosis of polycythemia have an increased risk for thrombosis and must be aware of the symptoms. Answers A, B, and C are not related to this disorder.

43. **Answer C is correct.** The client should strain all urine after the procedure and save any stones for examination. The statements in answers A, B, and D indicate a misunderstanding of how to provide proper self-care after the lithotripsy procedure.

44. **Answer A is correct.** The medication should be taken in the morning before food or other medications are ingested, with water as the only liquid. Answers B, C, and D are correct administrations. Answer B is an important choice for preventing esophageal problems with Fosamax administration.

45. **Answer B is correct.** Assessing for Tinel's sign is done to check for paresthesia in the median nerve. An abnormal result would be pain or tingling as this procedure is done. This test can also be performed by inflating a blood pressure cuff to the client's systolic pressure, resulting in pain and tingling. Answer A is another test in which the nurse asks the client to place the backs of the hands together and flex them at the same time. If the client experiences paresthesia within 60 seconds of performing the test, it is a positive result indicating carpel tunnel syndrome. Answers C and D are both assessment procedures for minengeal irritation.

46. **Answer D is correct.** A diet of mandarin orange salad, broiled chicken, and milk is the most balanced and best selection for promoting healing. Answers A, B, and C are not as inclusive of the food groups that promote healing.

47. **Answer D is correct.** Vomiting would be contraindicated with an acid, alkaline, or petroleum product. Answers A, B, and C do not contain any of these solutions, so vomiting would be a possible treatment.

48. **Answer A is correct.** Clients with AIDS who are experiencing diarrhea should avoid bowel irritants such as raw vegetables, nuts, and fatty and fried foods. Answers B, C, and D would not serve as irritants to the bowels.

49. **Answer B is correct.** The nurse should prioritize these clients and decide to see the client with the shortness of breath because this could be a possible alteration in breathing. The client in answer A has an abnormal PCO_2 (normal 35–45), but this would be expected in a client with COPD. The client's condition in answer C can be corrected by pain medication that someone else could administer. Answer D is incorrect because a temperature elevation of this level would not be a reason for great concern in a client after gallbladder surgery.

50. **Answer D is correct.** A malignant mass is usually firm and hard, typically is located in one breast, is not movable, and has an irregular shape. Answers A, B, and C are not characteristics of a malignancy.

51. **Answer B is correct.** The client has an open fracture, so the priority would be to cover the wound and prevent further contamination. Swelling usually occurs with a fracture, making answer C incorrect. Manual traction should not be attempted, as in answer A. Placing the client in the prone position, as in answer D, provides excessive movement and is an inappropriate action.

52. **Answer A is correct.** The drug can be mixed with D5W only. Mixing with normal saline can cause precipitates to form. The answers in B, C, and D are appropriate implementations for administering amphoteracin B, so they are incorrect.

53. **Answer A is correct.** This clinical manifestation is due to the hemolysis of the red blood cells in the kidney. Answer B occurs with a febrile reaction. A rash or urticaria occurs with an allergic reaction, making answer C incorrect. Answer D is incorrect because this clinical manifestation usually occurs with circulatory overload.

54. **Answer B is correct.** Hypercalcemia is a common occurrence with cancer of the bone. Clinical manifestations of hypercalcemia include mental confusion and an elevated blood pressure. The potassium level in answer A is elevated, but this is not related to the diagnosis. Answers C and D are both normal levels.

55. **Answer C is correct.** The client is at risk for an air embolus. Placing the client in a left lateral decubitus position will displace air from the right ventricle. Answers B and D would not help, and answer A would not be done first.

56. **Answer B is correct.** A catheter will allow urine elimination without disrupting the implant. There is usually no restriction on TV or phone use, as in answer A. The client is placed on a low-residue diet, not a high-fiber diet, as stated in answer C. Even though the implant is internally placed, neither the patient nor her secretions are radioactive, but the applicator is. Because secretions are not radioactive, answer D is incorrect.

57. **Answer A is correct.** Normal ICP is 10–20. A reading of 66 is high, and the physician should be notified. Answers C and D would not be appropriate actions. Answer B would be the action if the reading was normal.

58. **Answer A is correct.** Doxorubicin (Adriamycin) can cause cardiotoxicity exhibited by changes in the ECG and congestive heart failure. Rales and distended neck veins are clinical manifestations of congestive heart failure. Answer B is incorrect because the reddish discoloration of the urine is a harmless side effect of doxorubicin. Answer D is not specific to this drug, and answer C is common and not a reason to immediately notify the physician.

59. **Answer A is correct.** Clients with diabetes insipidous have excessive urinary output because they lack an antidiuretic hormone. Answers B, C, and D are not exhibited with diabetes insipidous.

60. **Answer D is correct.** Platelets deal with the clotting of blood and a lack of platelets can cause bleeding. Answers A, B, and C do not directly relate to platelets.

61. **Answer B is correct.** Spasmodic eye winking could indicate a toxicity or overdose of the drug Carbidopa/levodopa (Sinemet) and should be reported to the physician. Other signs of toxicity include involuntary twitching of muscles, facial grimaces, and severe tongue protrusion. Answers A, C, and D are side effects but do not indicate toxicity of the drug.

62. **Answer B is correct.** With neutropenia, the client is at risk for infection; therefore, this client would need to avoid crowds and people who are ill. Answer A would not be appropriate, and answers C and D correlates with a risk for bleeding.

63. **Answer C is correct.** D10W is the preferred solution to prevent complications from a sudden lack of glucose. Answers A, B, and D do not have glucose.

64. **Answer A is correct.** Vaginal bleeding or spotting is a common symptom of cervical cancer. Nausea, vomiting, and foul-smelling discharge, in answers B and C, are not specific or common to cervical cancer. Hyperthermia, in answer D, is not related to the diagnosis.

65. **Answer C is correct.** Clients with myasthenias can have problems with the muscular activity of breathing. Although answers A, B, and D are important, they are not priorities.

66. **Answer C is correct.** A bone marrow aspiration is usually done by the physician with specimens obtained from the sternum or the iliac crest. The high Fowler's position is the best position in which to obtain a specimen from the client's sternum. Answers A, B, and D are inappropriate positions for getting a bone marrow biopsy.

67. **Answer A is correct.** Hyperventilation is utilized to decrease the PCO_2 to 27–30, producing cerebral blood vessel constriction. Answers B, C, and D can decrease cerebral edema, but not by constriction of cerebral blood vessels.

68. **Answer B is correct.** The client is experiencing autonomic hyperreflexia, which can be caused by a full bowel or bladder or a wrinkled sheet. Answer A is not the appropriate action before performing the assessment of the bladder; answers C and D are not appropriate actions in this situation.

69. **Answer A is correct.** Plavix is an antiplatelet. Bleeding could indicate a severe effect. Answers B, C, and D are not associated with the undesired effects of Plavix.

70. **Answer D is correct.** Papilledema is a hallmark symptom of increased intracranial pressure. Answers A, B, and C are not as conclusive.

71. **Answer A is correct.** Imitrex results in cranial vasoconstriction to reduce pain, but it can also cause vasoconstrictive effects systemically. Therefore, it is contraindicated in clients with angina, and the physician should be notified. Answers B and D are inappropriate actions from the information given. Answer C is appropriate, but answer A is the most appropriate.

72. **Answer C is correct.** The pH is an accurate indicator of acute ventilatory failure and a need for mechanical ventilation. An elevated PCO_2, as in answer A, is not an adequate criterion for instituting ventilator support. Answer B, oxygen saturation of 90, would not be very abnormal for a COPD client. Answer D is normal.

73. **Answer C is correct.** The absence of breath sounds and subcutaneous air, increased heart rate, dyspnea, and restlessness indicate a pneumothorax, which would require immediate intervention. Answer A could occur with the pulmonary contusion and would be expected. Answer D would be expected with fractured ribs. Answer B is not a cause for great concern because the midline trachea is a normal finding.

74. **Answer D is correct.** A position of sitting or high Fowler's is the best choice for assisting the client to use respiratory muscles to breathe and lift the diaphragm from the abdominal area. Answer A is contraindicated, and answers B and C would not help as much as answer D for breathing.

75. **Answer C is correct.** This client is exhibiting symptoms of heart failure that happen commonly in clients with a COPD disorder. The client in answer A is being discharged, and the client in answer D with a PO_2 of 85 would not be cause for alarm in a COPD client. The client in answer B would not require immediate attention.

76. **Answer A is correct.** The occipital lobe is the visual lobe. If the client were having problems with the occipital lobe, it would mean that the edema and bleeding were increasing in that area. Answers B, C, and D are not related to the occipital lobe.

77. **Answer C is correct.** Flushing of the line is required when giving Dilantin IV push because Dilantin crystallizes in the tubing if D5W is present. Answers A, B, and D would not be appropriate or necessary for this procedure.

78. **Answer C is correct.** Lasix and Mannitol are given for their diuretic effects in decreasing cerebral edema. Answers A, B, and D are not the effects of the drugs in this situation.

79. **Answer C is correct.** Cyanosis and loss of consciousness will occur later as the obstruction worsens. Answers B and D are both earlier symptoms of obstruction, and answer A is not a definite clinical manifestation of obstruction.

80. **Answer D is correct.** O negative blood type is universal blood type for females of childbearing age. Answers A, B, and C are not to be given to females of childbearing age if this is not their blood type. A blood type of O positive is given to males and postmenopausal women in emergencies.

81. **Answer C is correct.** An MRI uses a powerful magnetic force; therefore, any metal or jewelry should be removed before this test. Answers A, B and D are not appropriate for this test.

82. **Answer C is correct.** The nurse should pay particular attention to any complaints of a headache when it is described in this way. The client could have a cerebral aneurysm. Pain medications are contraindicated in an undiagnosed neurological clients, so answer A is not appropriate. No criterion in the stem makes answers B or D appropriate.

83. **Answer D is correct.** An acoustic neuroma tumor is one of the eighth cranial nerve that deals with balance, hearing, and coordination, making the client at risk for injury from falls. Answers A, B, and C are not appropriate priorities with the information given.

84. **Answer D is correct.** The nurse should further assess the client for the cause of the symptoms, usually a pneumothorax. Answer A is another type of chest trauma not associated with the symptoms. Answer B is simply a term used to describe the symptoms, and answer C is not an appropriate assessment for these symptoms.

85. **Answer C is correct.** The calculated dosage of Atropine is 1.0mL, and the calculated dosage of Demerol is 1.5mL, making a total of 2.5mL the correct answer. Answers A, B, and D are incorrect calculations.

86. **Answer A is correct.** Nimotop is a calcium channel blocker and is used to prevent calcium influx. The etiology of vasospasm of the blood vessel has been thought to relate to this calcium influx; therefore, the drug is given to prevent this. Answers B, C, and D do not describe the action of this drug.

87. **Answer C is correct.** A simple partial seizure is characterized by jerking of extremities, twitching of the face, and mental alertness. Answers A, B, and D are not characterized with these clinical manifestations. Answer B is differentiated by the client's awareness of the seizure.

88. **Answer C is correct.** The essential piece of equipment is the ambu bag. Ventilator clients must always have another means of ventilation in case of a problem, such as a power failure. Answers A and B are needed, but not as much as answer C. Answer D is inappropriate for a client on the ventilator.

89. **Answer D is correct.** If the ventilator is set for 8 breaths per minute and the client's rate is 13 per minute, subtract 8 from 13 to find that the client is actually breathing 5 breaths on his own. Answers A, B, and C are incorrect information for the description provided in the stem, so they are wrong.

90. **Answer C is correct.** Contracting the abdominal muscles with exhalation is the proper technique for pursed-lip breathing. Answers A, B, and D are all incorrect techniques. The goal is to increase the exhalation phase.

91. **Answer C is correct.** A level of 15ug/mL is within the normal therapeutic theophylline level of 10–20ug/mL. Answers A, B, and D are not within the therapeutic range.

92. **Answer C is correct.** Readings of pH 7.35, PO_2 85, PCO_2 55, and HCO_3 27 represent compensated respiratory acidosis with increased PCO_2 (normal 35–45), low pH of less than 7.4 (normal 7.35–7.45), and high HCO_3 with compensation (normal 22–26). Answers A, B, and D are not reflected in the blood gas results listed in the stem.

93. **Answer A is correct.** Closed chest drainage is not usually used because it is helpful for serous fluid to accumulate in the space to prevent mediastinal shift. Answers B, C, and D are all involved in care on a client with lung surgery.

94. **Answer B is correct.** Any posterior craniotomy requires the client to lie flat and on one side as in answer A, rather than with the head of the bed elevated, as stated in answer B. A posterior fossa procedure would be at the lower back of the head. Answer C would not be contraindicated, and answer D would help to decrease intracranial pressure.

95. **Answer C is correct.** Raw or cooked vegetables are not allowed on a low-residue diet. Answers A, B, and D are all allowed foods.

96. **Answer C is correct.** A client with diverticulitis should avoid high-fiber foods containing seeds or nuts. Other foods to avoid include corn, popcorn, celery, figs, and strawberries. Answers A, B, and D are foods that do not
contain nuts or seeds and would not need to be avoided.

97. **Answer C is correct.** Asking the client about his usual diet is the least helpful information in identifying the problem. Answer A is important because the pain sometimes decreases as obstruction worsens. The distention in answer D indicates obstruction, and answer B is useful because a description of the vomit can help differentiate the type of obstruction.

98. **Answer C is correct.** Tegretol can cause bone marrow depression, which is evident by the low WBC of 4,000 (normal 5,000–10,000). It can also cause problems with the liver that would raise the BUN (normal 5–25mg/dL). Answers A, B, and D are not related to the adverse effects of this drug.

99. **Answer C is correct.** The parietal lobe deals with sensation; therefore, anyone with a problem in this area of the brain can have problems with sensation. Answers A, B, and D are not directly associated with this part of the brain.

100. **Answer B is correct.** Every nurse must know military times, Parkland formula, and how to calculate the amount of fluid needed for replacement therapy. The Parkland formula is 4mL × Weight in kilograms × Percentage of body surface area burned = Amount of fluid to be given in 24 hours. The nurse is to give half this amount in the first 8 hours.

    4mL × 68kg × 50% BSA = 13,600ml (amount to be given in 24 hours)

    Give half this amount in the first 8 hours.
    13,600 ÷ 2 = 6,800
    Answers A, C, and D are incorrect calculations.

101. **Answer D is correct.** A loss of pulse could indicate an occlusion in the graft that requires surgical intervention. Answers A and C are expected post-operative occurrences with this surgical procedure, which makes them incorrect. Answer B is not an immediate concern, so it is incorrect.

102. **Answer A is correct.** ECG changes associated with hypokalemia are peaked P waves, flat T waves, depressed ST segments, and prominent U waves. Answers B, C, and D are not associated with low potassium levels, so they are incorrect.

103. **Answer B is correct.** Inspect, auscultate, palpate, and percuss is the correct sequence of assessing the abdomen. The initial step is to inspect the abdomen. Auscultation must be accomplished before touching because movement could make auscultation inaccurate. Answers A, C, and D are incorrect assessment sequences.

104. **Answer C is correct.** Left Sim's position is the best position because it follows the natural direction of the colon. In answer A, the client would be placed on the abdomen. In answers B and D, the client would be placed on the back, so these answers are incorrect.

105. **Answer B is correct.** Trachea shift differentiates this clinical manifestation as a tension pneumothorax. When a person has a tension pneumothorax, air enters but cannot escape, causing a pressure buildup and shifting of the great vessels, the heart, and the trachea to the unaffected side. Answer A correlates with a pulmonary contusion, so it is incorrect. Answers C and D are associated with a pneumothorax; this makes them nonspecific for a tension pneumothorax and, thus, incorrect.

106. **Answer C is correct.** A client with an open pneumothorax is in distress and should be seen by the nurse first. The key word in this correct response is *unstable*. The clients in answers A, B, and D are more stable clients or those that are not as severely ill as the client in C, so they are incorrect.

107. **Answer A is correct.** Accolate should be taken 1 hour before or 2 hours after eating, to prevent slow absorption of the drug when taken with meals; therefore, this statement is incorrect and requires further teaching by the nurse. Answers B, C, and D are all true statements regarding this drug and are correct statements made by the client.

108. **Answer C is correct.** The assessment finding that causes the most concern is the one indicating a possible stroke. Right-sided weakness would mean that there is a loss of muscular functioning on the side opposite the surgical procedure. Answers A, B, and D might indicate a need for reassessments but are not a cause for immediate concern or intervention, so they are incorrect.

109. **Answer B is correct.** This client is the least stable of the ones listed. The key term in this answer is the word *new*. Bleeding would also give this client a priority status because of the possible deficit in maintaining circulation. The clients in answers A, C, and D are more stable, so they can be assigned to other personnel.

110. **Answer C is correct.** A needs assessment reveals that the brain tissue perfusion is most important. Answers A, B, and D are all important nursing diagnoses for a stroke client, but not as important as answer C, so they are incorrect.

111. **Answer A is correct.** Vitamin K decreases the effects of Coumadin. The client should be taught to avoid green, leafy vegetables, such as broccoli, cabbage, turnip greens, and lettuce. Answers B, C, and D are food choices that are low in vitamin K, so they are incorrect.

112. **Answer C is correct.** The clinical manifestation of clubbing of the fingers takes time, indicating that the condition is chronic and not acute. Answers A, B, and D are all nonspecific for chronicity, so they are incorrect.

113. **Answer A is correct.** Ambulating the client should help to pass the air. The air is used during the surgical procedure to assist in performance of the surgery. Answers B and C would not help, and answer D is not necessary or appropriate at this time.

114. **Answer D is correct.** Assessment is not within the role of a nurse's assistant, which makes this the least appropriate of the tasks listed. Answers A, B, and C are all appropriate tasks for an assistant, so they are incorrect.

115. **Answer B is correct.** An NG is inserted to decrease the secretion of pancreatic juices and assist in pain relief. Answer A is incorrect because these clients are held NPO. Clients are placed in semi-Fowler's position, which makes answer C incorrect. Answer D is not appropriate because the wastes are not contaminated.

116. **Answer B is correct.** To test for vagus nerve problems, the nurse uses a tongue blade and depresses the back of the throat to elicit a gag reflex. Another way to test for damage to the vagus nerve is to have the client say "Ah" while observing for uniform rising of the uvula and the soft palate. The absence of this reflex could indicate damage to the X cranial nerve. Answers A, C, and D are not tested in this manner, so they are incorrect.

117. **Answer D is correct.** The next step after calling for help is to open the airway to ventilate the client. Answers A and B are not performed until after answer D, so they are incorrect. Answer C is not a correct procedure for this situation.

118. **Answer D is correct.** Questran works by binding the bile acid in the GI tract and eliminating it, decreasing the itching associated with jaundice. Answers A, B, and C are not how Questran works to decrease itching.

119. **Answer D is correct.** Careful cleansing is necessary to prevent skin breakdown and skin irritation. Answer A is not an intervention used for illeostomies. Clients should avoid the high-fiber and gas-producing foods in answer B. Answer C is incorrect because these clients are not on fluid restriction.

120. **Answer B is correct.** Lomotil's desired effect is to decrease GI motility and the number of diarrhea stools. Answers A and D do not occur with the use of Lomotil. The drug should decrease cramping instead of increasing it, as in answer C.

121. **Answer A is correct.** During chest tube removal this procedure prevents air entrance into the chest cavity. Answers B and C are inappropriate actions for chest tube removal. Answer D could allow the air to enter the thoracic cavity, so it is incorrect.

122. **Answer B is correct.** Tremors are an extrapyramidal side effect that can occur when taking Haldol. Answers A, C, and D are not side or adverse effects of Haldol so are incorrect.

123. **Answer C is correct.** The pulmonic area is found in the second intercostal space, left of the sternum. Answer B is the correct location of the tricuspid area. Answers A and D are not assessment locations for heart auscultation.

124. **Answer B is correct.** A side effect of Aricept is dizziness; therefore, the client should be reminded to move slowly when rising from a lying or sitting position. Answer A is incorrect because it should be taken at bedtime, with no regard to food. Increasing the number of pills can increase the side effects, so answer C is incorrect. Another effect of the drug is bradycardia, making answer D incorrect.

125. **Answer A is correct.** Protein is a necessary component of wound healing. An inadequate amount of protein would correlate with the client's wound not healing properly. Answers B, C, and D do not directly relate to wound healing, so they are incorrect.

126. **Answer A is correct.** The first step is to assess the client, noting any signs or symptoms of a fluid volume deficit. Answers B, C, and D might all be required interventions at some point, but assessment is needed before any other actions, so they are incorrect.

127. **Answer C is correct.** All of the tests listed can be used to diagnose an ulcer, but an endoscopic exam is the only way to obtain accurate visual evidence. Answers A, B, and D are not as accurate or reliable, which makes them incorrect.

128. **Answer C is correct.** The parathyroid gland can be inadvertently removed or injured with thyroid removal. This can cause hypocalcemia and symptoms of tetany, which requires notifying the physician. Answers A and B are ineffective for treating or obtaining treatment for hypocalcemia, and answer D would allow the condition to progress; thus, these are incorrect.

129. **Answer C is correct.** PEEP can compress thoracic blood vessels, resulting in a decreased cardiac output and low BP. Answers A, B, and D don't relate to PEEP and are not the result of increased thoracic pressure.

130. **Answer B is correct.** This is the accurate instruction for application of the condom. The condom can be used once, so answer A is incorrect. K-Y jelly and glycerin are the only solutions that can be safely used with condoms, making answer C incorrect. Answer D is incorrect because the air should be squeezed out and nothing should be in the tip of the condom before application.

131. **Answer B is correct.** Immediate goals are to decrease body temperature and heart rate, which gives answer B priority. These clients might have mental status changes, but they do not have a problem with brain perfusion, as stated in answer C. Answers A and D are not a primary focus in the clinical picture of clients in thyroid crisis, so they are incorrect.

132. **Answer A is correct.** Clients with face and neck burns and singed nasal hairs are more serious because of the likely respiratory and airway involvement. The clients in answers B and C are more stable. The danger of heart damage from an electrical burn occurs more often when the current enters and leaves on opposite sides of the body, which makes answer D incorrect.

133. **Answer A is correct.** A vagal nerve stimulator is inserted surgically to treat seizure activity. If the device is working properly, the client will notice a voice change when the device is active. Answers B, C, and D do not occur with the operation of the device.

134. **Answer B is correct.** The client with the most risk factors for pulmonary complications is the 45-year-old with an open cholecystectomy. These include abdominal surgery and prolonged bed rest. The clients in answers A, C, and D do not have as high of a risk factor, so these are incorrect.

135. **Answer C is correct.** The hallmark symptom of carbon monoxide poisoning is the cherry red color. The answers in A, B, and D are not specific to carbon monoxide poisoning.

136. **Answer A is correct.** When a person is in the compensatory stage of shock, the BP remains within normal limits. Increased heart rate occurs, allowing cardiac output to be maintained. The client also exhibits confusion and cold, clammy skin. Answer B correlates with the progressive stage of shock, so it is incorrect. Answers C and D both indicate that the client is past compensation, so they are incorrect.

137. **Answer B is correct.** Airway clearance is necessary for oxygenation, which makes it a priority. Answers A, C, and D are all problems that can occur post-op laryngectomy, but airway is the priority concern.

138. **Answer B is correct.** Burn clients need large veins to administer the volume of fluid necessary for fluid-replacement therapy. Answer A is contraindicated because of the area burned. Answer C is an area that is not recommended because of the possibility of deep vein thrombosis. The vein in the forearm is smaller than the antecubital; therefore, answer D is incorrect.

139. **Answer D is correct.** Shortness of breath signifies an adverse reaction to the transplant procedure. Answers A and C can occur with the transplant process but do not signify an adverse reaction. Answer B is a normal finding with the bone marrow transplant.

140. **Answer D is correct.** Palms of the hands and soles of the feet are areas in dark-skinned clients where skin cancer is more likely to develop because of the decreased pigmentation found in these areas. Answers A, B, and C are not areas where low pigmentation occurs, so they are incorrect.

141. **Answer B is correct.** It is important to clamp the tube while auscultating because the sound from the suction interferes with the auscultation process. Answer A is one measure used to determine whether the NG is in the stomach. Answers C and D are not the correct procedure for assessing bowel sounds, so they are incorrect.

142. **Answer A is correct.** A culture result that shows minimal bacteria is a favorable outcome. The answers in B, C, and D are abnormal and negative outcomes, so they are incorrect.

143. **Answer B is correct.** The client should wait at least 5 minutes before instilling a second eye medication. Answers A, C, and D are correct procedures for eyedrop administration, so there is no need for further instruction with these observations.

144. **Answer C is correct.** Erythromycin is the only drug listed that is not penicillin based. Answers A, B, and D are in the same family as penicillin, so they are not as safe to administer; this makes them incorrect.

145. **Answer A is correct.** A normal potassium level is 3.5–5.0. Severe life-threatening complications can occur with hyperkalemia, requiring physician notification of any abnormality. Answers B, C, and D are normal results, making them incorrect.

146. **Answer C is correct.** Pulling the pinna down and back is correct for administering ear drops to a child because a child's ear canal is short and straight. The pinna is pulled up and back for adults. Answers A and B are improper techniques that would make it harder for the drops to be administered. Answer D would be incorrect because this is not a necessary part of the administration of ear drops, even though irrigation might be done to cleanse the ear before assessment.

147. **Answer B is correct.** The picture that follows depicts the percentages.

These percentages total 100% of the body surface area. 4.5%, 9%, and 9% equal to 22.5%, with the closest estimate at 23%. The answers in A, C, and D are not correctly calculated sums of the burned areas.

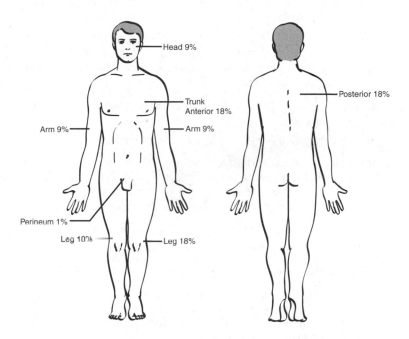

Head 9%

Trunk
Anterior 18%

Arm 9%

Arm 9%

Posterior 18%

Perineum 1%

Leg 10%

Leg 18%

148. **Answer D is correct.** Acute renal failure can occur with a lack of functioning in filtration when the MAP drops below 80. The mean arterial pressures in answers A, B, and C allow for proper functioning of the kidneys, which makes them incorrect.

149. **Answer C is correct.** An increase in head growth is used as a diagnostic gauge for hydrocephalus. Answers A and B can also occur with hydrocephalus, but they are not as specific or diagnostic as head circumference. Answer D is not related to hydrocephalus, so it is incorrect.

150. **Answer C is correct.** Two-thirds of the clients with chronic lymphocytic leukemia are older than 60 years of age at diagnosis. The answers in A, B, and D do not occur more often in the elderly.

151. **Answer C is correct.** Oxygen saturation is the best indicator of respiratory status because it is more objective. Answers A, B, and D are subjective and nonspecific, so they are incorrect.

152. **Answer B is correct.** Because of the moisturized air inhaled with swimming, it is an ideal sport for children with respiratory conditions. Answers A, C, and D can trigger an attack with asthma and would not be recommended.

153. **Answer A is correct.** Clients requiring low-bacteria foods cannot have raw fruits and vegetables. These types of foods must be cooked. Answers B, C, and D are raw fruits and vegetables, so they are incorrect.

154. **Answer C is correct.** The child weighs 24kg and should receive 5 units/kg, or 120 units every 4 hours. This would be 720 units in 24 hours. The answers in A, B, and D are incorrect dosages.

155. **Answer A is correct.** Hyponatremia can result from anorexia and nausea and vomiting caused by chemotherapy drugs. Normal sodium is 135–145mEq, so 50mg/dL is a low blood level that should be reported. Answers B, C, and D are normal or near-normal readings, so they are incorrect.

156. **Answer A is correct.** CBC results would indicate an elevated WBC count with leukemia. Answers B and D would not assist with the diagnosis, and answer C would be utilized to confirm leukemia; thus, they are incorrect.

157. **Answer C is correct.** Radial pulse differences over 10bpm are findings that relate to the location of the subclavian artery. Obstruction of the artery would also show a decrease in radial heart rate on the side of the obstruction. Answers A, B, and D are related to neurological problems as deficits, which makes them incorrect.

158. **Answer D is correct.** Everyone should wear sunscreen when going outside, to protect them from ultraviolet exposure. Answer A is not necessary. Answer B is the period of day when the sun's rays are most detrimental to the skin. Answer C is incorrect because only moles that are suspicious require removal and biopsy.

159. **Answer B is correct.** Normal pulmonary arterial wedge pressure is 4–12. This reading is elevated, indicating hypervolemia. The nurse should further assess for other indications of volume excess. Answers A and D correlate with hypovolemia. Answer C does not relate to the wedge pressure result.

160. **Answer B is correct.** Applying baby oil could help soothe the itchy skin. Answers A, C, and D would increase dryness and worsen the itching.

161. **Answer C is correct.** If a client has a curvature of less than 20°, it is considered mild, with no treatment required. If after re-evaluation the curve is progressing, treatment might be necessary. Answers A and B are done with curvatures of more than 20°, so they are incorrect. Answer D might be required with curvatures greater than 40°, making it incorrect.

162. **Answer A is correct.** Homocysteine levels are increased when a client has B12 deficiency. The answers in B, C, and D are incorrect because homocysteine levels are not increased by these disorders.

163. **Answer C is correct.** The pneumonia client is the most stable of the four. The clients in answers A and B are recent arrivals to the unit, indicating extensive assessments. The client in answer D is in danger of fluid volume deficit, requiring RN interventions.

164. **Answer B is correct.** The calculated dosage is 0.8mL. Answers A, C, and D are inaccurate dosages for the amount of medication ordered, making them incorrect.

165. **Answer B is correct.** The misuse and overuse of laxatives can cause serious fluid and electrolyte imbalances in the elderly. Answers A and D can be normal occurrences associated with the physiological changes of aging. Answer C is an incorrect response because the client states that increased fluid intake is not a new occurrence.

166. **Answer B is correct.** The normal sodium level is 135–145mEq/L. When hypernatremia occurs, the client can exhibit manic and hyperactivity behaviors. Other symptoms of increased sodium include restlessness, twitching, seizures, and hyperreflexia. Answers A, C, and D are not symptoms of high sodium levels. Answer D is associated with low sodium levels.

167. **Answer A is correct.** It is not a nursing responsibility to give detailed information about surgical procedures. The nurse can reinforce, but if the nurse feels that the client is not adequately informed, she can serve as an advocate and request that the surgeon visit the client to explain the procedure. Answer B is not the role of the nurse, so this is incorrect. Answers C and D are not appropriate and will not help in increasing or verifying patient understanding.

168. **Answer D is correct.** Safety and prevention of aspiration is the first priority. Answers A, B, and C would not be priority removals, so they are incorrect.

169. **Answer B is correct.** The client is asked to void before the procedure to prevent blurring of the pelvic bones. Answer A is incorrect because, although the client does need fluids to distribute and eliminate the isotope, this is not necessary 24 hours before the procedure. Answers C and D are not appropriate actions for the bone scan exam.

170. **Answer B is correct.** There will be a sensation of pulling during the aspiration. This feeling is painful. Answer A is incorrect because the position is inappropriate for bone marrow aspiration. Answer D is not a required preprocedure diet change. Although the client might receive a local anesthetic and/or pain medication, amnesic medications such as Versed are not usually administered, so answer C is incorrect.

171. **Answer C is correct.** It is most important to identify the pulses pre-operatively to have a baseline for post-operative evaluation. The answers in A, B, and D are not priorities for the client pre-operatively.

172. **Answer A is correct.** Excessive vagal stimulation causes bradycardia because of parasympathetic stimulation. Answers B, C, and D are not common arrhythmias associated with suctioning, so they are incorrect.

173. **Answer C is correct.** The client must be able to check the heart rate and report any rate that differs from the preset rate. Answers A and D are not required or have no effect on the pacemaker. Answer B would be contraindicated because the lack of movement could cause an inability to move the shoulder.

174. **Answer C is correct.** Diarrhea is not associated with esophageal cancer. Answers A, B, and D are clinical manifestations of esophageal cancer, so they are incorrect. The nurse would also assess for weight loss, regurgitation, and vomiting associated with esophageal cancer.

175. **Answer D is correct.** Perineal wound drainage is important to prevent abscess formation and infection. Answer A is incorrect because illeostomies produce liquid stools and do not require irrigation. Answer B cannot be done, and answer C would be inappropriate.

176. **Answer B is correct.** The client could have a mucus plug, so tracheal suctioning is the initial action most indicated. If suctioning doesn't work, notifying the doctor, as in answer A, is the next appropriate action. Answer C would not help, and answer D would be appropriate after the suctioning is done, to see if there has been any improvement.

177. **Answer C is correct.** High Fowler's is the best position for facilitating breathing. The nurse would suspect an allergic reaction to the shrimp. Answers B and D would both require an order from the physician. Answer A would worsen the client's respiratory efforts, so it is incorrect.

178. **Answer C is correct.** A measurement that reveals a numerical value would be the most accurate to detect changes in the size of the abdomen. Answers A, B, and D are less objective, so they are incorrect.

179. **Answer B is correct.** The stem gives objective assessment data that indicates a fluid volume deficit, a low BP with an elevated heart rate. Answer A is incorrect because of the lack of objective information that supports this nursing diagnosis. Answers C and D have no supportive data, so they are incorrect.

180. **Answer D is correct.** A client with an enlarged spleen has an increased risk for rupture; therefore, heavy lifting is contraindicated. Answers A, B, and C are not a cause for concern with an enlarged spleen.

181. **Answer D is correct.** A client who is immuno-suppressed is not allowed fresh fruit. Answers A, B, and C would still allow the client to eat raw fruit, which makes them incorrect.

182. **Answer B is correct.** The nurse must provide a water seal. Answer A could cause a tension pneumothorax if the client had no escape for the air. Answer C serves no purpose, and answer D would not allow maintenance of a sterile system.

183. **Answer A is correct.** An INR greater than 6.0 could result in spontaneous bleeding, so this would be a priority. Answers B, C, and D are not associated with the high INR result, so they are incorrect.

184. **Answer D is correct.** The highest calcium level is in the bagel with jam and skim milk. The client also needs to know that calcium in combination with high fiber and caffeine decreases the absorption; therefore, answers A, B, and C are incorrect.

185. **Answer C is correct.** Hemorrhage can occur with liver biopsies. The client is positioned on the right side to keep pressure on the area and prevent bleeding. Answers A, B, and D are not correct positions because of the location of the liver.

186. **Answer C is correct.** Hypernatremia is not an expected finding because hyponatremia is the likely occurrence when sodium moves out of the cell during the "fluid shift" phase of burn injury. The answers in A, B, and D are more of a priority for this client, which makes them incorrect.

187. **Answer C is correct.** Increased weight is the most objective answer. Answers A, B, and D also show evidence of anorexia nervosa but are not as objective, making them incorrect.

188. **Answer C is correct.** Gram negative infection invasion reveals clinical manifestations of severe diarrhea, hypothermia, and hypotension. Answer A is incorrect because the symptoms are abnormal. The infections identified in answers B and D are not consistent with the clinical manifestations identified in the question, so they are incorrect.

189. **Answer C is correct.** A 250mL infusion of packed cells to infuse over 2 hours is calculated by 250 divided by 2 = 125mL/hr. The answers in A, B, and D are incorrect calculations for infusion of the blood in 2 hours.

190. **Answer D is correct.** The nurse observes for sluggishness or lethargy, for early indications of increased ICP. A change in vital signs and papillary changes, as in answers A, B, and C, are late signs of increased ICP.

191. **Answer B is correct.** There is an increased risk for kidney stones with the use of topiramate (Topamax), so fluids are an important part of problem prevention. The drug is administered without regard to food and is not an hour-of-sleep medication, making answers A and D incorrect. Answer C is not required with the use of this medication.

192. **Answer C is correct.** The nurse responds appropriately by answering the question honestly and attempting to assess for more information, allowing the person to ventilate feelings. Answer A is an appropriate response but not as appropriate as answer C. Answers B and D are nontherapeutic communication techniques.

193. **Answer C is correct.** The PPD is administered by a mantoux test to determine infection with the TB bacillus. The correct procedure is to administer the test in the inner aspect of the forearm, approximately 4 inches below the elbow. The nurse uses a 26- to 27-gauge needle, and a wheal or bleb should be visible at the area. It is not administered IM, in the upper arm, or with a $1\frac{1}{2}$-inch needle, as stated in answers A, B, and D.

194. **Answer C is correct.** The initial action is to test the drainage for glucose because this could indicate the presence of cerebrospinal fluid. The next action is to notify the physician, as stated in answer B. Answers A and D are contraindicated, so they are incorrect.

195. **Answer B is correct.** The aspirate of gastric content should be green, brown, clear, or colorless, with a gastric pH of between 1 and 5. Answer A would likely be from the lungs, so it is incorrect. Answers C and D are not as accurate as color and pH for confirming gastric location, so they are incorrect.

196. **Answer D is correct.** A slight elevation in temperature would be expected from surgical intervention and would not be a cause for concern. Answers A, B, and C could indicate a progressing complication, so they are incorrect.

197. **Answer D is correct.** Pork has more thiamine than beef, fish, or chicken, which makes answers A, B, and C incorrect.

198. **Answer B is correct.** The client is exhibiting symptoms of respiratory depression from the use of a narcotic and requires an antagonist to reverse the effects. Answer A is a narcotic that would increase the negative effects the client is experiencing. Answers C and D are antianxiety and antipsychotic drugs, not narcotic-reversal agents.

199. **Answer A is correct.** The normal reading for central venous pressure is 3–8cm of H_2o. The doctor should be notified of any abnormal readings. Answer B is incorrect because a sterile technique should be utilized. Answer C is incorrect because of the 90° angle; the angle should be supine up to 45°. The zero should align at the phlebostatic axis, fourth intercostals space midaxillary, instead of the right clavicle, so answer D is incorrect.

200. **Answer D is correct.** The statement in answer D reflects the use of denial as a means of coping with the illness. Answers A, B, and C are defense mechanisms not reflected by the statement.

201. **Answer C is correct.** The Allen test is performed by having the client make a fist while the radial and ulnar arteries are compressed. When the hand blanches, the client is asked to release the fist while the nurse maintains pressure on the radial artery. Patency is indicated by the hand turning pink. Answers A, B, and D are incorrect for the Allen test procedure.

202. **Answer A is correct.** Clamping various areas of the tube allows the nurse to assess for a leak in the tubing. When the bubbling stops, the leak has been located. Answers B and C are assessed by reading the suction gauge and observing the bubbling in the suction-control chamber. Answer D is a diagnosis confirmed by client symptoms and x-ray not related to the chest tube system.

203. **Answer C is correct.** Respiratory depression is a sign of overdose. Other symptoms of overdose include seizures, shock, coma, and cardiovascular collapse. Answers A, B, and D lack any symptoms of overdose, so they are incorrect.

204. **Answer A is correct.** Vomiting, a heart rate of 120, and chest pain are symptoms of drinking alcohol while taking Antabuse. Additional symptoms include severe headache, nausea, cardiac collapse, respiratory collapse, convulsions, and death. Answers B, C, and D contain incomplete or inaccurate clinical signs of the combination of alcohol and Antabuse.

205. **Answer C is correct.** LDL has a harmful effect on the arterial wall. A high LDL is a modifiable risk factor that can be decreased by diet, exercise, and/or medication. Answers A, B, and D cannot be changed, so they are incorrect.

206. **Answer A is correct.** Symmetrel is the drug used for addiction to cocaine. It is classified as an anti-Parkinsonian drug and gives clients with this addiction a substitute for the neurotransmitter dopamine. Answer B is used for opioid addiction. Answer C is marijuana and is not used for replacement therapy. Answer D is used for alcohol abuse.

207. **Answer D is correct.** Troponin, T or I, is a protein found in the myocardium. Testing for protein is frequently used to identify an acute myocardial infarction. Answers A, B, and C return to normal in less than 4 days, which makes them incorrect.

208. **Answer B is correct.** The correct response uses the therapeutic technique of identifying the client's feelings. Answers A, C, and D are nontherapeutic, closed statements that reflect judgment and opinions by the nurse, so they are incorrect.

209. **Answer A is correct.** The most appropriate response is to answer the request of the client's spouse and define blackouts. Answers B, C, and D are not accurate definitions of blackouts, so they are incorrect.

210. **Answer B is correct.** Closing the doors can prevent shadows and help with the client's paranoia and hallucinations. A darkened room, as in answer A, would increase the client's anxiety. Answer C is an inappropriate intervention that does not usually occur with DTs, and vital signs would be assessed more frequently than in answer D.

211. **Answer B is correct.** Nothing should be put in the mouth of a client during a seizure. Answers A, C, and D are important nursing interventions to maintain a patent airway and prevent injury during a seizure, so they are incorrect.

212. **Answer C is correct.** Lethargy could indicate hepatatoxicity. The nurse should also observe for jaundice, nausea and vomiting, anorexia, facial edema, and unusual bleeding or bruising. Answers A, B, and D are not clinical manifestations of adverse effects of the drug Depakene.

213. **Answer A is correct.** Body image is a primary focus for children at this age; therefore, rehabilitation emphasis is on preventing scarring. Answers B, C, and D are important nursing diagnoses, but because of this client's age and body areas burned, answer A is the priority.

214. **Answer B is correct.** Adequate output would be an accurate assessment of fluid volume. If the client was hypovolemic, the body would compensate by retaining fluids and decreasing the urinary output. Answers A, C, and D do not relate to the fluid volume, and heart rate increase occurs with fluid volume deficit, so they are incorrect.

215. **Answer B is correct.** The therapeutic theophylline level is 10–20mcq/mL; therefore, notifying the physician is most appropriate. Answers A and D are not appropriate actions at this time, and answer C is a narcotic antagonist that is not used to reverse the effects of theophylline.

216. **Answer A is correct.** Sulfamylon is the topical agent of choice for electrical burns because of its ability to penetrate thick eschar. Answers B, C, and D have little or no penetration through eschar tissue, making them incorrect.

217. **Answer A is correct.** Fluid restriction is part of the treatment plan for clients with SIADH. This prescription gives the client too much fluid volume; therefore, the nurse should question this order. Answer B is a common medication for these clients. The weight and I and O are closely monitored, making answers C and D incorrect.

218. **Answer C is correct.** A change in the normal pattern of bleeding could indicate a problem in postpartum recovery. The normal pattern is lochia rubra, serosa, then alba. Answer A is a normal pulse rate. Diuresis and diaphoresis occur normally to rid the body of retained fluids, making answers B and D incorrect.

219. **Answer D is correct.** Before taking any action, an assessment is necessary to further investigate the situation. Answers A and B are appropriate actions, but not initially. Assessing the perineum, as in answer C, will not help the client to void or help assess for bladder distention, so it is incorrect.

220. **Answer A is correct.** A coup type of injury occurs when the brain damage is directly under the site of impact. When the injury is opposite the side of impact, it is identified as contrecoup, as in answer B. Answers C and D relate to the movement of brain tissue inside the head, not an impact.

221. **Answer B is correct.** Abruptly discontinuing seizure medications can cause status epilepticus to occur. This disorder is life threatening, so this would be most important to tell the client. Answers A, C, and D are not correct statements about Dilantin, so they are incorrect.

222. **Answer A is correct.** The nurse should try to find out more information to assist in determining the diagnosis. Answers B and D contain a diagnosis of which the nurse is not aware, and answer C is nontherapeutic because it is accusatory.

223. **Answer B is correct.** CSF evaluations are utilized to diagnose GB. An elevated protein without an increase in other cells is indicative of GB, which makes answers A, C, and D incorrect.

224. **Answer D is correct.** The normal CVP is 3–8cm of water. An elevation in CVP indicates a fluid volume excess. Answers A, B, and C indicate that the reading is normal or low, so they are incorrect.

225. **Answer A is correct.** A change in a client's neurological status requires further immediate intervention to prevent rapid deterioration. Answers B, C, and D would not be a cause for immediate concern.

226. **Answer C is correct.** The correct location of the fundus for this time period is 1 fingerbreadth above the umbilicus. Answer B occurs on the fourth day post-delivery, and answer A is the location for 12 hours after delivery. Answer D could indicate a distended bladder; therefore, answers A, B, and D are incorrect.

227. **Answer C is correct.** A normal finding is for the light to shine through the tissues and appear as a reddish glow. Answers B and D could also be true, but the best interpretation is that pus or fluid is present. Answer A is incorrect because it is not normal for the light to fail to penetrate the tissue.

228. **Answer A is correct.** The client with COPD uses hypoxemia as a stimulus to breathe. Raising the client's O_2 blood level can suppress the respiratory drive; therefore, this is the prescription the nurse should question. Answers B, C, and D are correct physician prescriptions for COPD clients and would not need to be questioned.

229. **Answer B is correct.** A decreased WBC count can occur with the application of Silvadene. The nurse would need to assess the laboratory test results for this adverse effect. Decreased potassium, sodium, and platelets are not associated with Silvadene administration, which makes answers A, C, and D incorrect.

230. **Answer B is correct.** The client most likely to experience complications is the one with the short delivery time due to the possible trauma and lacerations of the birth canal; therefore, she should be seen first. The clients in answers A, C, and D lack the criteria to make them a priority-level visit requirement.

231. **Answer A is correct.** Tactile fremitus is checked by asking the client to repeat terms such as *one*, *two*, *three* as the nurse's hands move down the thorax. Air does not conduct sound as well as a solid substance, so fremitus is increased with a solid substance and decreased when air is present, as with emphysema. Answers B and D are solid-tissue illnesses that would result in increased, not decreased, tactile fremitus. Answer C is incorrect because bronchopneumonia usually develops with tuberculosis, causing increased fremitus.

232. **Answer A is correct.** Zyban and Wellbutrin are classified as antidepressants and have been proven to increase long-term smoking abstinence. Answers B and C are bronchodilator drugs and are not used for smoking cessation. Answer D is a short-acting benzodiazepine and is not used for smoking-cessation therapy.

233. **Answer D is correct.** Pitocin is administered post-delivery to contract the uterus, resulting in a firm uterus and less chance of hemorrhage. Answers A and C are not desired effects of this drug. The contraction of the uterus is painful, which makes answer B incorrect.

234. **Answer A is correct.** Arterial blood gas PO_2 of 98 indicates adequate oxygenation and a favorable outcome. Answers B, C, and D are undesirable negative assessment findings, which makes them incorrect.

235. **Answer C is correct.** Asthma is the only disorder that is reversible with treatment or spontaneously after the attack. Answers A, B, and D can produce permanent damage to parts of the respiratory system, so they are incorrect.

236. **Answer B is correct.** The client's respirations would be assessed before administering morphine because morphine can cause respiratory depression. Answers C and D have no correlation with morphine administration, so they are incorrect. Answer A would be the next action after the assessment of a normal respiratory rate, but it would not be the first action.

237. **Answer A is correct.** The main cause of death after the immediate post-burn time frame is sepsis; therefore, preventing infection is a priority for this time period. Answer B would be emphasized earlier, and answer D requires a healed wound before it can be implemented. Answer C would be a necessary intervention during care, but it is not the primary focus.

238. **Answer B is correct.** The nurse should keep the stoma open until a sterile tracheostomy can be inserted. Answer A could eliminate the airway, answer C would possibly contaminate the airway with bacteria, and answer D would not be effective because the airway is via the stoma.

239. **Answer B is correct.** If there is any bleeding, new bruising, or pain at the puncture site, the physician should be notified. The information in answers A, C, and D are correct discharge teaching statements, so these answers are incorrect.

240. **Answer A is correct.** The nurse suspects congestive heart failure and anticipates an order for a diuretic to remove excess fluid. Answer B has insufficient data to support the need. Answer C would increase the client's fluid volume. Lowering the head, in answer D, would be an expectation for a client with a fluid volume deficit.

241. **Answer A is correct.** The suction source should not exceed 120mmHg when performing trachial suctioning. Answers B, C, and D exceed this amount and could cause damage to the trachea, so they are incorrect.

242. **Answer A is correct.** Bleeding at the site requires pressure to stop it. Answers B and C would be correct actions to take, but eliminating the bleeding process would take priority. Answer D is an inappropriate action, and the movement could increase the bleeding, so it is incorrect.

243. **Answer B is correct.** The systemic analysis of the electrocardiogram shows the information in the question as criteria for sinus tachycardia. Answer A would reveal an irregular rhythm and an early or different P wave. Answer C is incorrect because the P waves would be saw-toothed and the P: QRS ratio would be 2:1, 3:1, or 4:1. Answer D requires an unidentifiable P wave and a PR interval of less than 0.12 seconds, so it is incorrect.

244. **Answer A is correct.** The focus of treatment is to increase the heart rate to maintain cardiac output. Atropine is the first treatment of choice for this disorder. Answer B treats atrial arrhythmias, but side effects include bradycardia and heart blocks, which makes it incorrect. Answers C and D are used for ventricular arrhythmias.

245. **Answer D is correct.** Cigarette smoking directly affects the sweeping action of the cilia, which interferes with the ability to remove mucus and clear the airway. Answers A and B are accurate statements but do not relate to emphysema. Answer C is not a direct effect of smoking.

246. **Answer A is correct.** The increase in venous pressure causes the jugular veins to distend. Other symptoms of right-sided heart failure include ascites, weakness, anorexia, dependent edema, and weight gain. Answers B, C, and D result from the left ventricle's inability to pump blood out of the ventricle to the body and are specific for left-sided, not right-sided, heart failure.

247. **Answer D is correct.** The client might be asked to cough and breathe deeply at certain times during the procedure. Answer A is incorrect because fluids are encouraged, to increase urine output and flush out the dye. The client will receive mild to moderate sedation, which makes answer B incorrect. Assessment of the site and pedal pulses are performed every 15 minutes for the first hour and then every 1–2 hours until pulses are stable, which makes answer C incorrect.

248. **Answer B is correct.** Theophylline should be taken with food to prevent GI irritation. Because this drug can cause tachycardia, answer A is incorrect. The IV drug is aminophylline and may not be ordered with worsening symptoms, so answer C is incorrect. Answer D is incorrect because the client should continue to take the drug when symptoms get better.

249. **Answer D is correct.** The delivery of oxygen is the best measure to correct hypoxia. Answers A, B, and C should also improve the client's hypoxia, but oxygen is the prescription that would deliver immediate relief.

250. **Answer C is correct.** Delivering an anticoagulant to a client with a hemorrhagic stroke is contraindicated because of the likelihood of increasing the bleed and worsening the client's condition. Answers A, B, and D are necessary positive treatments for clients with strokes, so they would not be questioned.

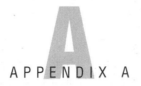

What's on the CD-ROM?

The CD features a state-of-the-art exam preparation engine from ExamForce. This uniquely powerful program will identify gaps in your knowledge and help you turn them into strengths. In addition to the ExamForce software, the CD includes an electronic version of this book in Portable Document Format (PDF) format and the Adobe Acrobat Reader used to display these files.

The CramMaster Engine

This innovative exam engine systematically prepares you for a successful test. Working your way through CramMaster is the fastest, surest route to a successful exam. The presentation of questions is weighted according to your unique requirements. Your answer history determines which questions you'll see next. It determines what you don't know and forces you to overcome those shortcomings. You won't waste time answering easy questions about things you already know.

Multiple Test Modes

ExamForce's CramMaster test engine has three unique testing modes to systematically prepare you for a successful exam.

Pretest Mode

Pretest mode is used to establish your baseline skill set. Train CramMaster by taking two or three pretests. There is no review or feedback on answers in this mode. View your topic-by-topic skill levels from the History menu on the main screen. Then, effective exam preparation begins by attacking your weakest topics first in Adaptive Drill mode.

Adaptive Drill Mode

Adaptive Drill mode enables you to focus on specific exam objectives. CramMaster learns the questions you find difficult and drills you until you master them. As you gain proficiency in one area, it seeks out the next with which to challenge you. Even the most complex concepts of the exam are mastered in this mode.

Simulated Exam Mode

Simulated Exam mode approximates the real NCLEX-RN® CAT exam. By the time you reach this level, you've already mastered the exam material. This is your opportunity to exercise those skills while building your mental and physical stamina.

Installing CramMaster for the NCLEX-RN® Exam

The following are the minimum system requirements for installation:

▶ Windows 98, Me, NT 4, 2000, or XP

▶ 128MB of RAM

▶ 38MB of disk space

NOTE

If you need technical support, please contact ExamForce at 1-800-845-8569 or email support@examforce.com. Additional product support can be found at www.examforce.com.

To install the CramMaster product from the CD-ROM, follow these instructions:

1. Close all applications before beginning this installation.

2. Insert the CD into your CD-ROM drive. If the setup starts automatically, go to step 6. If the setup does not start automatically, continue with step 3.

3. From the Start menu, select Run.

4. Click Browse to locate the CramMaster CD. From the Look in drop-down list in the Browse dialog box, select the CD-ROM drive.

5. In the Browse dialog box, double-click on the `fscommand` directory and then double-click `Setup.exe`. In the Run dialog box, click OK to begin the installation.

6. On the Welcome screen, click Next.

7. Select I Agree to the End User License Agreement (EULA), and then click Next.

8. On the Choose Destination Location screen, click Next to install the software to C:\Program Files\CramMaster.

9. On the Select Program Manager Group screen, verify that the Program Manager group is set to CramMaster, and click Next.

10. On the Start Installation screen, click Next.

11. On the Installation Complete screen, click Finish.

12. For your convenience, a shortcut to CramMaster is created automatically on your desktop.

Using CramMaster for the NCLEX-RN® Exam

An introductory slideshow starts when CramMaster first launches. It teaches you how to get the most out of this uniquely powerful program. Uncheck the Show on Startup box to suppress the Introduction from showing each time the application is launched. You can review it at any time from the Help menu on the main screen. Tips on using other CramMaster features can be found there, as well.

Customer Support

If you encounter problems installing or using CramMaster for the NCLEX-RN® exam, please contact ExamForce at 1-800-845-8569 or email support@examforce.com. Support hours are from 8:30 a.m. to 5:30 p.m. EST Monday through Friday. Additional product support can be found at www.examforce.com.

If you would like to purchase additional ExamForce products, call 1-800-845-8569 or visit www.examforce.com.

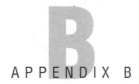

APPENDIX B

Need to Know More?

The National Council Exam for Licensed Practical Nurses

 http://www.ncsbn.org—The website for the National Council of State Boards of Nursing

Pharmacology

 http://www.accessdata.fda.gov

 http://www.druginfonet.com

 http://www.globalrph.com

 http://www.mosbysdrugconsult.com

 http://www.needymeds.com

 http://www.nlm.nih.gov/medlineplus

 http://www.nursespdr.com

 Deglin, J. and A. Vallerand. *Davis's Drug Guide for Nurses, 9th Edition*. Philadelphia: F. A. Davis, 2001.

The Respiratory System

 http://www.aaai.org—The website for the American Academy of Allergy, Asthma, and Immunology

 http://www.cdc.gov—The website for the Centers for Disease Control and Prevention

http://www.lpn220.topcities.com/resp./lowerrespiratory

 http://www.lungusa.org—The website for the American Lung Association

 http://www.nursing.uiowa.edu

 http://www.um.edu.respiratory/diseases.htm

 Ignatavicius, Donna D. and M. Linda Workman. *Medical-Surgical Nursing: Critical Thinking for Collaborative Care, Fourth Edition.* Philadelphia: W. B. Saunders Company, 2002.

 O'Connell, Suzanne C. Smeltzer, et al. (eds.). *Brunner and Suddarth's Textbook of Medical-Surgical Nursing, 10th Edition.* Philadelphia: Lippincott, Williams, and Wilkins, 2004.

 Sredl, D. "SARS: Here Today, Gone Tomorrow." *Nursing Made Incredibly Easy*, Nov.–Dec. 2003, 28–35.

The Renal and Genitourinary System

 http://www.drugmonitor.com/RIT97.html

 http://www.edu/urology-info/cancer.htm

 http://www.healthinfonet.ecu.edu

 http://www.nephron.com/preesrd.html

 http://www.umed.utah.edu/ms2/renal

 Ignatavicius, Donna D. and M. Linda Workman. *Medical-Surgical Nursing: Critical Thinking for Collaborative Care, Fourth Edition.* Philadelphia: W. B. Saunders Company, 2002.

O'Connell, Suzanne C. Smeltzer, et al. (eds.). *Brunner and Suddarth's Textbook of Medical-Surgical Nursing, 10th Edition.* Philadelphia: Lippincott, Williams, and Wilkins, 2004.

The Hematopoietic System

 http://www.americanhs.org—The website for the American Hemochromatosis Society

 http://www.aplastic.org—The website for the Aplastic Anemia and MDS International Foundation

 http://www.emedicine.com/med/topic3387.htm

http://www.hemophilia.org—The website for the National Hemophilia Foundation

 http://www.lpn220.topcity.com/BloodLymph/Blood/

 http://www.marrow.org

 http://www.nci.nih.gov—The website for the National Cancer Institute Information Center

 http://www.ons.org—The website for the Oncology Nursing Society

 http://www.sicklecelldisease.org—The website for the Sickle Cell Disease Association of America, Inc.

 Ignatavicius, Donna D. and M. Linda Workman. *Medical-Surgical Nursing: Critical Thinking for Collaborative Care, Fourth Edition*. Philadelphia: W. B. Saunders Company, 2002.

 O'Connell, Suzanne C. Smeltzer, et al. (eds.). *Brunner and Suddarth's Textbook of Medical-Surgical Nursing, 10th Edition*. Philadelphia: Lippincott, Williams, and Wilkins, 2004.

Fluid and Electrolyte Balance and Acid/Base Balance

 http://www.enursescribe.com

 http://www.globalph.com

 http://www.jcjc.cc.ms.us/depts/adn/Respacidbase.htm

 http://www.umed.utah.edu/ms2/renal

 Ignatavicius, Donna D. and M. Linda Workman. *Medical-Surgical Nursing: Critical Thinking for Collaborative Care, Fourth Edition*. Philadelphia: W. B. Saunders Company, 2002.

 O'Connell, Suzanne C. Smeltzer, et al. (eds.). *Brunner and Suddarth's Textbook of Medical-Surgical Nursing, 10th Edition*. Philadelphia: Lippincott, Williams, and Wilkins, 2004.

Burns

 Ignatavicius, Donna D. and M. Linda Workman. *Medical-Surgical Nursing: Critical Thinking for Collaborative Care, Fourth Edition*. Philadelphia: W. B. Saunders Company, 2002.

O'Connell, Suzanne C. Smeltzer, et al. (eds.). *Brunner and Suddarth's Textbook of Medical-Surgical Nursing, 10th Edition*. Philadelphia: Lippincott, Williams, and Wilkins, 2004.

Sensorineural Disorders

http://www.afb.org—The website for the American Foundation for the Blind

http://www.leweb.loc.gov.his—The website for the National Library Services for the Blind and Physically Handicapped

Ignatavicius, Donna D. and M. Linda Workman. *Medical-Surgical Nursing: Critical Thinking for Collaborative Care, Fourth Edition*. Philadelphia: W. B. Saunders Company, 2002.

O'Connell, Suzanne C. Smeltzer, et al. (eds.). *Brunner and Suddarth's Textbook of Medical-Surgical Nursing, 10th Edition*. Philadelphia: Lippincott, Williams, and Wilkins, 2004.

Cancer

http://www.abta.org—The website for the American Brain Tumor Association

http://www.cancer.gov—The website for the National Cancer Institute

http://www.cancer.org—The website for the American Cancer Society

http://www.komen.org—The website for the Susan G. Komen Breast Cancer Foundation

http://www.leukemia.org

http://www.leukemia-research.org

http://www.leukemialymphoma.org—The website for the Leukemia and Lymphoma Society

http://www.npcc.org—The website for the National Prostate Cancer Coalition

http://www.ons.org—The website for the Oncology Nursing Society http://www.skincancer.org—The website for the Skin Cancer Foundation

 Ignatavicius, Donna D. and M. Linda Workman. *Medical-Surgical Nursing: Critical Thinking for Collaborative Care, Fourth Edition.* Philadelphia: W. B. Saunders Company, 2002.

 O'Connell, Suzanne C. Smeltzer, et al. (eds.). *Brunner and Suddarth's Textbook of Medical-Surgical Nursing, 10th Edition.* Philadelphia: Lippincott, Williams, and Wilkins, 2004.

The Gastrointestinal System

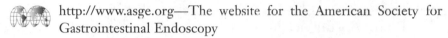 http://www.asge.org—The website for the American Society for Gastrointestinal Endoscopy

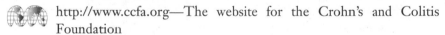 http://www.ccfa.org—The website for the Crohn's and Colitis Foundation

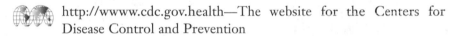 http://wwww.cdc.gov.health—The website for the Centers for Disease Control and Prevention

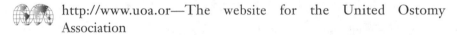 http://www.uoa.or—The website for the United Ostomy Association

Durston, S. "The ABCs and More of Hepatitis." *Nursing Made Incredibly Easy*, July–Aug. 2004, 22–31.

Ignatavicius, Donna D. and M. Linda Workman. *Medical-Surgical Nursing: Critical Thinking for Collaborative Care, Fourth Edition.* Philadelphia: W. B. Saunders Company, 2002.

O'Connell, Suzanne C. Smeltzer, et al. (eds.). *Brunner and Suddarth's Textbook of Medical-Surgical Nursing, 10th Edition.* Philadelphia: Lippincott, Williams, and Wilkins, 2004.

The Musculoskeletal System

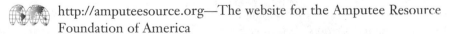 http://amputeesource.org—The website for the Amputee Resource Foundation of America

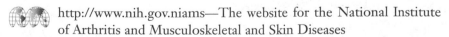 http://www.nih.gov.niams—The website for the National Institute of Arthritis and Musculoskeletal and Skin Diseases

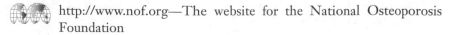 http://www.nof.org—The website for the National Osteoporosis Foundation

http://www.orthonurses.org—The website for the National Association of Orthopaedic Nurses

 Ignatavicius, Donna D. and M. Linda Workman. *Medical-Surgical Nursing: Critical Thinking for Collaborative Care, Fourth Edition.* Philadelphia: W. B. Saunders Company, 2002.

 O'Connell, Suzanne C. Smeltzer, et al. (eds.). *Brunner and Suddarth's Textbook of Medical-Surgical Nursing, 10th Edition.* Philadelphia: Lippincott, Williams, and Wilkins, 2004.

The Endocrine System

 http://www.cdc.gov/diabetes—The website for the Centers for Disease Control and Prevention

 http://www.diabetes.org—The website for the American Diabetes Association

 http://www.diabetesnet.com—The website for the American Association of Diabetes Educators

 http://www.eatright.org—The website for the American Dietetic Association

 http://www.endo-society.org—The website for the National Endocrine Society

 http://www.medhelp.org/nadf—The website for the National Adrenal Disease Foundation

 http://www.niddk.nih.gov—The website for the National Diabetes Clearing House

 http://www.pancreasfoundation.org—The website for the National Pancreas Foundation

 http://www.thyroid.org—The website for the American Thyroid Association

 Ignatavicius, Donna D. and M. Linda Workman. *Medical-Surgical Nursing: Critical Thinking for Collaborative Care, Fourth Edition.* Philadelphia: W. B. Saunders Company, 2002.

 O'Connell, Suzanne C. Smeltzer, et al. (eds.). *Brunner and Suddarth's Textbook of Medical-Surgical Nursing, 10th Edition.* Philadelphia: Lippincott, Williams, and Wilkins, 2004.

The Cardiovascular System

 http://www.americanheart.org—The website for the American Heart Association

 http://www.nursebeat.com—The website for the *Nurse Beat: Cardiac Nursing Electronic Journal*

 Ignatavicius, Donna D. and M. Linda Workman. *Medical-Surgical Nursing: Critical Thinking for Collaborative Care, Fourth Edition.* Philadelphia: W. B. Saunders Company, 2002.

 O'Connell, Suzanne C. Smeltzer, et al. (eds.). *Brunner and Suddarth's Textbook of Medical-Surgical Nursing, 10th Edition.* Philadelphia: Lippincott, Williams, and Wilkins, 2004.

 Woods, A. "An ACE Up Your Sleeve and an ARB in Your Back Pocket," *Nursing Made Incredibly Easy*, Sept.–Oct. 2003, 36–42.

The Neurological System

 http://www.apdaparkinson.com—The website for the American Parkinson's Disease Association

 http://www.biausa.org—The website for the Brain Injury Association

 http://www.epilepsyfoundation.org—The website for the Epilepsy Foundation

 http://www.guillain-barre.com/—The website for the Guillain-Barré Syndrome Foundation

 http://www.nmss.org—The website for the National Multiple Sclerosis Society

 http://www.parkinson.org—The website for the National Parkinson's Foundation

 http://www.stroke—The website for the American Stroke Association

 Ignatavicius, Donna D. and M. Linda Workman. *Medical-Surgical Nursing: Critical Thinking for Collaborative Care, Fourth Edition.* Philadelphia: W. B. Saunders Company, 2002.

 O'Connell, Suzanne C. Smeltzer, et al. (eds.). *Brunner and Suddarth's Textbook of Medical-Surgical Nursing, 10th Edition.* Philadelphia: Lippincott, Williams, and Wilkins, 2004.

Psychiatric Disorders

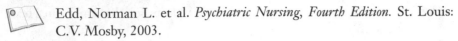 Edd, Norman L. et al. *Psychiatric Nursing, Fourth Edition.* St. Louis: C.V. Mosby, 2003.

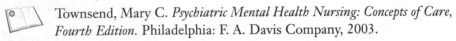 Townsend, Mary C. *Psychiatric Mental Health Nursing: Concepts of Care, Fourth Edition.* Philadelphia: F. A. Davis Company, 2003.

Maternal/Infant

Loudermilk, Deitra Leonard, et al. (eds.). *Maternity and Women's Health Care, Seventh Edition.* St. Louis: C.V. Mosby, 2000.

McKinney, Emily Slone, et al. (eds.). *Maternal-Child Nursing, Second Edition.* St. Louis: W. B. Saunders Company, 2005.

Wong, Donna L., et al. (eds.). *Maternal-Child Nursing Care, Second Edition.* St. Louis: C.V.Mosby, 2002.

Pediatrics

McKinney, Emily Slone, et al. (eds.). *Maternal-Child Nursing, Second Edition.* St. Louis: W. B. Saunders Company, 2005.

Wong, Donna L., et al. (eds.). *Maternal-Child Nursing Care, Second Edition.* St. Louis: C.V.Mosby, 2002.

Cultural Practices Influencing Nursing Care

Ignatavicius, Donna D. and M. Linda Workman. *Medical-Surgical Nursing: Critical Thinking for Collaborative Care, Fourth Edition.* Philadelphia: W. B. Saunders Company, 2002.

O'Connell, Suzanne C. Smeltzer, et.al. (eds.). *Brunner and Suddarth's Textbook of Medical-Surgical Nursing, 10th Edition.* Philadelphia: Lippincott, Williams, and Wilkins, 2004.

Potter, Patricia A and and Anne Griffin Perry. *Fundamentals of Nursing, Sixth Edition.* St. Louis: C.V. Mosby, 2005.

Legal Issues in Nursing Practice

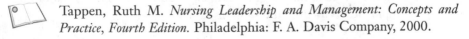 Tappen, Ruth M. *Nursing Leadership and Management: Concepts and Practice, Fourth Edition.* Philadelphia: F. A. Davis Company, 2000.

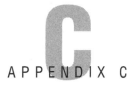

APPENDIX C

Alphabetical Listing of Nursing Boards in the United States and Protectorates

This appendix contains contact information for nursing boards found throughout the United States. The information found here is current as of this writing, but be aware that names, phone numbers, and websites do change. If the information found here is not completely current, most likely some of the information will be useful enough for you to still make contact with the organization. If all the information is incorrect, a helpful hint is to use an Internet search engine, such as Yahoo! or Google, and enter the name of the nursing board you are trying to contact. Most likely, you'll find some contact information. Also, if you don't have access to the Internet, contact your state government because they should be able to help you find the information you need.

Alabama Board of Nursing
770 Washington Avenue
RSA Plaza, Suite 250
Montgomery, AL 36130-3900

Phone: 334-242-4060
Fax: 334-242-4360

Contact person: N. Genell Lee, MSN, JD, RN, Executive Officer
Website: http://www.abn.state.al.us/

Alaska Board of Nursing
550 West Seventh Avenue, Suite 1500
Anchorage, AK 99501-3567

Phone: 907-269-8161
Fax: 907-269-8196

Contact person: Dorothy Fulton, MA, RN, Executive Director
Website: http://www.dced.state.ak.us/occ/pnur.htm

American Samoa Health Services
Regulatory Board
LBJ Tropical Medical Center
Pago Pago, AS 96799

Phone: 684-633-1222
Fax: 684-633-1869

Contact person: Etenauga Lutu, RN, Executive Secretary

Arizona State Board of Nursing
1651 E. Morten Avenue, Suite 210
Phoenix, AZ 85020

Phone: 602-889-5150
Fax: 602-889-5155

Contact person: Joey Ridenour, MN, RN, Executive Director
Website: http://www.azboardofnursing.org/

Arkansas State Board of Nursing
University Tower Building
1123 S. University, Suite 800
Little Rock, AR 72204-1619

Phone: 501-686-2700
Fax: 501-686-2714

Contact person: Faith Fields, MSN, RN, Executive Director
Website: http://www.state.ar.us/nurse

California Board of Registered Nursing
400 R Street, Suite 4030
Sacramento, CA 95814-6239

Phone: 916-322-3350
Fax: 916-327-4402

Contact person: Ruth Ann Terry, MPH, RN, Executive Officer
Website: http://www.rn.ca.gov/

California Board of Vocational Nurses and Psychiatric Technicians
2535 Capitol Oaks Drive, Suite 205
Sacramento, CA 95833

Phone: 916-263-7800
Fax: 916-263-7859

Contact person: Teresa Bello-Jones, JD, MSN, RN, Executive Officer
Website: http://www.bvnpt.ca.gov/

Colorado Board of Nursing
1560 Broadway, Suite 880
Denver, CO 80202

Phone: 303-894-2430
Fax: 303-894-2821

Contact person: Nancy L. Smith, PhD, RN, BC, FAANP, Program Director
and Education Consultant
Website: http://www.dora.state.co.us/nursing/

Connecticut Board of Examiners for Nursing
Dept. of Public Health
410 Capitol Avenue, MS# 13PHO
P.O. Box 340308
Hartford, CT 06134-0328

Phone: 860-509-7624
Fax: 860-509-7553

Contact person: Jan Wojick, Board Liaison; Nancy L. Bafundo, BSN, MS, RN, Board President
Website: http://www.state.ct.us/dph/

Delaware Board of Nursing
861 Silver Lake Boulevard
Cannon Building, Suite 203
Dover, DE 19904

Phone: 302-739-4522
Fax: 302-739-2711

Contact person: Iva Boardman, MSN, RN, Executive Director
Website: http://www.professionallicensing.state.de.us/boards/nursing/index.shtml

District of Columbia Board of Nursing
Department of Health
825 N. Capitol Street, N.E., 2nd Floor
Room 2224
Washington, DC 20002

Phone: 202-442-4778
Fax: 202-442-9431

Contact person: Karen Scipio-Skinner, MSN, RNC, Executive Director
Website: http://www.dchealth.dc.gov/

Florida Board of Nursing
Mailing address:
4052 Bald Cypress Way, BIN C02
Tallahassee, FL 32399-3252

Street address:
4042 Bald Cypress Way, Room 120
Tallahassee, FL 32399

Phone: 850-245-4125
Fax: 850-245-4172

Contact person: Dan Coble, RN, PhD, Executive Director
Website: http://www.doh.state.fl.us/mqa/

Georgia Board of Nursing
237 Coliseum Drive
Macon, GA 31217-3858

Phone: 478-207-1640
Fax: 478-207-1660

Contact person: Sylvia Bond, RN, MSN, MBA, Executive Director
Website: http://www.sos.state.ga.us/plb/rn

Georgia State Board of Licensed Practical Nurses
237 Coliseum Drive
Macon, GA 31217-3858

Phone: 478-207-1300
Fax: 478-207-1633

Contact person: Jacqueline Hightower, JD, Executive Director
Website: http://www.sos.state.ga.us/plb/lpn

Guam Board of Nurse Examiners
Regular mailing address:
P.O. Box 2816
Hagatna, Guam 96932

Street address for FedEx and UPS:
651 Legacy Square Commercial Complex
South Route 10, Suite 9
Mangilao, Guam 96913

Phone: 671-735-7406 or 671-725-7411
Fax: 671-735-7413

Contact person: Lillian Perez-Posadas, Interim Executive Officer

Hawaii Board of Nursing
King Kalakaua Building
335 Merchant Street, 3rd Floor
Honolulu, HI 96813

Phone: 808-586-3000
Fax: 808-586-2689

Contact person: Kathleen Yokouchi, MBA, BBA, BA, Executive Officer
Website: http://www.state.hi.us/dcca/pvl/areas_nurse.html

Idaho Board of Nursing
280 N. 8th Street, Suite 210
P.O. Box 83720
Boise, ID 83720

Phone: 208-334-3110
Fax: 208-334-3262

Contact person: Sandra Evans, MA.Ed, RN, Executive Director
Website: http://www.state.id.us/ibn/ibnhome.htm

Illinois Department of Professional Regulation
James R. Thompson Center
100 West Randolph, Suite 9-300
Chicago, IL 60601

Phone: 312-814-2715
Fax: 312-814-3145

Contact person: Mary Ann Alexander, PhD, Nursing Act Coordinator
Website: http://www.dpr.state.il.us/

Indiana State Board of Nursing
Health Professions Bureau
402 W. Washington Street, Room W066
Indianapolis, IN 46204

Phone: 317-234-2043
Fax: 317-233-4236

Contact person: Kristen Kelley, Director of Nursing
Website: http://www.state.in.us/hpb/boards/isbn/

Iowa Board of Nursing
RiverPoint Business Park
400 S.W. 8th Street, Suite B
Des Moines, IA 50309-4685

Phone: 515-281-3255
Fax: 515-281-4825

Contact person: Lorinda Inman, MSN, RN, Executive Director
Website: http://www.state.ia.us/government/nursing/

Kansas State Board of Nursing
Landon State Office Building
900 S.W. Jackson, Suite 1051
Topeka, KS 66612

Phone: 785-296-4929
Fax: 785-296-3929

Contact person: Mary Blubaugh, MSN, RN, Executive Administrator
Website: http://www.ksbn.org/

Kentucky Board of Nursing
312 Whittington Parkway, Suite 300
Louisville, KY 40222

Phone: 502-329-7000
Fax: 502-329-7011

Contact person: Sharon Weisenbeck, MS, RN, Executive Director
Website: http://www.kbn.ky.gov/

Louisiana State Board of Practical Nurse Examiners
3421 N. Causeway Boulevard, Suite 505
Metairie, LA 70002

Phone: 504-838-5791
Fax: 504-838-5279

Contact person: Claire Glaviano, BSN, MN, RN, Executive Director
Website: http://www.lsbpne.com/

Louisiana State Board of Nursing
3510 N. Causeway Boulevard, Suite 501
Metairie, LA 70002

Phone: 504-838-5332
Fax: 504-838-5349

Contact person: Barbara Morvant, MN, RN, Executive Director
Website: http://www.lsbn.state.la.us/

Maine State Board of Nursing
158 State House Station
Augusta, ME 04333

Phone: 207-287-1133
Fax: 207-287-1149

Contact person: Myra Broadway, JD, MS, RN, Executive Director
Website: http://www.maine.gov/boardofnursing/

Maryland Board of Nursing
4140 Patterson Avenue
Baltimore, MD 21215

Phone: 410-585-1900
Fax: 410-358-3530

Contact person: Donna Dorsey, MS, RN, Executive Director
Website: http://www.mbon.org/

Massachusetts Board of Registration in Nursing
Commonwealth of Massachusetts
239 Causeway Street, Suite 500
Boston, MA 02114

Phone: 617-727-9961
Fax: 617-727-1630

Contact person: Rula Faris Harb, MS, RN, Acting Executive Director
Website: http://www.state.ma.us/reg/boards/rn/

Michigan/DCH/Bureau of Health Professions
Ottawa Towers North
611 W. Ottawa, 1st Floor
Lansing, MI 48933

Phone: 517-335-0918
Fax: 517-373-2179

Contact person: Diane Lewis, MBA, BA, Policy Manager for Licensing Division
Website: http://www.michigan.gov/healthlicense

Minnesota Board of Nursing
2829 University Avenue SE
Minneapolis, MN 55414

Phone: 612-617-2270
Fax: 612-617-2190

Contact person: Shirley Brekken, MS, RN, Executive Director
Website: http://www.nursingboard.state.mn.us/

Mississippi Board of Nursing
1935 Lakeland Drive, Suite B
Jackson, MS 39216-5014

Phone: 601-987-4188
Fax: 601-364-2352

Contact person: Delia Owens, RN, JD, Executive Director
Website: http://www.msbn.state.ms.us/

Missouri State Board of Nursing
3605 Missouri Boulevard
P.O. Box 656
Jefferson City, MO 65102-0656

Phone: 573-751-0681
Fax: 573-751-0075

Contact person: Lori Scheidt, BS, Executive Director
Website: http://pr.mo.gov/nursing.asp

Montana State Board of Nursing
301 South Park
P.O. Box 200513
Helena, MT 59620-0513

Phone: 406-841-2340
Fax: 406-841-2343

Contact person: Vacant, Executive Director
Website: http://www.discoveringmontana.com/dli/bsd/license/
bsd_boards/nur_board/board_page.htm

Nebraska Department of Health and Human Services Regulation and Licensure
Nursing and Nursing Support
301 Centennial Mall South
Lincoln, NE 68509-4986

Phone: 402-471-4376
Fax: 402-471-1066

Contact person: Charlene Kelly, PhD, RN, Executive Director
Nursing and Nursing Support
Website: http://www.hhs.state.ne.us/crl/nursing/nursingindex.htm

Nevada State Board of Nursing
Administration, Discipline & Investigations
5011 Meadowood Mall #201
Reno, NV 89502-6547

Phone: 775-688-2620
Fax: 775-688-2628

Contact person: Debra Scott, MS, RN, Executive Director
Website: http://www.nursingboard.state.nv.us/

New Hampshire Board of Nursing
21 South Fruit Street, Suite 16
Concord, NH 03301-2341

Phone: 603-271-2323
Fax: 603-271-6605

Contact person: Margaret Walker, MBA, BSN, RN, Executive Director
Website: http://www.state.nh.us/nursing/

New Jersey Board of Nursing
P.O. Box 45010
124 Halsey Street, 6th Floor
Newark, NJ 07101

Phone: 973-504-6586
Fax: 973-648-3481

Contact person: George Hebert, Executive Director
Website: http://www.state.nj.us/lps/ca/medical.htm

New Mexico Board of Nursing
6301 Indian School Road, NE
Suite 710
Albuquerque, NM 87110

Phone: 505-841-8340
Fax: 505-841-8347

Contact person: Allison Kozeliski, RN, Executive Director
Website: http://www.state.nm.us/clients/nursing

New York State Board of Nursing
Education Bldg.
89 Washington Avenue
2nd Floor West Wing
Albany, NY 12234

Phone: 518-474-3817, extension 280
Fax: 518-474-3706

Contact person: Barbara Zittel, PhD, RN, Executive Secretary
Website: http://www.nysed.gov/prof/nurse.htm

North Carolina Board of Nursing
3724 National Drive, Suite 201
Raleigh, NC 27602

Phone: 919-782-3211
Fax: 919-781-9461

Contact person: Polly Johnson, MSN, RN, Executive Director
Website: http://www.ncbon.com/

North Dakota Board of Nursing
919 South 7th Street, Suite 504
Bismarck, ND 58504

Phone: 701-328-9777
Fax: 701-328-9785

Contact person: Constance Kalanek, PhD, RN, Executive Director
Website: http://www.ndbon.org/

Northern Mariana Islands
Commonwealth Board of Nurse Examiners
P.O. Box 501458
Saipan, MP 96950

Phone: 670-664-4812
Fax: 670-664-4813

Contact person: Rosa M. Tuleda, Associate Director of Public Health & Nursing

Ohio Board of Nursing
17 South High Street, Suite 400
Columbus, OH 43215-3413

Phone: 614-466-3947
Fax: 614-466-0388

Contact person: John Brion, RN, MS, Executive Director
Website: http://www.nursing.ohio.gov/

Oklahoma Board of Nursing
2915 N. Classen Boulevard, Suite 524
Oklahoma City, OK 73106

Phone: 405-962-1800
Fax: 405-962-1821

Contact person: Kimberly Glazier, M.Ed., RN, Executive Director
Website: http://www.youroklahoma.com/nursing

Oregon State Board of Nursing
800 NE Oregon Street, Box 25
Suite 465
Portland, OR 97232

Phone: 503-731-4745
Fax: 503-731-4755

Contact person: Joan Bouchard, MN, RN, Executive Director
Website: http://www.osbn.state.or.us/

Pennsylvania State Board of Nursing
P.O. Box 2649
Harrisburg, PA 17105-2649

Phone: 717-783-7142
Fax: 717-783-0822

Contact person: Laurette D. Keiser, RN, MSN, Executive Secretary/Section Chief
Website: http://www.dos.state.pa.us/bpoa

Commonwealth of Puerto Rico Board of Nurse Examiners
800 Roberto H. Todd Avenue
Room 202, Stop 18
Santurce, PR 00908

Phone: 787-725-7506
Fax: 787-725-7903

Contact person: Roberto Figueroa, RN, MSN, Executive Director of the
Office of Regulations and Certifications of Health Care Professions

Rhode Island Board of Nurse Registration and Nursing Education
105 Cannon Building
Three Capitol Hill
Providence, RI 02908

Phone: 401-222-5700
Fax: 401-222-3352

Contact person: Jean Marie Rocha, MPH, RN, Executive Officer
Website: http://www.healthri.org/hsr/professions/nurses.htm

South Carolina State Board of Nursing
110 Centerview Drive, Suite 202
Columbia, SC 29210

Phone: 803-896-4550
Fax: 803-896-4525

Contact person: Martha Bursinger, RN, MSN, Executive Director
Website: http://www.llr.state.sc.us/pol/nursing

South Dakota Board of Nursing
4305 South Louise Avenue, Suite 201
Sioux Falls, SD 57106-3115

Phone: 605-362-2760
Fax: 605-362-2768

Contact person: Gloria Damgaard, RN, MS, Executive Secretary
Website: http://www.state.sd.us/doh/nursing/

Tennessee State Board of Nursing
425 Fifth Avenue North
1st Floor - Cordell Hull Building
Nashville, TN 37247

Phone: 615-532-5166
Fax: 615-741-7899

Contact person: Elizabeth Lund, MSN, RN, Executive Director
Website: http://www.tennessee.gov/health

Texas Board of Nurse Examiners
333 Guadalupe, Suite 3-460
Austin, TX 78701

Phone: 512-305-7400
Fax: 512-305-7401

Contact person: Katherine Thomas, MN, RN, Executive Director
Website: http://www.bne.state.tx.us/

Utah State Board of Nursing
Heber M. Wells Bldg., 4th Floor
160 East 300 South
Salt Lake City, UT 84111

Phone: 801-530-6628
Fax: 801-530-6511

Contact person: Laura Poe, MS, RN, Executive Administrator
Website: http://www.commerce.state.ut.us/

Vermont State Board of Nursing
81 River Street
Heritage Building
Montpelier, VT 05609-1106

Phone: 802-828-2396
Fax: 802-828-2484

Contact person: Anita Ristau, MS, RN, Executive Director
Website: http://www.vtprofessionals.org/opr1/nurses/

Virgin Islands Board of Nurse Licensure
Veterans Drive Station
St. Thomas, VI 00803

Phone: 340-776-7397
Fax: 340-777-4003

Contact person: Winifred Garfield, CRNA, RN, Executive Secretary

Virginia Board of Nursing
6603 West Broad Street
5th Floor
Richmond, VA 23230-1712

Phone: 804-662-9909
Fax: 804-662-9512

Contact person: Jay Douglas, RN, MSM, CSAC, Executive Director
Website: http://www.dhp.state.va.us/

Washington State Nursing Care Quality Assurance Commission
Department of Health
HPQA #6
310 Israel Road SE
Tumwater, WA 98501-7864

Phone: 360-236-4700
Fax: 360-236-4738

Contact person: Paula Meyer, MSN, RN, Executive Director
Website: https://wws2.wa.gov/doh/hpqa-licensing/HPS6/Nursing/
default.htm

West Virginia Board of Examiners for Registered Professional Nurses
101 Dee Drive
Charleston, WV 25311

Phone: 304-558-3596
Fax: 304-558-3666

Contact person: Laura Rhodes, MSN, RN, Executive Director
Website: http://www.wvrnboard.com/

West Virginia State Board of Examiners for Licensed Practical Nurses
101 Dee Drive
Charleston, WV 25311

Phone: 304-558-3572
Fax: 304-558-4367

Contact person: Lanette Anderson, RN, BSN, JD, Executive Director
Website: http://www.lpnboard.state.wv.us/

Wisconsin Department of Regulation and Licensing
1400 E. Washington Avenue, Room 173
Madison, WI 53708

Phone: 608-266-0145
Fax: 608-261-7083

Contact person: Kimberly Nania, PhD, MA, BS, Director, Bureau of Health
Service Professions
Website: http://www.drl.state.wi.us/

Wyoming State Board of Nursing
2020 Carey Avenue, Suite 110
Cheyenne, WY 82002

Phone: 307-777-7601
Fax: 307-777-3519

Contact person: Cheryl Lynn Koski, MN, RN, CS, Executive Director
Website: http://nursing.state.wy.us/

Register this book!

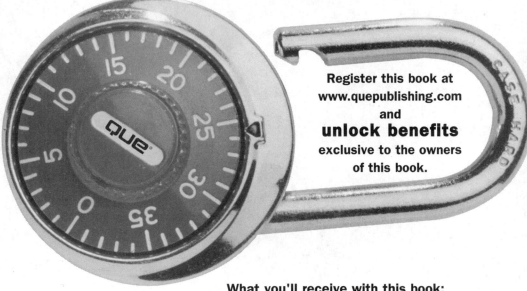

Register this book at
www.quepublishing.com
and
unlock benefits
exclusive to the owners
of this book.

What you'll receive with this book:

- ▶ Hidden content
- ▶ Additional content
- ▶ Book errata
- ▶ New templates, spreadsheets, or files to download
- ▶ Increased membership discounts
- ▶ Discount coupons
- ▶ A chance to sign up to receive content updates, information on new editions, and more

Book registration is free and only takes a few easy steps.

1. Go to www.quepublishing.com/bookstore/register.asp.
2. Enter the book's ISBN (found above the barcode on the back of your book).
3. You will be prompted to either register for or log-in to Quepublishing.com.
4. Once you have completed your registration or log-in, you will be taken to your "My Registered Books" page.
5. This page will list any benefits associated with each title you register, including links to content and coupon codes.

**The benefits of book registration vary with each book, so be sure to register
every Que Publishing book you own to see what else you might
unlock at Quepublishing.com!**